T0226495

Genitourinary Pathology

Editor

SEAN R. WILLIAMSON

SURGICAL PATHOLOGY CLINICS

www.surgpath.theclinics.com

Consulting Editor
JASON L. HORNICK

December 2018 • Volume 11 • Number 4

ELSEVIER

1600 John F. Kennedy Boulevard • Suite 1800 • Philadelphia, Pennsylvania, 19103-2899

http://www.theclinics.com

SURGICAL PATHOLOGY CLINICS Volume 11, Number 4
December 2018 ISSN 1875-9181, ISBN-13: 978-0-323-64219-4

Editor: Stacy Eastman
Developmental Editor: Donald Mumford

© **2018 Elsevier Inc. All rights reserved.**

This periodical and the individual contributions contained in it are protected under copyright by Elsevier, and the following terms and conditions apply to their use:

Photocopying
Single photocopies of single articles may be made for personal use as allowed by national copyright laws. Permission of the Publisher and payment of a fee is required for all other photocopying, including multiple or systematic copying, copying for advertising or promotional purposes, resale, and all forms of document delivery. Special rates are available for educational institutions that wish to make photocopies for non-profit educational classroom use. For information on how to seek permission visit www.elsevier.com/permissions or call: (+44) 1865 843830 (UK)/(+1) 215 239 3804 (USA).

Derivative Works
Subscribers may reproduce tables of contents or prepare lists of articles including abstracts for internal circulation within their institutions. Permission of the Publisher is required for resale or distribution outside the institution. Permission of the Publisher is required for all other derivative works, including compilations and translations (please consult www.elsevier.com/permissions).

Electronic Storage or Usage
Permission of the Publisher is required to store or use electronically any material contained in this periodical, including any article or part of an article (please consult www.elsevier.com/permissions). Except as outlined above, no part of this publication may be reproduced, stored in a retrieval system or transmitted in any form or by any means, electronic, mechanical, photocopying, recording or otherwise, without prior written permission of the Publisher.

Notice
No responsibility is assumed by the Publisher for any injury and/or damage to persons or property as a matter of products liability, negligence or otherwise, or from any use or operation of any methods, products, instructions or ideas contained in the material herein. Because of rapid advances in the medical sciences, in particular, independent verification of diagnoses and drug dosages should be made.

Although all advertising material is expected to conform to ethical (medical) standards, inclusion in this publication does not constitute a guarantee or endorsement of the quality or value of such product or of the claims made of it by its manufacturer.

Surgical Pathology Clinics (ISSN 1875-9181) is published quarterly by Elsevier Inc., 360 Park Avenue South, New York, NY 10010. Months of issue are March, June, September, and December. Business and Editorial Office: Elsevier Inc., 1600 John F. Kennedy Blvd., Ste. 1800, Philadelphia, PA 19103-2899. Accounting and Circulation Offices: Elsevier Inc., 3251 Riverport Lane, Maryland Heights, MO 63043. Periodicals postage paid at New York, NY and at additional mailing offices. Subscription prices are $206.00 per year (US individuals), $279.00 per year (US institutions), $100.00 per year (US students/residents), $258.00 per year (Canadian individuals), $318.00 per year (Canadian Institutions), $258.00 per year (foreign individuals), $318.00 per year (foreign institutions), and $120.00 per year (international & Canadian students/residents). Foreign air speed delivery is included in all *Clinics'* subscription prices. All prices are subject to change without notice. **POSTMASTER:** Send address changes to *Surgical Pathology Clinics*, Elsevier, 3251 Riverport Lane, Maryland Heights, MO 63043. **Customer Service: 1-800-654-2452 (US). From outside the United States, call 1-314-447-8871. Fax: 1-314-447-8029. E-mail: JournalsCustomerServiceusa@elsevier.com (for print support) and JournalsOnlineSupport-usa@elsevier.com (for online support).**

Reprints. For copies of 100 or more, of articles in this publication, please contact the Commercial Reprints Department, Elsevier Inc., 360 Park Avenue South, New York, NY 10010-1710. Tel. 212-633-3874; Fax: 212-633-3820; E-mail: reprints@elsevier.com.

Surgical Pathology Clinics of North America is covered in *MEDLINE/PubMed (Index Medicus).*

Contributors

CONSULTING EDITOR

JASON L. HORNICK, MD, PhD
Director of Surgical Pathology and
Immunohistochemistry, Brigham and
Women's Hospital, Professor of Pathology,
Harvard Medical School, Boston,
Massachusetts

EDITOR

SEAN R. WILLIAMSON, MD
Senior Staff Pathologist, Department of
Pathology and Laboratory Medicine, Henry
Ford Health System, Henry Ford Hospital,
Clinical Associate Professor of Pathology,
Department of Pathology and Laboratory
Medicine, Wayne State University School of
Medicine, Detroit, Michigan

AUTHORS

HIKMAT AL-AHMADIE, MD
Department of Pathology, Memorial
Sloan Kettering Cancer Center, New York,
New York

ALEX BORCHERT, MD
Vattikuti Urology Institute, Henry Ford Health
System, Detroit, Michigan

BETH L. BRAUNHUT, MD
Department of Pathology and Laboratory
Medicine, University of Miami Miller School of
Medicine, Miami, Florida

YING-BEI CHEN, MD, PhD
Assistant Attending Pathologist, Department of
Pathology, Memorial Sloan Kettering Cancer
Center, New York, New York

BONNIE CHOY, MD
Surgical Pathology Fellow, Department of
Pathology, The University of Chicago, Chicago,
Illinois

ALEXANDER J. GALLAN, MD
Genitourinary Pathology Fellow, Department
of Pathology, The University of Chicago,
Chicago, Illinois

BRYCE SHAWN HATFIELD, MD
Fellow, Surgical Pathology, Department
of Pathology, Virginia Commonwealth
University School of Medicine, Richmond,
Virginia

CLARA HWANG, MD
Senior Staff Physician, Department of Internal
Medicine, Division of Hematology and
Oncology, Henry Ford Cancer Institute, Henry
Ford Health System, Clinical Assistant
Professor, Department of Internal Medicine,
Wayne State University, Detroit, Michigan

KENNETH A. ICZKOWSKI, MD
Professor, Department of Pathology,
Medical College of Wisconsin, Milwaukee,
Wisconsin

MUHAMMAD T. IDREES, MD, MBBS
Associate Professor, Pathology and
Laboratory Medicine, Indiana University
School of Medicine, Indianapolis, Indiana

GOPA IYER, MD
Department of Medicine, Genitourinary
Oncology Service, Memorial Sloan Kettering
Cancer Center, New York, New York

CHIA-SUI KAO, MD
Department of Pathology, Stanford University
School of Medicine, Stanford, California

OLEKSANDR N. KRYVENKO, MD
Departments of Pathology and Laboratory
Medicine, and Urology, Sylvester
Comprehensive Cancer Center, University
of Miami Miller School of Medicine, Miami,
Florida

MARTIN J. MAGERS, MD
Fellow, Pathology and Laboratory Medicine,
Indiana University School of Medicine,
Indianapolis, Indiana

ANDRES MATOSO, MD
Departments of Pathology, Urology, and
Oncology, The Johns Hopkins Medical
Institutions, The Johns Hopkins Hospital,
Baltimore, Maryland

MARK CAMERON MOCHEL, MD
Assistant Professor, Department of Pathology,
Virginia Commonwealth University School of
Medicine, Richmond, Virginia

KELLY L. MOONEY, MD
Department of Pathology, Stanford University
School of Medicine, Stanford, California

GLADELL P. PANER, MD
Associate Professor, Departments of
Pathology and Surgery, Section of
Urology, The University of Chicago,
Chicago, Illinois

YU-CHING PENG, MD, PhD
Genitourinary Pathology Fellow, Department of
Pathology, Memorial Sloan Kettering Cancer
Center, New York, New York

SANOJ PUNNEN, MD
Department of Urology, Sylvester
Comprehensive Cancer Center, University
of Miami Miller School of Medicine, Miami,
Florida

M. RUHUL QUDDUS, MD
Department of Pathology, Women & Infants
Hospital of Rhode Island, Providence, Rhode
Island

CRAIG G. ROGERS, MD
Director of Renal Surgery and Urologic
Oncology, Vattikuti Urology Institute, Henry
Ford Health System, Detroit, Michigan

SAMEH SAMAAN, MD
Department of Pathology, The Johns Hopkins
Medical Institutions, The Johns Hopkins
Hospital, Baltimore, Maryland

STEVEN CHRISTOPHER SMITH, MD, PhD
Associate Professor, Director of Genitourinary
and Soft Tissue Pathology, Department of
Pathology, Virginia Commonwealth University
School of Medicine, Richmond, Virginia

KANIKA TANEJA, MD
Resident in Anatomic and Clinical Pathology,
Department of Pathology and Laboratory
Medicine, Henry Ford Health System, Henry
Ford Hospital, Detroit, Michigan

SEAN R. WILLIAMSON, MD
Senior Staff Pathologist, Department of
Pathology and Laboratory Medicine, Henry
Ford Health System, Henry Ford Hospital,
Clinical Associate Professor of Pathology,
Department of Pathology and Laboratory
Medicine, Wayne State University School of
Medicine, Detroit, Michigan

Contents

Large-gland proliferations of the prostate have gained considerable attention in the past decade. The differential diagnosis is quite broad but can be refined using histologic criteria and, sometimes, immunostains. Pathologists have come to realize that cribriform and intraductal as well as ductal carcinomas are particularly aggressive patterns, and should name them in diagnostic reporting when present.

Urothelial carcinoma is a morphologically and genomically heterogeneous disease that exhibits a wide spectrum of morphologic features and molecular alterations and subtypes. Classic urothelial carcinoma (not otherwise specified) is the most common tumor type that develops in the urinary bladder but many, well-documented, variant histologies are commonly encountered in approximately one-third of invasive urothelial carcinoma, including squamous, glandular, micropapillary, sarcomatoid, small cell/neuroendocrine, clear cell, lymphoepithelioma-like, and plasmacytoid types, among others. In this review, we provide an update on the molecular advances in urothelial carcinoma and some of its variant histologies.

A heightened understanding of hereditary renal cancer syndromes and their molecular basis has led to an increased awareness and recognition of these renal neoplasms by pathologists. Because a diagnosis of hereditary renal cell carcinoma has a profound impact on the patient and family members, when and how to raise such a suspicion via pathologic assessment has become an important yet very challenging task. This review discusses key clinicopathologic, immunohistochemical, and genetic characteristics of hereditary renal cancer syndromes, and important differential diagnostic challenges, emphasizing recent pathologic and molecular advances.

This article provides a comprehensive review of non–germ cell tumors of the testis and paratestis in adults, incorporating the latest 2016 World Health Organization updates. Clinical features, gross pathologic findings, key morphologic details, immunohistochemical profiles, and differential diagnoses are covered, with an emphasis on how to resolve commonly encountered, and sometimes difficult, differential diagnoses.

Since its development between 1966 and 1977, the Gleason grading system has remained one of the most important prognostic indicators in prostate cancer. The grading system was first majorly revised in 2005 and again in 2014. With the publication of the 8th edition of the American Joint Committee on Cancer TNM staging manual in 2018, the classification of prostate cancer and its reporting have further evolved and are now included as part of staging criteria. This article reflects the aspects that are most influential on daily practice. A brief summary of 3 ancillary commercially available genomic tests is also provided.

Grading and staging of urothelial neoplasm are the most crucial factors in risk stratification and management; both necessitate optimal accuracy and consistency. Several updates and recommendations have been provided though recent publications of the 4th edition of the World Health Organization classification, the 8th edition of the American Joint Committee on Cancer staging system, and the International Consultation on Urological Diseases–European Association of Urology updates on bladder cancer. Updates and recent studies have provided better insights into and approaches to the challenging scenarios in grading and staging of urothelial neoplasm; however, there remain aspects that need further investigation and refinement.

The most important prognostic parameter in renal cell carcinoma is tumor stage. Although pathologic primary tumor (pT) categories are influenced by tumor size (pT1–pT2), critical elements ($\geq$pT3) are dictated by invasion of structures, including renal sinus, perinephric fat, and the renal vein or segmental branches. Because this invasion can be subtle, awareness of the unique characteristics of renal cell carcinoma is critical for the pathologist to aid in clinical decision making. This review addresses challenges in pathologic stage and grade reporting and updates to the World Health Organization and American Joint Commission on Cancer classification schemes.

The American Joint Committee for Cancer eighth edition staging manual incorporated several critical changes regarding staging of testis germ cell tumors, and these changes are summarized and discussed in this article. Further challenges, however, remain, and these are also highlighted.

Certain tumors are more difficult to recognize when they present in an unusual location. Within the urinary tract, primary melanomas, carcinoid tumors, or epithelioid angiosarcoma could present diagnostic challenges due to their infrequent occurrence. This article emphasizes the clinical and histopathologic features of these entities and their differential diagnoses including the immunophenotype and their prognoses.

Mesenchymal neoplasms of the genitourinary (GU) tract often pose considerable diagnostic challenges due to their wide morphologic spectrum, relative rarity, and unexpected incidence at GU sites. Soft tissue tumors arise throughout the GU tract, whether from adventitia surrounding or connective tissues within the kidneys, urinary bladder, and male and female genital organs. This selected article focuses on a subset of these lesions, ranging from benign to malignant and encompassing a range of patterns of mesenchymal differentiation, where recent scholarship has lent greater insight into their clinical, molecular, or diagnostic features.

Pathologic variables play an important role in prognostication in urologic malignancies. Histologic subtype, histologic grade, and anatomic extent of disease (pathologic tumor and nodal staging) influence treatment decisions in both the adjuvant and metastatic settings. This article discusses treatment paradigms for the most common urologic malignancies, followed by the evidence base to support the relationship between pathologic assessment and decision making by the medical oncologist.

Prostate cancer, bladder cancer, and kidney cancer represent the 3 most common urologic malignancies, and form a heterogenous group of disease processes, with a wide range of pathologic features. As a urologist, a strong understanding of the pathologic features of urologic malignancies is essential to prognosticate and counsel patients and to determine the most effective course of treatment. This review discusses the pathologic features of prostate, bladder, and kidney cancer, and examines how detailed pathologic reporting is critical to today's practicing urologist.

SURGICAL PATHOLOGY CLINICS

THE CLINICS ARE AVAILABLE ONLINE!
Access your subscription at:
www.theclinics.com

Preface

Updates in Urologic Pathology: Emerging Areas, Staging, Grading, Unexpected Entities, and Clinical Significance

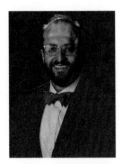

Sean R. Williamson, MD
Editor

The field of urologic pathology continues to evolve based on improved integration of histopathology, immunohistochemistry, and genetics of disease processes and tumors. Since the publication of the last issue of *Surgical Pathology Clinics* focusing on genitourinary pathology,[1] major updates to the field have included a new World Health Organization Classification of tumors,[2] widespread implementation of a new prostate cancer grading system,[3,4] a revised American Joint Commission on Cancer staging system,[5] and many individual studies revealing new insights into genetics and phenotypes of diseases and tumors. Clinical management of urologic cancers also continues to evolve, with growing roles for surveillance and adjuvant or neoadjuvant therapies. Considering this continually improving understanding, this issue contains a series of articles in genitourinary pathology, addressing four main themes. First, a series of articles addresses hot topics in urologic pathology with emerging areas of understanding, focusing on large glandular lesions of the prostate, hereditary renal cancer types, molecular subtypes of urothelial carcinoma, and non-germ-cell tumors of the testis. The second series of articles addresses the major changes to grading and staging in the major urologic cancers, including the novel prostate cancer grading system, staging and grading of renal cell carcinoma, staging and reporting of testicular cancer, and grading and staging of urothelial carcinoma. Two articles discuss interesting challenges in genitourinary pathology, including known entities occurring in an unexpected context (the "Man in Istanbul") and mesenchymal tumors in the genitourinary tract. Finally, two articles highlight the most relevant parameters in urologic pathology from the perspective of clinicians in urology and genitourinary medical oncology.

It has been a pleasure and honor to serve as Editor for this issue of *Surgical Pathology Clinics*, and I wish to extend my sincere thanks to all contributing authors for their time and invaluable expertise. We hope that this will serve as a helpful resource for pathologists of all experience levels and other biomedical professionals to recognize and navigate areas of change, challenge, and controversy in genitourinary pathology.

Sean R. Williamson, MD
Department of Pathology W615
Henry Ford Hospital
2799 West Grand Boulevard
Detroit, MI 48202, USA

E-mail address:
swilli25@hfhs.org

Surgical Pathology 11 (2018) ix–x
https://doi.org/10.1016/j.path.2018.09.001
1875-9181/18/© 2018 Published by Elsevier Inc.

REFERENCES

1. Hirsch MS. Preface. Surg Pathol Clin 2015;8:xi.
2. Moch H, Humphrey PA, Ulbright TM, et al, International Agency for Research on Cancer. WHO classification of tumours of the urinary system and male genital organs. Lyon (France): International Agency for Research on Cancer; 2016. p. 356.
3. Epstein JI, Amin MB, Reuter VE, et al. Contemporary Gleason grading of prostatic carcinoma: an update with discussion on practical issues to implement the 2014 International Society of Urological Pathology (ISUP) Consensus Conference on Gleason grading of prostatic carcinoma. Am J Surg Pathol 2017;41: e1–7.
4. Epstein JI, Egevad L, Amin MB, et al. The 2014 International Society of Urological Pathology (ISUP) Consensus Conference on Gleason Grading of Prostatic Carcinoma: definition of grading patterns and proposal for a new grading system. Am J Surg Pathol 2016;40:244–52.
5. Amin MB, Edge SB, Greene FL, et al. AJCC cancer staging manual. 8th edition. Switzerland: Springer; 2017.

Large-Gland Proliferations of the Prostate

Kenneth A. Iczkowski, MD

KEYWORDS

- Cribriform • Gleason grading • Prostate cancer • Morphology • Ductal • Intraductal

Key points

- Differential diagnosis of large-duct/gland spaces other than cancer includes the following: normal central zone epithelium, urothelium, seminal vesicle, basal cell hyperplasia, basal cell hyperplasia, and prostatic intraepithelial neoplasia.

- Large-gland cancers of nonprostatic origin that may be sampled in biopsy or resections include urothelial and rectal carcinomas.

- Prostatic-origin large-gland cancer includes intraductal carcinoma (IDC), ductal carcinoma, invasive cribriform (to papillary) carcinoma of Gleason grade 4; prostatic intraepithelial neoplasia–like, and invasive pseudohyperplastic carcinoma of Gleason grade 3.

- Pathologists should report in line diagnosis or on a template, the presence of invasive cribriform carcinoma when it is a component of high-grade cancer.

ABSTRACT

Large-gland proliferations of the prostate have gained considerable attention in the past decade. The differential diagnosis is quite broad but can be refined using histologic criteria and, sometimes, immunostains. Pathologists have come to realize that cribriform and intraductal as well as ductal carcinomas are particularly aggressive patterns, and should name them in diagnostic reporting when present. The somewhat overlapping entities of invasive cribriform carcinoma, intraductal, and ductal carcinoma, all associated with adverse outcome, can be distinguished from each other and from high-grade prostatic intraepithelial neoplasia using consensus criteria. The grading of large-gland prostate cancer patterns has been refined by International Society of Urologic Pathology (ISUP) consensus conferences. Rare forms of large-gland cancer include prostatic intraepithelial neoplasia (PIN)-like, pseudohyperplastic, adenoid cystic/basal cell, and squamous cell.

OVERVIEW

Large-gland proliferations of the prostate encompass several benign and malignant entities (Fig. 1). Both urothelial and colorectal cancer can produce large cancer glands and are sampled by some prostatic specimens. The somewhat overlapping entities of invasive cribriform carcinoma, intraductal, and ductal carcinoma, all associated with adverse outcome, can be distinguished from each

NONCANCER LARGE GLANDS

The epithelium of noncancer large-gland spaces in the prostate may be either 1-layered to 2-layered or multilayered. *Cystic atrophy* comprises dilated gland spaces with a nearly single-layered epithelium, with few and inconspicuous basal cells. Rarely, however, the single-layered epithelium can represent pseudoatrophic cancer, discussed later in this article. *Multilayered epithelium* is often a source of consternation for pathologists and residents, because it carries a 6-way differential diagnosis (Fig. 2).

Disclosure: The author has no commercial or financial conflict of interest. There is no funding source for this work.

Department of Pathology, Medical College of Wisconsin, 9200 West Wisconsin Avenue, Milwaukee, WI 53226, USA

E-mail address: kaiczkowski@mcw.edu

Surgical Pathology 11 (2018) 687–712
https://doi.org/10.1016/j.path.2018.07.001
1875-9181/18/© 2018 Elsevier Inc. All rights reserved.

surgpath.theclinics.com

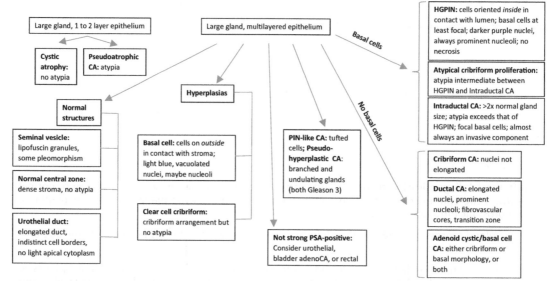

Fig. 1. Diagnostic decision tree: large-gland proliferation of prostate. CA, carcinoma.

DIFFERENTIAL DIAGNOSIS OF MULTILAYERED EPITHELIUM

High-grade PIN (HGPIN) (see **Fig. 2**A)[1] is a common type of large gland noted for its approximately 25% to 30% predictive value for cancer on repeat biopsy. HGPIN is most commonly tufted but also may be papillary, flat, or cribriform. Benign *hyperplastic* epithelium (see **Fig. 2**B) can be stratified. If nucleoli and nuclear enlargement are present in secretory cells, *HGPIN* is the diagnosis; these same features in basal cells constitute *basal cell hyperplasia* (BCH) (see **Fig. 2**C), frequently over-called as HGPIN. At low power, HGPIN "pops out" because of its hyperchromasia, whereas BCH tends not to because its nuclei are less hyperchromatic. The nuclear chromatin of HGPIN secretory cells is dark purple, as opposed to the light blue of the basal cells. Nuclear vacuolation is rare in HGPIN, frequent in BCH. Most importantly, HGPIN cells with nucleoli are in contact with the lumen, whereas BCH has cells arrayed around the periphery of the acinus, in contact with the stroma, never in contact with the lumen.

The prostate's *central zone* (see **Fig. 2**D) gets sampled in prostatectomy specimens, but less often in biopsy specimens. Located posterior to the verumontanum and superior to the transition zone, the central zone normally has tall nonatypical, cribriform, bridging, or papillary epithelium. Nuclei stream parallel to the glandular bridges, compared with the more rigid bridges in HGPIN or cancer.[2] The central zone's characteristic dense stroma and lack of nuclear atypia are keys

to preventing an overcall. Finally, both *urothelium* (see **Fig. 2**E) and *seminal vesicle* epithelium (see **Fig. 2**F) are stratified.

A rare variant of benign hyperplasia is *clear cell cribriform hyperplasia* (**Fig. 3**); this is the only type of hyperplasia that is cribriform. Situated in the transition zone, the very dark prominent basal layer, lack of nuclear atypia, clear cytoplasm, and background of nodular hyperplasia serve to distinguish this from cribriform HGPIN.

Seminal vesicle, or more commonly its intraprostatic portion, the ejaculatory duct, may be sampled on needle biopsy. Seminal vesicle atypia (**Fig. 4**) is a benign mimic of cancer, often with marked nuclear enlargement, more than usual for cancer, and prominent nucleoli. Clues to benignity include the presence of golden brown lipofuscin granules, and the branched, open morphology of the gland spaces.

PROSTATIC VERSUS NONPROSTATIC ADENOCARCINOMA

UROTHELIAL CARCINOMA

Urothelial carcinoma may involve the prostate via spread through prostatic ducts, a phenomenon observed in 15% to 48% of cystoprostatectomy specimens.[3–7] Less frequently, the tips of prostatic needle core biopsies can sample periurethral (transition zone) tissue. Therefore, regardless of how a specimen is labeled, when nearly solid proliferations of malignant cells are encountered, consideration must be given to the differential

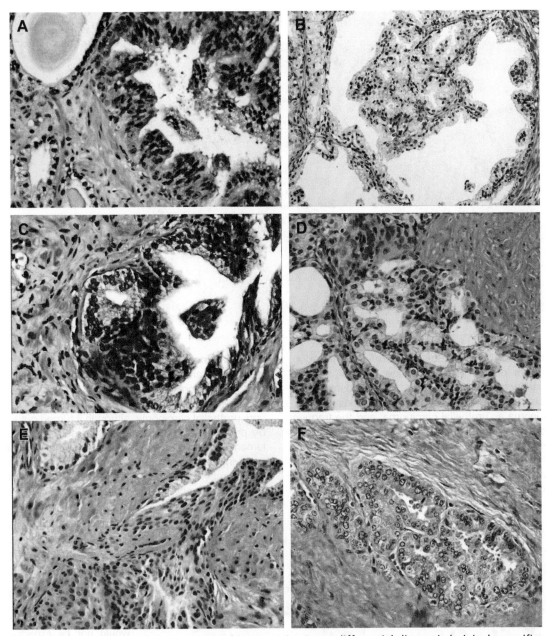

Fig. 2. Multilayered epithelium in prostatic biopsy carries 6-way differential diagnosis (original magnification ×20). (*A*) HGPIN. The hyperchromasia strongly contrasts with benign glands (*left*). Hyperchromatic secretory cells with macronucleoli have their cytoplasm in contact with the lumen. (*B*) Glandular hyperplasia. Heaped-up cell layers without atypia. (*C*) BCH. Stratified cells are somewhat hyperchromatic. Unlike HGPIN, their cytoplasm is in contact with the stroma, not the lumen. Nuclei are light and have chiseled/angulated contours; nuclear vacuolation may occur. (*D*) Central zone with normal cribriform epithelium. Anastomosing trabeculae of multilayered epithelium are without atypia. Dense stroma (*right*) reflects the proximity to the bladder neck detrusor muscle. Corpora amylacea are seen (*lower right*). (*E*) Urothelium of urothelial duct (*bottom*) is extending into a prostatic acinus (*top*). Urothelial cells have indistinct borders and lack a distinct, light apical cytoplasm, unlike prostatic cells. Urothelium is seen most frequently in specimens designated transition zone. (*F*) Intraprostatic seminal vesicle/ejaculatory duct epithelium may feature pleomorphic nuclei and macronucleoli, but its golden lipofuscin pigment and vesicular nuclei distinguish it from HGPIN. Specimens from the prostatic base are most likely to sample this epithelium.

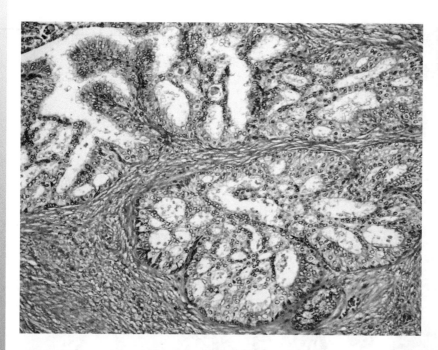

Fig. 3. Clear cell cribriform hyperplasia. Nuclei stream parallel to bridges (original magnification ×20).

diagnosis of large-duct (cribriform, solid, intraductal, or ductal) prostate cancer versus urothelial carcinoma. Unnecessary cystoprostatectomy can result from misdiagnosing prostatic adenocarcinoma as urothelial carcinoma, and the frequent overlap of their morphologies facilitates this error. Urothelial carcinoma is favored when cells have indistinct cell borders, more nuclear anaplasia with or without prominent nucleoli, and do not form gland lumens. Ductal prostatic adenocarcinoma (see later in this article) is favored when cells are columnar with focally prominent nucleoli and form gland spaces.

Shown is a case in which morphology alone favors urothelial carcinoma, although it turned out to be prostatic carcinoma. Growth is solid with no lumen spaces (**Fig. 5**). In this case, the normal overlying urothelium was the only clue that the cancer may not be urothelial. I have lost count of how many specimens I examined, submitted as

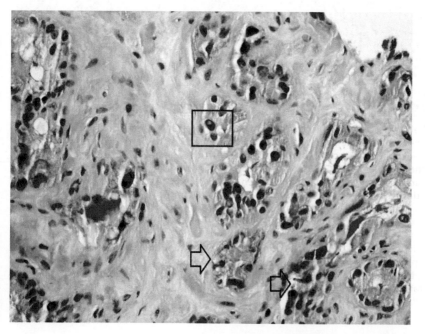

Fig. 4. Seminal vesicle (*square*). Normal seminal vesicle can display varying degrees of nuclear pleomorphism. The vacuolation of nuclei (*square*) and light golden lipofuscin pigment (*arrows*) would not be expected in cancer (original magnification ×40).

Fig. 5. (*A*) Prostatic adeno-carcinoma mimicking urothelial carcinoma. Suburothelial nodules growing in a solid pattern, and (*inset*) without obvious gland spaces or vacuoles, would seem to favor high-grade urothe-lial carcinoma, rather than acinar or ductal prostate cancer. This is despite the urothelium (*right*) being non-neoplastic. (*B*) PSA im-munostain of this tumor was, surprisingly, focally positive. (Benign urothe-lium is considered negative with "edge" effect.) Also, uroplakin II immunostain was negative (original magnification ×4).

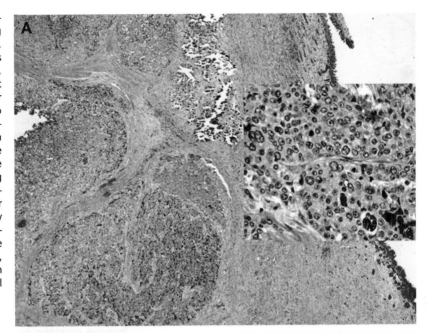

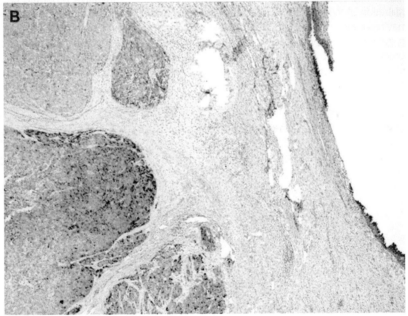

"bladder tumor," that turned out to be prostatic carcinoma. Thus, I maintain a low threshold for use of immunostains for tumors that are clinically periurethral or from the bladder neck (regardless of whether the transurethral resection was desig-nated prostate or bladder).

For *prostatic carcinoma*, prostate-specific anti-gen (PSA) is the most useful marker (**Fig. 6**); pros-tatic acid phosphatase and P501S may be added as second-line and third-line markers.[8] For *urothe-lial carcinoma*, uroplakin II and uroplakin III are often markers of choice. Uroplakin II is the more sensitive of the two.[9] GATA-3, not available in all laboratories, is a sensitive but less-specific urothe-lial carcinoma marker[8,10] that also marks breast carcinoma and several other malignancies. Other readily available second-line markers for urothelial carcinoma that discriminate it from prostatic carci-noma are p63, p40, thrombomodulin, cytokeratin 5/6, and high molecular weight cytokeratin clone 34βE12. Rarely, urothelial and prostatic carci-nomas coexist (**Figs. 7** and **8**).

Pitfalls

Prostatic Versus Other Carcinomas

! Unnecessary cystoprostatectomy can result from misdiagnosing prostatic adenocarcinoma as urothelial carcinoma, and the frequent overlap of their morphologies facilitates this error.

! Experts cannot tell the difference consistently from routine sections; thus, any bladder neck or urethral mass deserves immunostains.

! P504S is positive in almost all rectal and urothelial carcinomas and may rarely be negative in prostatic adenocarcinomas; thus, it cannot discriminate among these 3.

RECTAL ADENOCARCINOMA

Infiltration of the prostate by rectal adenocarcinoma may resemble a large-duct primary prostatic cancer. In some of the reported cases, no primary colorectal tumor was known before the prostatic biopsy specimen. Mucin, an asymmetric thinning of gland walls,

and "dirty" lumens with neutrophils and necrosis favor rectal origin. Positive staining for villin, CDX2, and cytokeratin 20 with negative reactivity for PSA and NKX3.1 can rule in rectal origin.[11] I recently encountered a case of rectal adenocarcinoma invading the prostate that was negative for CDX2 but positive for villin. Bladder adenocarcinoma would have goblet cells; some cases have weak focal PSA and prostatic acid phosphatase reactivity.

Overall diagnostic choices for nonprostatic carcinomas are shown (**Table 1**).

LARGE-GLAND PROSTATIC ADENOCARCINOMA

The past 5 years produced a revolution in our understanding of large-gland neoplasia of the prostate, including cribriform/papillary invasive carcinoma, intraductal carcinoma (IDC), and ductal carcinoma. The diagnostic criteria for each are shown (**Table 2**).

Invasive prostatic cancer acini should properly be called *pseudoacini*, because they are not functional acini. There is loss of function, as shown by decreased immunohistochemical PSA secretion per cell, in cancer compared with non-neoplastic acini. The main reason that cancer causes

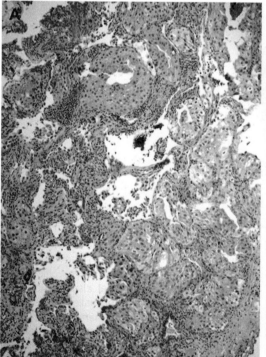
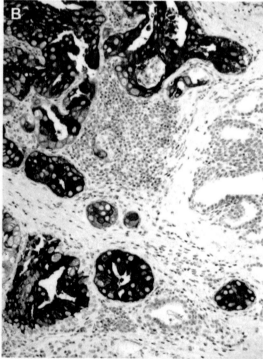

Fig. 6. Urothelial carcinoma of prostatic ducts (original magnification ×4). (*A*) *Left:* Large-duct proliferation with cells having indistinct cell borders and no prominent nucleoli. There is no obvious gland space formation. (*B*) *Right:* The uroplakin II stain is positive.

Fig. 7. Both urothelial (*top*) and prostatic (*bottom*) carcinomas coexist in this transurethral resection of bladder neck (original magnification ×4).

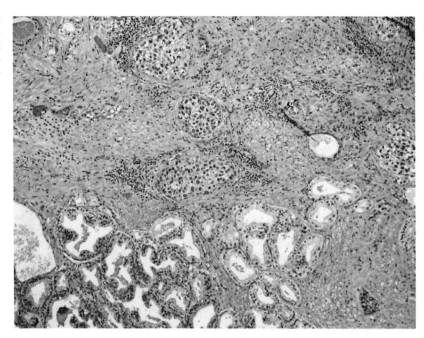

elevated serum PSA is that the PSA leaks from the pseudoacini into the stroma, rather than being secreted into the lumina. For convenience, we will henceforth use the term, *acini*.

P504S is a digestive enzyme overexpressed in prostate cancer, usually visualized by a red chromogen. Remember that whereas P504S should be positive in all 3 of these tumor types, it is not an infallible marker; technical optimization is tricky. Some obvious cancers have a weak pink signal, a common problem in many laboratories, even despite a strong signal in the control cancer tissue.

> ### *Pitfall*
>
> ! Immunoreactivity to P504S may be absent in 5% to 25% of typical prostate carcinomas.[8,12]

CURRENT GRADING OF LARGE-GLAND CANCER

Cancers presenting within large-gland spaces include not only cribriform, but also the glomeruloid variant (**Fig. 9**), the mucinous variant, and the rare adenoid cystic/basal cell carcinoma. The 2014 ISUP consensus set or refined Gleason grading criteria of all of these (**Table 3**).

PROGNOSTIC GRADE GROUPS

At its 2014 meeting, the ISUP also adopted a simplified patient-centric grading system comprising 5 grade groups[18] as proposed in 2013 based on data from Johns Hopkins and published in the World Health Organization Blue Book.[19] Grade groups 1 through 5 were designated as Gleason score (GS) 3 + 3 = 6, GS 3 + 4 = 7, GS 4 + 3 = 7, GS 8, and GS 9 to 10, respectively.[20] The partition of GS 3 + 4 = 7 from GS 4 + 3 = 7, and of GS 8 from GS 9 to 10, which were previously bundled together for prognostic and research purposes, are supported by studies showing significantly different outcomes.[21–23] Based on radical prostatectomy results, prognostic grade groups 2, 3, 4, and 5, carried biochemical recurrence hazard ratios, relative to group 1, of 1.9, 5.1, 8.0, and 11.7.[24]

However, mentioning the presence of cribriform cancer modifies the effect of the groups. The presence of cribriform cancer within grade group 4 (GS = 8) was an independent predictive factor that dichotomized cancer-free survival up to 36 months (P = .018).[23] Presence of cribriform cancer in biopsy specimens, likewise, can stratify Gleason 3 + 4 = 7 and predict upgrading and extraprostatic extension.[25,26]

TYPES OF LARGE-GLAND CANCER

INVASIVE LARGE-GLAND CARCINOMA (INCLUDING CRIBRIFORM AND PAPILLARY)

Those of us who took our pathology training before 2005 had learned to include the large-gland, cribriform pattern of invasive prostate cancer in the continuum of Gleason grade 3. As most such proliferations had rounded contours and were not

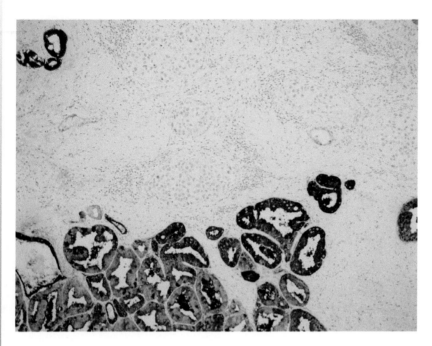

Fig. 8. Do not hesitate to immunostain high-grade cancer in bladder neck or transurethral resection specimens. PSA stain of **Fig. 7** shows reactivity in prostatic (*bottom*) but not urothelial (*top*) carcinoma (original magnification ×4).

confluent, we assigned these areas a GS of 3 + 3 = 6. All but the most cellular cribriform patterns were subsumed under "moderately differentiated" cancer, and this undoubtedly drove biochemical and metastatic recurrence rates for "Gleason 6" cancer higher than under current criteria.

Amin and colleagues[27] studied the use of basal cell markers to distinguish invasive cribriform carcinoma from cribriform prostatic intraepithelial neoplasia in 1994. The first indication that invasive cribriform carcinoma carried an elevated

biologic potential came in 1999 when Egevad and colleagues[28] noted that 40% of cribriform cancers were nondiploid, compared with only 12% of Gleason pattern 3 cancers. Further studies on patterns with respect to biochemical relapse were not pursued until a 2011 study.[29] In that study, 76 men undergoing prostatectomy who had subsequent PSA failure were matched to 77 men without failure, and 9 distinct patterns of cancer were digitally annotated on scanned whole-mount slides. A cribriform pattern (without necrosis) was present in 61% (46/76) of failures

Table 1
Differential diagnosis: nonprostatic carcinoma in prostate or bladder neck

	Prostatic Carcinoma	Urothelial Carcinoma	Rectal Carcinoma
Clinical	Prostate-specific antigen (PSA) elevated	PSA not elevated (unless coexistent prostate cancer)	PSA not elevated
Morphology	Cribriform, solid, intraductal, or ductal	Less likely to form gland spaces	Gland spaces with attenuated walls and "dirty" lumens with neutrophils and debris
Main positive immunostains[12]	PSA (PSA weak in high-grade cancer)	Uroplakin II, GATA-3	Villin, CDX2
Other positive immunostains	Prostatic acid phosphatase and P501S, NKX3.1	p63, p40, thrombomodulin, cytokeratin 5/6, and cytokeratin clone 34βE12	Cytokeratin 20
Negative immunostains	Uroplakin II, GATA-3	PSA	PSA and NKX3.1

Table 2
Differential diagnosis of large-gland prostate cancer

	Invasive Cribriform (to Papillary), Grade 4	Intraductal	Ductal
Clinical	Elevated prostate-specific antigen (PSA)	Elevated PSA (because is so frequently associated with acinar component)	Hematuria and bladder outlet obstruction
Cystoscopic/ Gross	Normal	Normal	Usually, exophytic mass protruding into urethra
Location	Peripheral > transition zone	Peripheral > transition zone	Transition zone/urethra
Basal cells	Absent	Present	Absent
Histology	No or mild duct distension; only as much nuclear enlargement as other invasive cancer; no necrosis	Distended and possibly branched duct space, more marked nuclear enlargement; possible necrosis	Distinctly columnar cells with stratified nuclei
Immunostains[12]	PSA, P504S+; no CK 34βE12 + or p63 + basal layer	PSA, P504S+; at least focal basal layer with 34βE12 + or p63+	PSA, P504S+; no CK 34βE12 + or p63 + basal layer
Metastasis	Lymph node, bone	Lymph node, bone	Routes similar to acinar adenocarcinoma[13]

but 16% (12/77) of nonfailures (P<.0001). Presence of cribriform cancer conferred a 5.9 odds ratio for PSA failure, the highest among histologic patterns studied. The amount of cribriform cancer dose-dependently raised the risk of failure, with a cumulative odds ratio of 1.173 per added square millimeter of cribriform pattern (P = .008), higher than for any other pattern. Cribriform carcinoma also held a strong association

(P = .001) with the individual cell pattern (grade 5) (**Fig. 10**). A separate category of "small cribriform," denoting acini not larger than benign ones in the same specimen (**Fig. 11**) or with thin, "collapsible" cell bridges (**Fig. 12**) shared the same predictive value for failure as large cribriform. Indeed, hypothetical regrading of all cribriform cancer as Gleason 5 improved the grade association with failure.[29]

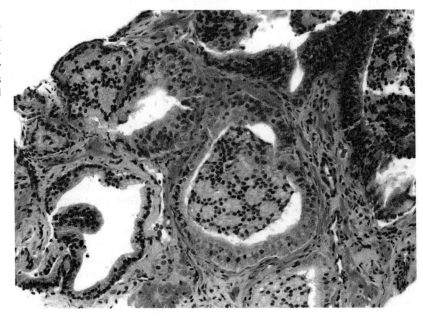

Fig. 9. Glomeruloid variant of prostate cancer is rare and resembles a renal glomerular tuft. This is, by consensus, graded as Gleason grade 4 (original magnification ×20).

Table 3
Grading of large-gland prostate cancer patterns

Histologic Pattern	2005 Consensus[14]	2014 Consensus[15]
Cribriform (according to the Gleason scheme, mostly a 3, sometimes a 4)	4, but rarely 3 if acini not much larger than benign, have "loose" cells, and acinus contours are round	Always 4; if comedonecrosis, then 5
Glomeruloid variant	No consensus, 3 vs 4	Always 4
Mucinous variant	No consensus; some said 4 + 4 = 8	Depends on growth pattern irrespective of the mucin background; can be 3, 4, or 5
Intraductal (when "isolated": no invasive carcinoma) – intraductal carcinoma	—	Do not grade
Ductal	4 + 4 = 8	—
Adenoid cystic/Basal cell carcinoma	Do not grade[16,17]	

Along these lines, in needle biopsy sets, cribriform cancer assumed an importance comparable to grade 5.[23] Among Gleason 8 cancers, the matter of whether the highest Gleason grade was 3 + 5 = 8 versus 4 + 4 = 8 proved only mildly predictive of recurrence. However, the presence of cribriform cancer dichotomized cancer-specific survival in Gleason 8 cancer (P = .018).[23] Moreover, the presence of cribriform growth in a biopsy proved to be more strongly predictive of biochemical recurrence than whether the highest Gleason grade was 3 + 5 = 8 versus 4 + 4 = 8.[23] Thus, many urologic pathologists now make a comment for each specimen or biopsy core with Gleason grade 4 cancer as to whether cribriform growth is present or absent; if the urologist performing the biopsy is not aware, the adverse prognostic implication of this finding should be added.

Radiologic Detection of Cribriform Cancer

In recent years, MRI to guide "targeted" biopsy sampling has come into use. It has become evident that this method best detects higher-grade cancer. Similarly, the number of cores with cribriform cancer as a percentage of total cores was higher with targeted biopsy than sextant biopsy (mean, 0.30 vs 0.05, P = .0002). Also, the number of cores with cribriform cancer as a fraction of total cancer cores was higher (0.38 vs 0.17, P = .0002).[30] The combination of targeted biopsy with sextant biopsy detects cribriform cancer better than either alone.[31] Interestingly, the b-value of the apparent diffusion coefficient (ADC) in MRI performed before prostatectomy can significantly predict cribriform pattern.[32]

Cribriform Cancer in Biopsy Predicts Adverse Pathology

Sixteen total articles since 2011, based on either biopsy or prostatectomy tissue,[26,29,31,33–45] have shown that cribriform cancer confers an elevated biologic potential compared with noncribriform Gleason 4 patterns, apparently regardless of the amount.[29,36,42] After 2014, evidence for the particularly adverse prognostic impact of cribriform invasive (and noninvasive, or intraductal) carcinoma accrued at an accelerating pace. My review article covers all the pertinent articles, including very recent data that remained in abstract form as of 2017.[46]

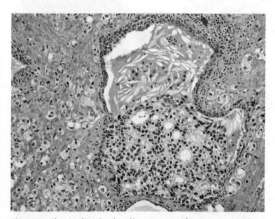

Fig. 10. The individual cell pattern of cancer, or Gleason grade 5 (*left*) is strongly and independently associated with cribriform growth (*right*) (original magnification ×10).

Fig. 11. Small cribriform cancer, with acini no larger than benign acini, shared the same prognostic implications as large cribriform cancer (original magnification ×10).

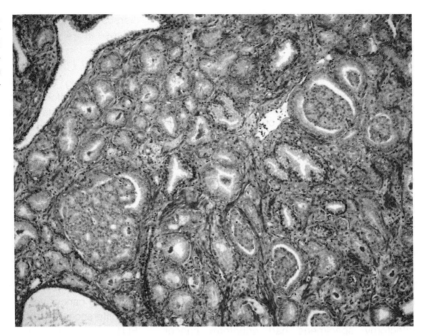

In biopsy specimens, several studies have linked clinicopathologic findings with the presence of a cribriform pattern.[46] Biopsied cancers with a cribriform component had significantly higher percent core involvement than did cancers without it.[30] The percentage of grade 4 cancer has limited ability to predict organ-confined cancer[47]; this prediction is greatly boosted by assessing cribriform cancer in the biopsies.[31,32,40,48]

Cribriform Cancer in Prostatectomy Predicts Outcome

Most studies of cribriform cancer have used radical prostatectomy specimens as source material. Following the consensus conferences of 2005 and 2014, assignment of GS 7 has risen,[49] and management of this cohort is less straightforward for urologists than with scores of 6 or 8 to 10. A contribution of cribriform cancer to Gleason 7

Fig. 12. Smaller acini with "collapsible" thin bridges and lower cellularity, shared the same prognostic implications as large cribriform cancer (original magnification ×20).

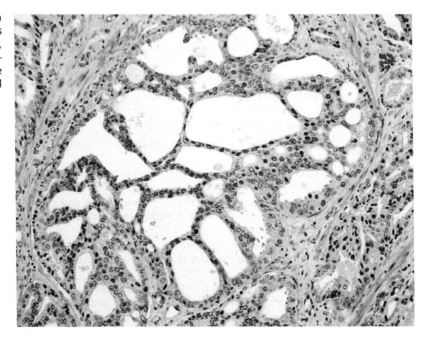

cancer could be pivotal. A recent meta-analysis of 14 publications determined an odds ratio of 11.37 for adverse outcome in cribriform cancer, including both clinical and pathologic findings.[50] Not only the cribriform pattern, but the number of high-grade morphologies at prostatectomy,[51] predicts recurrence. Thus, most urologic pathologists currently make a comment on the presence cribriform Gleason grade 4 cancer.

Studies using metastasis and death from prostate cancer as endpoints showed that cribriform pattern strongly predicted metastasis[34,41] and death.[40,41,46] Cribriform pattern was noted in 81% of cases with metastasis or death, versus 38% of controls ($P = .001$).[41]

Findings After Active Surveillance or Hormone Ablation

In a study of men undergoing delayed prostatectomy after a period of active surveillance (9–77 months, median 26), 22% of the patients' prostatectomy specimens had cribriform cancer. Specimens with cribriform cancer had on average 2 times the tumor volume of those with noncribriform grade 4 cancer. Rates of extraprostatic extension were 48% when cribriform cancer was present versus 9% for noncribriform.[52] Another study of cribriform cancer focused on men with cancer relapse after a course of abiraterone/gonadotropin-releasing hormone antagonist. Prostatectomy stage > ypT2 was noted in 80% of patients with cribriform/intraductal cancer versus 30% with absence of these patterns ($P<.0001$). The median tumor volume was 2.2

versus 0.2 mL in these groups and the rate of relapse at ≥4 years was 68% versus 27%.[53]

Molecular Profile

The accruing evidence for molecular changes unique to cribriform cancer provides a rationale for its aggressiveness (Table 4). The overall proliferative index measured by Ki67 in prostatectomy specimens with cribriform pattern was 3.8, versus 2.7 in noncribriform cancer.[54] Notably, the presence of cribriform pattern was associated with higher proliferation in Gleason grade 3 areas.[54] Also, in prostatectomy tissues meeting these criteria, the proliferative index was 5.8 for cribriform cancer versus 3.9 for fused and 3.9 for poorly formed acini; for Gleason grade 5 cancer the index was 12.9.[55]

A study using the The Cancer Genome Atlas public portal showed that mutations in SPOP and FOXA1 were more common among patients with cribriform cancer versus noncribriform Gleason 4. No differences were detected in ERG, ETV1/4, or FLI1.[56] Distinct DNA methylation alterations (specifically in APC, Ras1, T-box genes) are associated with cribriform carcinoma and IDC in Gleason pattern 4 prostate tumors, as opposed to noncribriform cancer.[56,57] Phosphatase and tensin homolog (PTEN) loss inactivates cell cycle inhibitor p27/Kip1, both prognostically adverse events. In our series of 52 prostate cases,[58] PTEN and p27 losses by immunostaining, normalized to benign acini, were greater for cribriform cancer than noncribriform grade 4. A biphenotypic cell population in cribriform structures was described, with more PTEN loss centrally and more p27 loss peripherally. Overall,[58]

Table 4
Molecular marker expression in cribriform cancer

Marker	Expression in Cribriform vs Noncribriform Cancer	Reference
Ki67	3.8 in prostatectomy cancers, Gleason score ≥7 with cribriform vs 2.7	Hwang et al,[54] 2016
Ki67	5.8 for cribriform cancer vs 3.9	Fu et al,[55] 2016
SPOP and FOXA1	More mutations (no difference in ERG, ETV1/4, or FLI1)	Elfandy et al,[56] 2017
APC, Ras1, T-box genes	Distinct DNA methylation alterations in cribriform and intraductal cancer	Elfandy et al,[56] 2017; Olkhov-Mitsel et al,[57] 2017
PTEN and p27	Losses were greater for cribriform cancer (RNA and protein); more PTEN loss centrally and more p27 loss peripherally	Ronen et al,[58] 2017
Copy number alterations	Increased genomic instability in cribriform and intraductal cancer; also, association with prostatic hypoxia	Elfandy et al,[56] 2017; Böttcher et al,[60] 2018
SChLAP1	Long noncoding RNA that is, an unfavorable biomarker; overexpressed in cribriform and intraductal	Chua et al,[59] 2017; Pressner et al,[61] 2013

PTEN loss compared with all other acini was significant for fused small acini, cribriform-central cells, small cribriform acini, and Gleason grade 5 cells. p27 loss compared with benign acini (mean 2.5 + on a 0–3 scale) was significant only for cribriform-peripheral cells (mean 1.5+); CD44v7/8 showed expression loss in cribriform-peripheral cells; other comparisons were not significant. By in situ hybridization, cribriform cancer had significant PTEN loss normalized to benign acini (P<.02), but the difference was not significant for other morphologies. Other studies have shown that cribriform/intraductal cancer was associated with increased genetic instability (percentage genomic alterations as determined by copy number alterations).[59,60] Affected genes included loss of *PTEN*, *CDH1*, and *BCAR1*, and gain of *MYC*, and with lesser frequency, point mutations in *TP53*, *SPOP*, and *FOXA1*.[60] There was an association with prostatic hypoxia, measured before therapy by transrectal needle piezoelectrode. Cribriform pattern was also associated with overexpression of the long noncoding RNA SChLAP1,[59] a finding of interest because SChLAP1 was previously shown to represent a biomarker for unfavorable cancer.[61]

Diagnostic Reproducibility

The diagnosis of cribriform cancer was more reproducible than that of other Gleason grade 4 patterns among 12 urologic pathologists surveyed. Their diagnostic concordance was 79% for cribriform, versus 61% for poorly formed acini and 36% for fused acini.[62] In another study, a definitive cribriform pattern had the strongest agreement of any pattern for prognostic assessment by 3 methods, including the 17-gene Genomic Prostate Score.[63] These findings support the ability of pathologists to diagnose cribriform cancer reliably.

Implications for Grading

The abundant and reproducible evidence described previously supports inclusion of cribriform morphology into grading practice. Whereas some dose-dependence is suggested by outcome data,[29] any quantity of it appears important,[29,33,35,39] even if it forms less than 5% of the cancer.[36] This has been acknowledged as an emerging issue.[46,64] Although all urologic pathologists[65] and probably most general surgical pathologists would specify the presence of IDC, the need to mention whether Gleason 4 is cribriform is less widely recognized. Anecdotally, many prominent urologic pathologists now specify whenever a cribriform pattern is present, either by a line diagnosis or synoptic template.

Pitfalls

! Some active surveillance protocols allow a limited amount of Gleason 4 cancer for eligibility

! Not specifying whether grade group 2 includes cribriform cancer could subject men to active surveillance who should not be candidates for it.[42]

A scheme for indicating the presence of cribriform pattern has been proposed. Subdivision of grade group 2 into cribriform (proposed grade group 2C) and noncribriform[46] would address the issue. Specifying cribriform cancer in groups 3 and 4 (possibly by using grades 3C and 4C)[46] may also be consequential for treatment choice, such as whether or not to perform pelvic lymphadenectomy. (This would be in addition to specifying the percentage of Gleason 4 cancer in grade group 2 or 3, a recommendation already in place.[66]) A small number of grade group 4 cancer in 1 core with cribriform pattern would suggest a worse outcome than exclusively noncribriform cancer. Notably, cribriform cancer with central comedonecrosis (**Fig. 13**) is already Gleason grade 5 by consensus,[15,64] thus cribriform designation is irrelevant.

Many pathologists do mention the percentage pattern 4[22]; although its effect is modest,[47] compared with the stronger effect of cribriform pattern. The presence of cribriform pattern actually shows a robust correlation with the percentage pattern 4.[63] In prostatectomy specimens graded as Gleason 6 from 2003 to 2007, when Gleason 4 cancer was found and was broken down by deciles of percentage, those deciles with ≥11% contained more than half of cases with a cribriform pattern.[63]

INTRADUCTAL CARCINOMA

The term IDC of the prostate was first used in 1972,[66] but since approximately 2005 it has gained acceptance as a separate entity.[67,68] Before that, the term IDC, along with "intraductal dysplasia," was largely subsumed by high-grade prostatic intraepithelial neoplasia.[68] Molecular evidence now points to retrograde cancerization of duct spaces by the invasive cancer as the origin of IDC.[69]

Clinical Features

The segregation of IDC and related entities from HGPIN was in recognition of the much higher

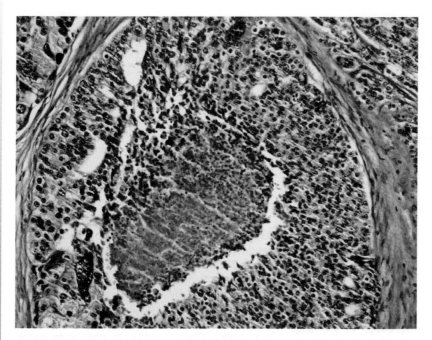

Fig. 13. Cribriform cancer may have central comedonecrosis, and more subtle forms of this exist. Because necrosis implies grade 5 by consensus, no adjustment to the grading system is needed for cancer with necrosis (original magnification ×40).

predictive value for cancer of isolated IDC compared with HGPIN's approximate currently accepted value of 20% to 25% (higher if ≥4 cores have HGPIN).[70]

Almost always occurring in association with invasive acinar cancer, IDC occurs as an isolated finding in only 2% of biopsy sets, where it poses both a diagnostic and therapeutic challenge. Some studies have chosen to group cribriform cancer with IDC of the prostate[36,42,53] (Fig. 14), a logical choice as most IDC is cribriform, and both lesions bear strong associations with adverse pathology. Molecular evidence points to retrograde colonization of duct spaces by the invasive cancer as the origin of IDC.[69]

Morphology

IDC criteria are as follows:

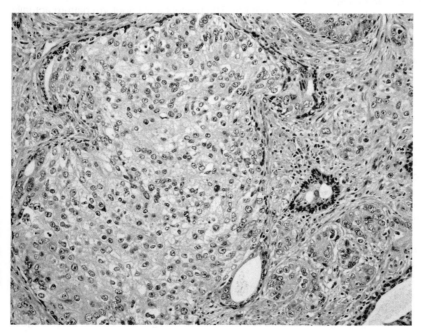

Fig. 14. IDC is an expansile proliferation of markedly atypical cells contained within a duct space that retains its basal layer. It is almost always accompanied by invasive carcinoma (*right*) (original magnification ×40).

- A lumen-spanning proliferation of neoplastic cells in distended, preexisting ducts

- Dense cribriform or partial solid growth pattern

- Nuclear atypia exceeds that of HGPIN (some say 6 times size of a benign nucleus) (**Fig. 15**)

- At least focal basal cells are preserved

- Branching of the distended duct spaces is diagnostically helpful (**Fig. 16**)

Differential Diagnosis and Reproducibility

Invasive cribriform carcinoma and HGPIN are the main differential diagnoses. IDC resembling invasive carcinoma (**Fig. 17**) is distinguished by retaining at least a patchy layer of basal cells (**Fig. 18**). Some pathologists use a category called "atypical cribriform proliferation,"[71] borderline,[72] or atypical "intraductal cribriform proliferation"[73] for diagnostic findings intermediate between HGPIN and IDC (**Fig. 19**).

The interobserver reproducibility for IDC remains modest,[65,74] probably because of its frequent admixture with invasive cribriform cancer. The presence of any amount of either cribriform cancer or IDC was associated with biochemical relapse (odds ratio 3, $P = .0002$).[36] The borderline[72] or atypical "intraductal cribriform proliferation"[72] category appears similar to IDC in molecular and clinicopathologic features such as frequency of ERG and PTEN positivity.[72] IDC and even atypical cribriform proliferation have both recently been proven to predict biochemical recurrence even after controlling for grade, stage, and margin status.[36,72,73] However, in the absence of concurrent invasive cancer or IDC, the significance of "borderline" is uncertain. If it is an isolated finding, it cannot be included in grading and is best communicated as a comment with recommended repeat biopsy.

We surveyed 39 urologic pathologists to assess the interobserver variability of an IDC diagnosis. We provided 38 images of HGPIN versus IDC versus invasive cancer. In 19 cases that were candidates for IDC, only 5 (26%) achieved at least a two-thirds consensus of IDC. Lack of consensus warrants the diagnosis of atypical cribriform proliferation (see **Fig. 19**). An example of a case achieving consensus for IDC is shown in **Fig. 20**. Nine more (47%) cases had a consensus for a combined category of "either borderline or IDC."[74] Findings that differed across diagnostic categories were lumen-spanning neoplastic cells ($P<.001$), 2 × benign duct diameters ($P<.001$), duct space contours (round, irregular, and branched) ($P<.001$), papillary growth ($P = .048$), dense cribriform or solid growth (both $P = .023$), and comedonecrosis ($P = .015$). Lack of IDC consensus was most often attributed to the image displaying loose ("collapsible") cribriform growth,

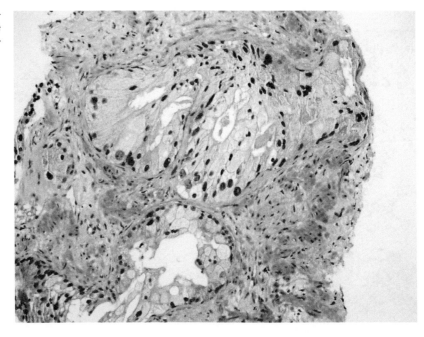

Fig. 15. The nuclear atypia of IDC should be marked (original magnification ×40).

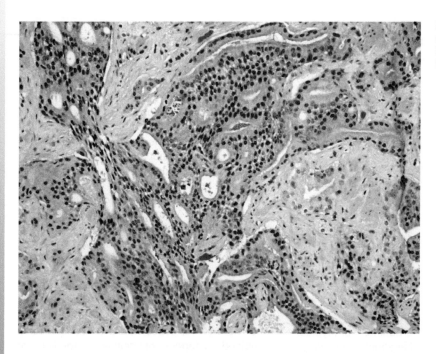

Fig. *16.* Branching of cribriform structures is a key finding of IDC (original magnification ×20).

central nuclear maturation, or central comedonecrosis.[74] Thus, subjectivity persists in the application of diagnostic criteria for IDC. Rarities not particular to IDC, such as vacuolar alteration (**Fig. 21**) and mucinous carcinoma, also may be found in IDC.

Molecular Profile

IDC has a unique molecular biologic profile (**Table 5**).[68] The rates of ERG fusion and PTEN loss in IDC are at least commensurate with those of invasive carcinoma, and exceed the corresponding rates for HGPIN. Fine and colleagues[75] found no difference in ERG translocation/deletion or copy number increase in tumors from men with or without IDC. Immunoreactivity for ERG protein, reflecting a TMPRSS2-ERG gene fusion, has been reported in 35% to 75%[68] of IDC but rarely or never in "atypical cribriform lesions" that fall short of IDC criteria. A topographic study using proximity to invasive cancer to discriminate IDC[76] provided a

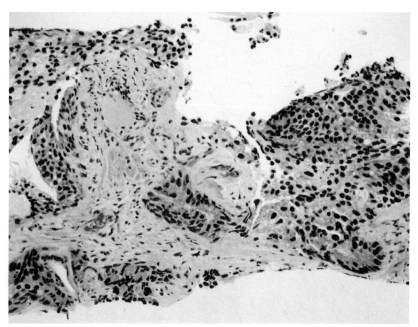

Fig. *17.* Diagnosis in this biopsy is between IDC and invasive cribriform carcinoma, but the branching nature of acini favors IDC (original magnification ×10).

Fig. 18. The cytokeratin 34βE12/p63/P504S immunostain of *Fig. 17* demonstrates at least a patchy basal cell layer is present, confirming IDC (original magnification ×10).

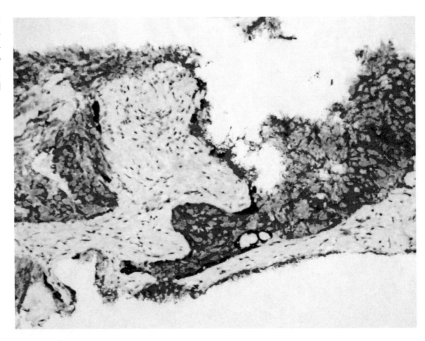

molecular justification for topography being discriminatory. Schneider and Osunkoya[77] found that the presence or absence of ERG reactivity in IDC always matched that of the acinar carcinoma; but the 35% rate of expression of the invasive carcinoma associated with IDC was less than that separate from IDC, suggesting that when IDC is present, the accompanying invasive component tends to have a unique phenotype. ERG

immunostaining may be diagnostically useful in select cases. Cytoplasmic PTEN loss has been suggested as a marker to distinguish IDC from HGPIN, being observed in 84% of IDC and 100% of lesions intermediate between IDC and HGPIN, but never in HGPIN.[78] Nuclear reactivity for PTEN may be retained in IDC. IDC's rate of PTEN loss exceeds the 35% to 45% rates reported for acinar carcinoma[79–82] but is similar to the significantly

Fig. 19. Atypical cribriform proliferation. This is ambiguous for IDC. It is a loose cribriform formation. Differential diagnosis includes HGPIN. Gleason grading does not apply (original magnification ×10).

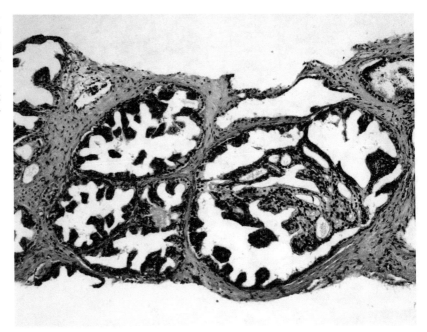

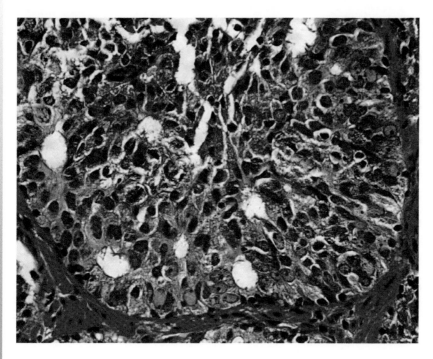

Fig. 20. IDC. Unambiguous findings with duct space enlargement, dense cribriform to solid cells, and 6× nuclear enlargement (original magnification ×40).

higher PTEN loss in Gleason grades 4 to 5 cancer,[78] supporting the aggressiveness of IDC.

DUCTAL CARCINOMA

Clinical Features

Previously termed "endometrioid carcinoma,"[13] this large-glandular growth occurs in 3% of prostate cancer and is most frequent in the transition zone. In all but 0.2% to 0.4% of cases, there is admixed acinar carcinoma. An exophytic mass usually protrudes into the urethra, thus common symptoms are hematuria and bladder outlet obstruction. To the urologist performing urethroscopy, ductal carcinoma can mimic a urothelial carcinoma of the prostatic or

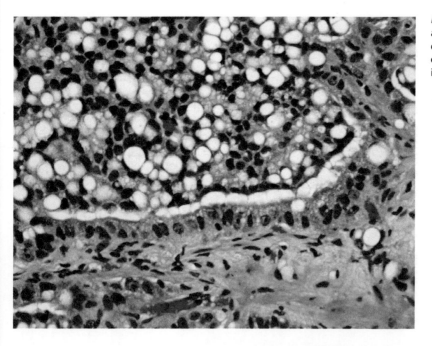

Fig. 21. Vacuolar alteration of IDC. An invasive carcinoma component coexists (*bottom*) (original magnification ×40).

Table 5
Molecular markers to discriminate IDC from high-grade prostatic intraepithelial neoplasia (HGPIN)

Marker	Intraductal Carcinoma	HGPIN	Reference
ERG fusion	No difference in ERG translocation, deletion or copy number		Fine et al,[75] 2010
ERG fusion	Immunoreactivity for ERG in 35%–75% but none or rare in "atypical cribriform lesion"	<35%	Zhou,[68] 2018
ERG fusion	Rate of positivity matched that of invasive carcinoma		Schneider et al,[77] 2013
PTEN loss (cytoplasmic)	84% of IDC and 100% of "atypical cribriform lesion"	Never	Yoshimoto et al,[78] 2013
PTEN loss (cytoplasmic)	IDC PTEN loss exceeds the 35%–45% rate in most acinar carcinoma	—	Reid et al,[79] 2010; Bhalla et al,[80] 2013; Chaux et al,[81] 2012; Lotan et al,[82] 2011
Loss of heterozygosity for microsatellite markers	60% of cases (exceeds 29% for grade 4 cancer)	9% of cases	Dawkins et al,[76] 2000

membranous urethra. Because tumor cells secrete their PSA into the urethra instead of the bloodstream, serum PSA may not be elevated; if PSA is elevated, it is attributable to an admixed acinar component.[13] Ductal carcinoma metastasizes along routes similar to acinar adenocarcinoma.[13]

Ductal carcinoma, by ISUP consensus, should be graded as Gleason 4; any presence of comedonecrosis raises the grade to Gleason 5 (see **Table 4**). By virtue of its constant, higher Gleason grade, ductal carcinoma on average carries a higher stage, tumor volume, and more aggressive behavior than acinar adenocarcinoma.

Fig. 22. Low power view of ductal prostate cancer from a mass at the floor of the bladder (original magnification ×4).

Morphology

Ductal carcinoma criteria are as follows:

- Large-gland spaces
- Mainly papillary pattern, verging on cribriform (**Figs. 22** and **23**)
- Presence of true fibrovascular cores
- Tall columnar cytologically malignant cells line the cores
- Nuclei are stratified, usually elongated

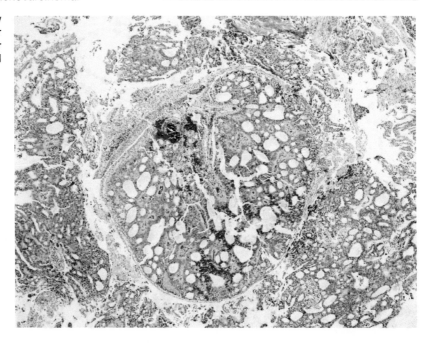

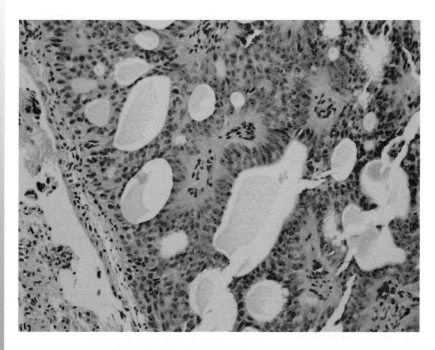

Fig. 23. Ductal prostate cancer at high power shows elongated, crowded nuclei lining cribriform structures (original magnification ×10).

In an interobserver study using 21 photomicrographs distributed to 20 urologic pathologists, a two-thirds consensus was reached in 76% of cases comprising 52% consensus for ductal carcinoma and 24% against it.[83] Differential diagnoses included IDC and HGPIN. More than 80% of cases featured papillary architecture and stratification of nuclei, making these the 2 most distinguishing features. More than 50% featured tall columnar epithelium and elongated nuclei.[83]

If the definition of ductal carcinoma were broadened to cribriform as well as papillary proliferations 5 mm in extent, regardless of the presence of columnar cells with stratified nuclei or a periurethral location, the incidence

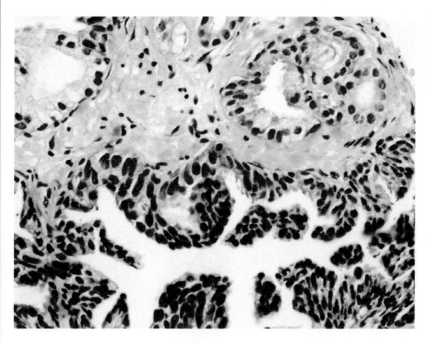

Fig. 24. PIN-like carcinoma has a tufted stratified epithelium. A small acinar component accompanies it (*top*) (original magnification ×40).

would top 5%.[84] This might produce better inter-observer reproducibility, but it would change ductal carcinoma's fundamental definition.

LESS COMMON LARGE-GLAND CARCINOMAS

PSEUDOHYPERPLASTIC AND PROSTATIC INTRAEPITHELIAL NEOPLASIA–LIKE

Pseudohyperplastic cancer was noted in 11% of radical prostatectomy specimens and 2% of needle biopsy specimens.[85,86] This diagnostic pitfall is a mimic of benign nodular hyperplasia. Pseudohyperplastic cancer comprises large or dilated acinar spaces with papillary infoldings, undulated lumens, and branching.

Another large-gland cancer is PIN-like carcinoma, a mimic of HGPIN (**Fig. 24**). Both of these cancers should be graded as a large acinar type of Gleason grade 3.[15] Constant findings are nuclear enlargement, prominent nucleoli, and (in radical prostatectomy specimens) a transition to usual small acinar carcinoma. P504S is negative in 23% to 30% of cases of the pseudohyperplastic carcinoma variant[85] (described in the next section[86,87]). A *microcystic* variant[88] has been described, including gland spaces 0.4 to 0.9 cm, with an 11.2% prevalence in prostatectomy specimens. This pattern strongly mimicked cystic atrophy, and basal markers/P504S were diagnostic.

PSEUDOATROPHIC CARCINOMA

This entity resembles atrophy on low power, with dilated lumen spaces and a thin epithelium. P504S is negative in 30% of *pseudoatrophic carcinoma*.[85,86]

ADENOID CYSTIC/BASAL CELL CARCINOMA

This histologic variant features an adenoid cystic-like pattern similar to its salivary gland counterpart.

Clinical Features

Two studies reported 48 cases of this special type of prostate cancer, 34 with clinical outcome.[17,89] Patients ranged in age from 42 to 89 years, and all but one presented with urinary obstruction and were diagnosed by transurethral resection, suggesting a predilection for the transition zone. Four patients had concurrent acinar adenocarcinoma. Eight metastases and 2 deaths were documented among the 34 patients who had follow-up in the 2 studies. Thus, adenoid cystic/basal cell carcinoma (ACBCC) is a potentially aggressive tumor requiring ablative therapy.

Morphology

The growth can be predominantly adenoid cystic (**Fig. 25**) or feature predominantly basaloid (**Fig. 26**) cancer cells. Immunohistochemically, the tumor

Fig. 25. ACBCC. Predominant adenoid pattern (original magnification ×20).

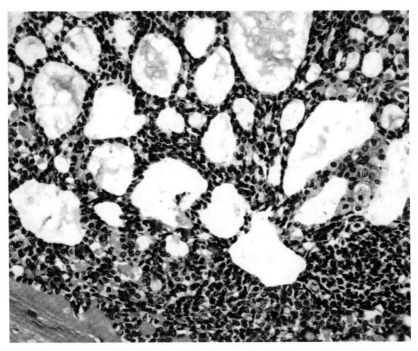

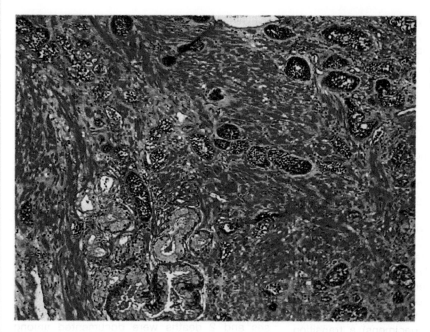

Fig. 26. ACBCC. Proliferation of basaloid nests of cancer cells fills most of the field, with conventional acinar carcinoma seen at lower left (original magnification ×4).

cells of ACBCC were immunoreactive for p63, and cytokeratins 7 and 34βE12 but not cytokeratin 20. This basaloid phenotype overlaps with urothelial carcinoma. Interestingly, the tumors were positive for Her2Neu, predominantly in inner cell nests, unlike acinar carcinoma.[90] Extraprostatic extension was noted in a combined 10 of 12 patients who underwent prostatectomy. Some reported cases invaded skeletal muscle of the bladder neck.

Extraprostatic Spread

A case of aggressive ACBCC has been reported, apparently distal to the prostate and involving the membranous urethra and penis as well as the prostate. The prostate also had high-grade acinar adenocarcinoma. This ACBCC was reactive for cytokeratin 7 and p63[91]; however, the close proximity to the prostate as well as presence of concurrent prostatic acinar adenocarcinoma suggest contiguous spread from a prostatic primary.

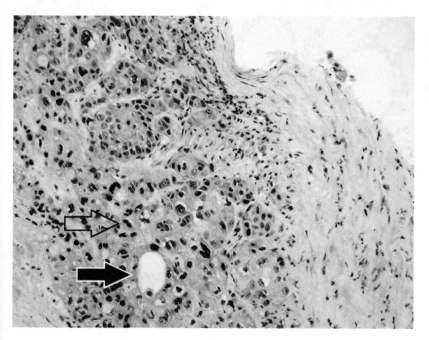

Fig. 27. Squamous cell carcinoma of the prostate. Dyskeratotic cell (*open arrow*) and rare lumen formation (*dark arrow*) (original magnification ×20).

SQUAMOUS CELL CARCINOMA

Squamous cell carcinoma can result in large-gland spaces and usually arises after androgen deprivation therapy. We have reported a case arising in the absence of androgen deprivation, with a small admixed component of acinar adenocarcinoma (**Fig. 27**).[92] Large cells with intracellular keratin and intercellular bridges are key to the diagnosis.

REFERENCES

1. Bostwick DG, Cheng L. Precursors of prostate cancer. Histopathology 2012;60:4–27.
2. Srodon M, Epstein JI. Central zone histology of the prostate: a mimicker of high grade prostatic intraepithelial neoplasia. Hum Pathol 2002;33:518–23.
3. Knoedler JJ, Karnes RJ, Thompson RH, et al. The association of tumor volume with mortality following radical prostatectomy. Prostate Cancer Prostatic Dis 2014;17:144–8.
4. Lerner SP, Shen S. Pathologic assessment and clinical significance of prostatic involvement by transitional cell carcinoma and prostate cancer. Urol Oncol 2008;26:481–5.
5. Revelo MP, Cookson MS, Chang SS, et al. Incidence and location of prostate and urothelial carcinoma in prostates from cystoprostatectomies: implications for possible apical sparing surgery. J Urol 2008; 179(5 Suppl):S27–32.
6. Wood DP, Montie JE, Pontes JE, et al. Transitional cell carcinoma of the prostate in cystoprostatectomy specimens removed for bladder cancer. J Urol 1989; 141:346–9.
7. Mazzucchelli R, Barbisan F, Scarpelli M, et al. Is incidentally detected prostate cancer in patients undergoing radical cystoprostatectomy clinically significant? Am J Clin Pathol 2009;131:279–83.
8. Epstein JI, Egevad L, Humphrey PA, et al, Members of the ISUP Immunohistochemistry in Diagnostic Urologic Pathology Group. Best practices recommendations in the application of immunohistochemistry in the prostate: report from the International Society of Urologic Pathology consensus conference. Am J Surg Pathol 2014; 38:e6–19.
9. Smith SC, Mohanty SK, Kunju LP, et al. Uroplakin II outperforms uroplakin III in diagnostically challenging settings. Histopathology 2014;65:132–8.
10. Tian W, Guner G, Miyamoto H, et al. Utility of Uroplakin II expression as a marker of urothelial carcinoma. Hum Pathol 2015;46:58–64.
11. Osunkoya AO, Netto GJ, Epstein JI. Colorectal adenocarcinoma involving the prostate: report of 9 cases. Hum Pathol 2007;38:1836–41.
12. Varma M, Jasani B. Diagnostic utility of immunohistochemistry in morphologically difficult prostate cancer: review of current literature. Histopathology 2005;47:1–16.
13. Bostwick DG, Kindrachuk RW, Rouse RV. Prostatic adenocarcinoma with endometrioid features. Clinical, pathologic, and ultrastructural findings. Am J Surg Pathol 1985;9:595–609.
14. Epstein JI, Allsbrook WC, Amin MB, et al, and the ISUP Grading Committee. The International Society of Urological Pathology (ISUP) consensus conference on Gleason grading of prostatic carcinoma. Am J Surg Pathol 2005;29:1228–42.
15. Epstein JI, Egevad L, Amin MB, et al. The 2014 International Society of Urological Pathology (ISUP) consensus conference on Gleason grading of prostatic carcinoma: definition of grading patterns and proposal for a new grading system. Am J Surg Pathol 2016;40:244–52.
16. Kryvenko ON, Epstein JI. Prostate cancer grading: a decade after the 2005 modified Gleason system. Arch Pathol Lab Med 2016;140:1140–52.
17. Iczkowski KA, Ferguson KL, Grier DD, et al. Adenoid cystic carcinoma of the prostate: clinicopathologic findings in 19 cases. Am J Surg Pathol 2003;27:1523–9.
18. Kryvenko ON, Epstein JI. Changes in prostate cancer grading: Including a new patient-centric grading system. Prostate 2016;76:427–33.
19. Moch H, Humphrey PA, Ulbright TM, et al, editors. WHO classification of tumours of the urinary system and male genital organs. 4th edition. Lyon (France): International Agency for Research on Cancer; 2016.
20. Egevad L, Delahunt B, Evans AJ, et al. International Society of Urologic Pathology (ISUP) grading of prostate cancer. Am J Surg Pathol 2016;40:858–61.
21. O'Kelly F, Elamin S, Cahill A, et al. Characteristics of modern Gleason 9/10 prostate adenocarcinoma: a single tertiary centre experience within the Republic of Ireland. World J Urol 2014;32:1067–74.
22. Tsao CK, Gray KP, Nakabayashi M, et al. Patients with biopsy Gleason 9 and 10 prostate cancer have significantly worse outcomes compared to patients with Gleason 8 disease. J Urol 2015;194:91–7.
23. Harding-Jackson N, Kryvenko ON, Whittington EE, et al. Outcome of Gleason 3+5=8 prostate cancer diagnosed on needle biopsy: prognostic comparison with Gleason 4+4=8. J Urol 2016;196:1076–81.
24. Epstein JI, Zelefsky MJ, Sjoberg DD, et al. A contemporary prostate cancer grading system: a validated alternative to the Gleason score. Eur Urol 2016;69:428–35.
25. Flood TA, Schieda N, Keefe DT, et al. Utility of Gleason pattern 4 morphologies detected on transrectal ultrasound (TRUS)-guided biopsies for prediction of upgrading or upstaging in Gleason score 3 + 4 = 7 prostate cancer. Virchows Arch 2016;469:313–9.
26. Kweldam CF, Kümmerlin IP, Nieboer D, et al. Prostate cancer outcomes of men with biopsy Gleason

score 6 and 7 without cribriform or intraductal carcinoma. Eur J Cancer 2016;66:26–33.

27. Amin MB, Schultz DS, Zarbo RJ. Analysis of cribriform morphology in prostatic neoplasia using antibodies to high-molecular-weight cytokeratins. Arch Pathol Lab Med 1994;118:260–4.

28. Egevad L, Engstrom K, Wester K, et al. Heterogeneity of DNA ploidy in prostate cancer. J Urol Pathol 1999;10:23–37.

29. Iczkowski KA, Torkko KC, Kotnis GR, et al. Digital quantification of five high-grade prostate cancer patterns, including the cribriform pattern, and their association with adverse outcome. Am J Clin Pathol 2011;136:98–107.

30. Wang Y, Deng F, Huang H, et al. MRI-targeted prostate biopsy detects more cribriform prostate carcinoma than standard sextant biopsy, [abstract]. Mod Pathol 2017;30:266A.

31. Truong M, Feng C, Hollenberg G. A comprehensive analysis of cribriform morphology on magnetic resonance imaging/ultrasound fusion biopsy correlated with radical prostatectomy specimens. J Urol 2018; 199:106–13.

32. Hurrell SL, McGarry SD, Kaczmarowski A, et al. Optimized b-value selection for the discrimination of prostate cancer grades, including the cribriform pattern, using diffusion weighted imaging. J Med Imaging (Bellingham) 2018;51:011004.

33. Wang Y, Deng F, Huang H, et al. Gleason score 7 and 8 prostate cancer with cribriform morphology diagnosed in prostate biopsy is more likely to have seminal vesicle invasion and pelvic lymph node metastasis in radical prostatectomy, [abstract]. Mod Pathol 2017;30:266A.

34. Kryvenko ON, Gupta NS, Virani N, et al. Gleason score 7 adenocarcinoma of the prostate with lymph node metastases: analysis of 184 radical prostatectomy specimens. Arch Pathol Lab Med 2013;137: 610–7.

35. Dong F, Yang P, Wang C, et al. Architectural heterogeneity and cribriform pattern predict adverse clinical outcome for Gleason grade 4 prostatic adenocarcinoma. Am J Surg Pathol 2013;37: 1855–61.

36. Trudel D, Downes MR, Sykes J, et al. Prognostic impact of intraductal carcinoma and large cribriform carcinoma architecture after prostatectomy in a contemporary cohort. Eur J Cancer 2014;50:1610–6.

37. Sarbay BC, Kir G, Topal CS, et al. Significance of the cribriform pattern in prostatic adenocarcinomas. Pathol Res Pract 2014;210:554–7.

38. Kir G, Sarbay BC, Gümüş E, et al. The association of the cribriform pattern with outcome for prostatic adenocarcinomas. Pathol Res Pract 2014;210:640–4.

39. Siadat F, Sykes J, Zlotta AR, et al. Not all Gleason pattern 4 prostate cancers are created equal: a study of latent prostatic carcinomas in a cystoprostatectomy and autopsy series. Prostate 2015;75:1277–84.

40. Keefe DT, Schieda N, El Hallani S, et al. Cribriform morphology predicts upstaging after radical prostatectomy in patients with Gleason score 3+4=7 prostate cancer at transrectal ultrasound (TRUS)-guided needle biopsy. Virchows Arch 2015;467:437–42.

41. Kweldam CF, Wildhagen MF, Steyerberg EW, et al. Cribriform growth is highly predictive for postoperative metastasis and disease-specific death in Gleason score 7 prostate cancer. Mod Pathol 2015;28: 457–64.

42. Kweldam CF, Kümmerlin IP, Nieboer D, et al. Disease-specific survival of patients with invasive cribriform and intraductal prostate cancer at diagnostic biopsy. Mod Pathol 2016;29:630–6.

43. Ross HM, Kryvenko ON, Cowan JE, et al. Do adenocarcinomas of the prostate with Gleason score (GS) ≤6 have the potential to metastasize to lymph nodes? Am J Surg Pathol 2012;36:1346–52.

44. Choy B, Pearce SM, Anderson BB, et al. Prognostic significance of percentage and architectural types of contemporary Gleason pattern 4 prostate cancer in radical prostatectomy. Am J Surg Pathol 2016;40: 1400–6.

45. McKenney JK, Wei W, Hawley S, et al. Histologic grading of prostatic adenocarcinoma can be further optimized: analysis of the relative prognostic strength of individual architectural patterns in 1275 patients from the Canary Retrospective Cohort. Am J Surg Pathol 2016;40:1439–56.

46. Iczkowski KA, van der Kwast TA, Paner GP. The new realization about cribriform prostate cancer. Adv Anat Pathol 2018;25:31–7.

47. Perlis N, Sayyid R, Evans A, et al. Limitations in predicting organ confined prostate cancer in patients with Gleason pattern 4 on biopsy: implications for active surveillance. J Urol 2017;197:75–83.

48. Hogan K, Robertson SJ, Schieda N, et al. Do specific Gleason pattern 4 morphologies detected on transrectal ultrasound guided biopsies predict upgrading or upstaging in Gleason score 3+4=7 prostate cancer?, [abstract]. Mod Pathol 2016;29:239A.

49. Danneman D, Drevin L, Robinson D, et al. Gleason inflation 1998-2011: a registry study of 97,168 men. BJU Int 2015;115:248–55.

50. Luo X, Jhala N, Khurana JS. The association of cribriform lesions with prostatic adenocarcinoma outcomes: a meta analysis [abstract]. Mod Pathol 2017;30:240A.

51. Flood TA, Schieda N, Sim J, et al. Evaluation of tumor morphologies and association with biochemical recurrence after radical prostatectomy in grade group 5 prostate cancer. Virchows Arch 2018; 472(2):205–12.

52. Troncoso P, Davis JW, Tapia E, et al. Prostate cancer Gleason grade 4 pattern heterogeneity in men on

active surveillance who undergo delayed prostatectomy, [abstract]. Mod Pathol 2016;29:267A.

53. Troncoso P, Li-Ning-Tapia E, Davis JW, et al. Cribriform/intraductal carcinoma, a candidate predictor of response to neoadjuvant treatment with novel androgen inhibitors in localized high risk prostate cancer, [abstract]. Mod Pathol 2017;30:264A.

54. Hwang M, Fu L, Adeniran A, et al. Proliferation index of Gleason grade 3 prostate adenocarcinoma with and without associated grade 4, [abstract]. Mod Pathol 2016;29:239A.

55. Fu L, Hwang M, Adeniran A, et al. Proliferation index of different Gleason grade 4 prostatic adenocarcinoma morphologies, [abstract]. Mod Pathol 2016; 29:230A.

56. Elfandy H, Pederzoli F, Pullman E, et al. Molecular characterization of prostatic adenocarcinoma Gleason 4, cribriform pattern, [abstract]. Mod Pathol 2017;30:222A.

57. Olkhov-Mitsel E, Siadat F, Kron K, et al. Distinct DNA methylation alterations (APC, Ras1, T-box genes) are associated with cribriform architecture and intraductal carcinoma in Gleason pattern 4 prostate tumors. Oncol Lett 2017;14:390–6.

58. Ronen S, Abbott DW, Abdelkader A, et al. PTEN and p27 loss differ among morphologic patterns of prostate cancer. Hum Pathol 2017;65:85–91.

59. Chua ML, Lo W, Pintilie M. A prostate cancer "Nimbosus": genomic instability and SChLAP1 dysregulation underpin aggression of intraductal and cribriform subpathologies. Eur Urol 2017;72:665–74.

60. Böttcher R, Kweldam CF, Livingstone J, et al. Cribriform and intraductal prostate cancer are associated with increased genomic instability and distinct genomic alterations. BMC Cancer 2018;18:8.

61. Pressner JR, Iyer MK, Sahu A. The long noncoding RNA SChLAP1 promotes aggressive prostate cancer and antagonizes the SWI/SNF complex. Nat Genet 2013;45:1392–8.

62. Li J, Shah R, Amin A, et al. Diagnostic accuracy of subpatterns of Gleason pattern 4 prostate cancer morphological subpatterns, [abstract]. Mod Pathol 2016;29:245A.

63. Falzarano SA, Klein EA, Magi-Galluzzi C, et al. Prostatic adenocarcinoma with poorly formed gland and cribriform morphology: grade group, Canary histologic analysis, and 17-gene expression assay comparison in 218 patients, [abstract]. Mod Pathol 2017; 30:224A.

64. Epstein JI, Amin MB, Reuter VE, et al. Contemporary Gleason grading of prostatic carcinoma: an update with discussion on practical issues to implement the 2014 International Society of Urological Pathology (ISUP) consensus conference on Gleason grading of prostatic carcinoma. Am J Surg Pathol 2017;41:e1–7.

65. Varma M, Egevad L, Algaba F, et al. Intraductal carcinoma of prostate reporting practice: a survey of expert European uropathologists, [abstract]. Mod Pathol 2015;28:266A.

66. Rhamy RK, Buchanan RD, Spalding MJ. Intraductal carcinoma of the prostate gland. Trans Am Assoc Genitourin Surg 1972;64:61–8.

67. Iczkowski KA. Intraductal carcinoma of the prostate: emerging support for a unique diagnostic entity. Pathol Case Rev 2014;19:178–83.

68. Zhou M. High-grade prostatic intraepithelial neoplasia, PIN-like carcinoma, ductal carcinoma, and intraductal carcinoma of the prostate. Mod Pathol 2018;31(S1):S71–9.

69. Haffner MC, Weier C, Xu MM, et al. Molecular evidence that invasive adenocarcinoma can mimic prostatic intraepithelial neoplasia (PIN) and intraductal carcinoma through retrograde glandular colonization. J Pathol 2016;238:31–41.

70. Tosoian J, Alam R, Ball M, et al. Managing high-grade prostatic intraepithelial neoplasia (HGPIN) and atypical glands on prostate biopsy. Nat Rev Urol 2018;15:55–66.

71. Shah RB, Magi-Galluzzi C, Han B, et al. Atypical cribriform lesions of the prostate: relationship to prostatic carcinoma and implication for diagnosis in prostate biopsies. Am J Surg Pathol 2010;34: 470–7.

72. Lotan TL, Gumuskaya B, Rahimi H, et al. Cytoplasmic PTEN protein loss distinguishes intraductal carcinoma of the prostate from high-grade prostatic intraepithelial neoplasia. Mod Pathol 2013;26: 587–603.

73. Hickman RA, Yu H, Li J, et al. Atypical intraductal cribriform proliferations of the prostate exhibit similar molecular and clinicopathologic characteristics as intraductal carcinoma of the prostate. Am J Surg Pathol 2017;41:550–6.

74. Iczkowski KA, Egevad L, Ma J, et al. Intraductal carcinoma of the prostate: interobserver reproducibility survey of 39 urologic pathologists. Ann Diagn Pathol 2014;18:333–42.

75. Fine SW, Gopalan A, Leversha MA, et al. TMPRSS2-ERG gene fusion is associated with low Gleason scores and not with high-grade morphological features. Mod Pathol 2010;23:1325–33.

76. Dawkins HJ, Sellner LN, Turbett GR, et al. Distinction between intraductal carcinoma of the prostate (IDC-P), high-grade dysplasia (PIN), and invasive prostatic adenocarcinoma, using molecular markers of cancer progression. Prostate 2000;44:265–70.

77. Schneider TM, Osunkoya AO. ERG expression in intraductal carcinoma of the prostate: comparison with adjacent conventional acinar prostatic adenocarcinoma. Mod Pathol 2013;25:247A.

78. Yoshimoto M, Ding K, Sweet JM, et al. PTEN losses exhibit heterogeneity in multifocal prostatic adenocarcinoma and are associated with higher Gleason score. Mod Pathol 2013;26:435–47.

79. Reid AH, Attard G, Ambroisine L, et al. Molecular characterisation of ERG, ETV1 and PTEN gene loci identifies patients at low and high risk of death from prostate cancer. Br J Cancer 2010;102:678–84.

80. Bhalla R, Kunju LP, Tomlins SA, et al. Novel dual-color immunohistochemical methods for detecting ERG-PTEN and ERG-SPINK1 status in prostate carcinoma. Mod Pathol 2013;26:835–48.

81. Chaux A, Peskoe SB, Gonzalez-Roibon N, et al. Loss of PTEN expression is associated with increased risk of recurrence after prostatectomy for clinically localized prostate cancer. Mod Pathol 2012;25:1543–9.

82. Lotan TL, Gurel B, Sutcliffe S, et al. PTEN protein loss: analytic validation and prognostic indicator for a high risk surgical cohort of prostate cancer patients. Clin Cancer Res 2011;17:6563–73.

83. Seipel AH, Delahunt B, Samaratunga H, et al. Diagnostic criteria for ductal adenocarcinoma of the prostate: interobserver variability among 20 expert uropathologists. Histopathology 2014;65:216–27.

84. Bock BJ, Bostwick DG. Does prostatic ductal adenocarcinoma exist? Am J Surg Pathol 1999;23:781–5.

85. Hameed O, Humphrey PA. Pseudoneoplastic mimics of prostate and bladder carcinomas. Arch Pathol Lab Med 2010;134:427–43.

86. Humphrey PA, Kaleem Z, Swanson PE, et al. Pseudohyperplastic prostatic adenocarcinoma. Am J Surg Pathol 1998;22:1239–46.

87. Kaleem Z, Swanson PE, Vollmer RT, et al. Prostatic adenocarcinoma with atrophic features: a study of 202 consecutive completely embedded radical prostatectomy specimens. Am J Clin Pathol 1998;109:695–703.

88. Yaskiv O, Cao D, Humphrey PA. Microcystic adenocarcinoma of the prostate: a variant of pseudohyperplastic and atrophic patterns. Am J Surg Pathol 2010;34:556–61.

89. Ali TZ, Epstein JI. Basal cell carcinoma of the prostate: a clinicopathologic study of 29 cases. Am J Surg Pathol 2007;31:697–705.

90. Iczkowski KA, Montironi R. Adenoid cystic/basal cell carcinoma of the prostate strongly expresses HER-2/neu. J Clin Pathol 2006;59:1327–30.

91. Zhang M, Pettaway C, Vikram R, et al. Adenoid cystic carcinoma of the urethra/Cowper's gland with concurrent high-grade prostatic adenocarcinoma: a detailed clinico-pathologic case report and review of the literature. Hum Pathol 2016;58:138–44.

92. Abbott D, Iczkowski KA. Squamous cell carcinoma of the prostate with concomitant adenocarcinoma in the absence of prior androgen deprivation therapy. Case Rev Clin Pathol 2016;3:60–3.

Updates on the Genetics and Molecular Subtypes of Urothelial Carcinoma and Select Variants

Hikmat Al-Ahmadie, MD[a],*, Gopa Iyer, MD[b]

KEYWORDS

- Urothelial carcinoma • Divergent differentiation • Variant histology • Squamous • Small cell
- Neuroendocrine • Plasmacytoid • Micropapillary

Key points

- Bladder cancer is morphologically and genomically heterogeneous.

- Urothelial carcinoma has high mutation burden associated with variable mutational signatures and variable clinical outcomes.

- Many molecular subtypes of urothelial carcinoma are present based on expression profiles.

- Some variants of urothelial carcinoma can be characterized by specific genetic aberrations.

- Most variant histologies harbor similar genetic alterations to those seen in classic urothelial carcinoma.

ABSTRACT

Urothelial carcinoma is a morphologically and genomically heterogeneous disease that exhibits a wide spectrum of morphologic features and molecular alterations and subtypes. Classic urothelial carcinoma (not otherwise specified) is the most common tumor type that develops in the urinary bladder but many, well-documented, variant histologies are commonly encountered in approximately one-third of invasive urothelial carcinoma, including squamous, glandular, micropapillary, sarcomatoid, small cell/neuroendocrine, clear cell, lymphoepithelioma-like, and plasmacytoid types, among others. In this review, we provide an update on the molecular advances in urothelial carcinoma and some of its variant histologies.

OVERVIEW

Urothelial carcinoma is the most common cancer that develops in the bladder and is mostly of classical or usual subtype (or not otherwise specified), but can invariably exhibit a wide spectrum of variant histologies. This classification has, historically, primarily relied on defined morphologic features, but recent technological advances have increased our knowledge of the genomic landscape of urothelial carcinoma and enhanced our understanding of the molecular features associated with this disease and some of its variant histologies. The purpose of this review is to highlight the diagnostic and molecular features of the major subtypes of bladder cancer and a subset of its variants whose molecular underpinnings have been recently investigated.

Disclosure Statement: This study funded in part by the Sloan Kettering Institute for Cancer Research Cancer Center Support Grant P30CA008748 and the Marie-Josée and Henry R. Kravis Center for Molecular Oncology.
[a] Department of Pathology, Memorial Sloan Kettering Cancer Center, 1275 York Avenue, New York, NY 10065, USA; [b] Department of Medicine, Genitourinary Oncology Service, Memorial Sloan Kettering Cancer Center, 1275 York Avenue, New York, NY 10065, USA
* Corresponding author.
E-mail address: alahmadh@mskcc.org

Surgical Pathology 11 (2018) 713–723
https://doi.org/10.1016/j.path.2018.07.011
1875-9181/18/© 2018 Elsevier Inc. All rights reserved.

UPDATES ON THE GENOMICS OF INVASIVE UROTHELIAL CARCINOMA (THE CANCER GENOME ATLAS EXPERIENCE)

Recently, The Cancer Genome Atlas (TCGA) bladder cancer group published a comprehensive genomic landscape of 412 muscle-invasive urothelial carcinomas of the bladder.[1] This comprehensive multiplatform analysis led to several findings. It identified a high mutation burden in this cohort, which is one of the highest among all cancer types, with a median of 5.8 per Mb and a mean of 7.9 per Mb in coding regions. Whole exome sequencing data analysis revealed that the main mutation signature within these tumors was derived from APOBEC mutagenesis, attributed to a family of enzymes known to contribute to cancer mutagenesis and the development of hypermutation phenotypes. The APOBEC family of enzymes catalyzes typical base changes within a trinucleotide context and 2 APOBEC-mediated mutation signatures are associated with 66% of the single nucleotide variants within muscle-invasive bladder cancer.[1–3] It was shown that the presence of APOBEC3-associated mutation signature is associated with better prognosis and improved 5-year overall survival in patients with muscle-invasive bladder cancer in the updated TCGA cohort. A second mutational signature associated with ERCC2 mutations is thought to cause approximately 20% of all single nucleotide variants. ERCC2 encodes a DNA helicase that has a central role in the nucleotide-excision repair pathway, a highly conserved DNA repair pathway. Mutations in ERCC2, as well as other genes involved in DNA damage response and repair, were shown to be associated with an improved response to cisplatin-based chemotherapy as well as immune checkpoint blockade and radiation therapy for advanced bladder cancer.[4–8] It was additionally shown that this mutational signature is associated with smoking independent of ERCC2 mutation status.[9] A third signature in the TCGA analysis was likely related to 5-methylcytosine deamination is and associated with 8% of single nucleotide variants. From a mutation signature activity standpoint, the TCGA cohort could be grouped into 4 mutational signature clusters (MSig1–4) with distinct mutation burdens and overall survival.[1]

Fifty-two significantly mutated genes representing several pathways involved in cell signaling and other canonical functions (cell cycle and chromatin regulation, receptor tyrosine kinase signaling, transcription, DNA repair, and others) were identified by analysis of TCGA. Examples include mutations in TP53 (48%), the most commonly altered gene, which were mutually exclusive with MDM2 amplifications (7%), both events resulting in dysregulation of the cell cycle. RB1 inactivating alterations were identified in 18% of tumors, whereas CDKN2A deletions were observed in 24% of specimens. Both genes are involved in the regulation of cell division. Oncogenic alterations within genes involved in cell signaling were noted, including hotspot activating FGFR3 and PIK3CA point mutations as well as FGFR3 fusions.

MOLECULAR TAXONOMY OF UROTHELIAL CARCINOMA

Although bladder tumors can be grouped based on significantly mutated genes, and this can also have therapeutic usefulness through the identification of potentially targetable alterations, several groups, including TCGA, have also identified RNA expression-based molecular subtypes of bladder cancer that may have both prognostic relevance and prediction for response to a variety of therapies. Over the last several years, different

---

Key Features
BLADDER CANCER GENOMICS

- Bladder cancer is genomically heterogeneous and is associated with a high mutation burden.

- The mutational signature strongly is associated with APOBEC activity.

- Different mutational signatures may be associated with different clinical outcomes.

Key Features
MOLECULAR TAXONOMY OF UROTHELIAL CARCINOMA

- Urothelial carcinoma can be grouped into distinct molecular subtypes based on expression profiles.

- Many classification systems exist for this molecular subtyping, with significant overlap among them.

- Some of the molecular subtypes may have predictive or prognostic significance.

- The stability of these subtypes within the same tumor and disease states is under investigation.

groups independently identified different subtypes based on RNA and/or immunohistochemical expression characteristics. Although the different classifications used different designations to label these different subtypes, significant overlap exists among them.[1,10–13] Efforts to harmonize and unify the terminology for these subtypes are currently underway to try to classify them into distinct and clinically relevant entities.[14] The most comprehensive of these classifications are the ones proposed by the Lund University group and that of the TCGA.[1,13] One of the earliest studies by the Lund University group was reported by Lindgren and colleagues,[15] who initially described 2 molecular subtypes of bladder cancer, MS1 and MS2, based on genome-wide gene expression analysis of 144 tumors, including both muscle-invasive and non–muscle-invasive bladder tumors. These 2 subtypes correlated with stage (MS1 tumors were primarily Ta whereas MS2 tumors were ≥T2). MS2 tumors were also characterized by high grade as compared with MS1. FGFR3 mutations were enriched within MS1 tumors (55% vs 7% in MS2; $P<.05$) and TP53 mutations were more common in MS2 tumors. Sjödahl and colleagues[13] subsequently expanded this analysis by performing gene expression profiling and immunohistochemical expression on a larger cohort of tumors and identified 5 discrete molecular subtypes: urobasal A, characterized by KRT5 and FGFR3 overexpression and a favorable prognosis; genomically unstable, harboring TP53 mutations and ERBB2 overexpression and enriched with muscle-invasive high-grade tumors; a squamous cell carcinoma-like subtype typified by squamous differentiation, overexpression of basal keratins, and a poor prognosis; urobasal B tumors, which shared features of the other 3 subtypes; and infiltrated tumors, with infiltration of immunologic cells and extracellular matrix gene expression.[12,13,16] The Lund group continues to refine their classification and modify or add more details to their existing subtypes. For example, they currently include a small cell/neuroendocrine-like subtype in their classification, which shares features of the genomically unstable subtype but additionally expresses higher levels of neuroendocrine markers such as chromogranin, synaptophysin, neuron-specific enolase (NSE, ENO2) and NCAM1 (CD56).[16,17] They also identified a mesenchymal-like subtype characterized by high expression of mesenchymal markers such as vimentin and ZEB2 and differed from other subtypes by showing low expression of FOXA1, GATA3, KRT5, and KRT14.

The TCGA analysis confirmed the presence of 2 major luminal and basal subtypes and provided additional discrimination into these 2 major categories. The basal and luminal subtyping of muscle-invasive bladder cancer was initially proposed after the perceived similarities to the molecular subtypes of breast cancer and was defined based on distinct expression signatures. Basal tumors express basal type keratins KRT5, KRT14, and KRT6A/B/C, whereas luminal tumors are characterized by high expression of FGFR3; the transcription factors PPARG, GATA3, FOXA1, and ELF3; the uroplakin genes found in umbrella cells; and KRT20.[10,11,18] The TCGA analysis further expanded and refined this classification and identified 3 subgroups within the luminal subtype along with a basal-squamous subtype as well a distinct neuronal cluster (for a total of 5 subtypes). This process identified subgroups within the luminal subtype; luminal–papillary, luminal–infiltrated, and luminal. The luminal–papillary cluster was enriched in tumors with papillary morphology and lower stage and was enriched with FGFR3 overexpression associated with FGFR3 mutations, amplification, and FGFR3-TACC3 fusions. The luminal-infiltrated subtype was distinguished from other luminal subtypes by lower purity that was derived from lymphocytic infiltrates and the presence of smooth muscle and myofibroblast gene signatures. A similar expression signature has been previously reported to be associated with chemoresistance and characterized by a wild-type p53 signature,[10] but was also reported to derive most benefit from anti-PDL1 treatment.[19] Tumors included in this subtype had increased expression of several immune markers, including CD274 (PD-L1) and PDCD1 (PD-1). The luminal subtype had the highest expression levels of uroplakins UPK1A and UPK2 as well as genes that are highly expressed in terminally differentiated umbrella cells such as KRT20 (CK20). The basal subtype contained nearly all the tumors that exhibited squamous differentiation by histopathologic review and was, thus, called basal–squamous. This subtype was associated with high expression of basal and stemlike markers (CD44, KRT5, KRT6A, and KRT14, **Fig. 1**) and squamous differentiation markers such as desmocollins (DSC1-3) and desmogleins (DSG1-4), TGM1 (transglutaminase 1), and PI3 (elafin). It was also enriched in TP53 mutations, was more common in females, and showed a strong immune gene signature expression as well as lymphocytic infiltrates.

The neuronal subtype included 3 cases of neuroendocrine/small cell histology, but also 17 additional tumors that had no histopathologic features suggestive of neuroendocrine differentiation. All 20 tumors showed a relatively high expression

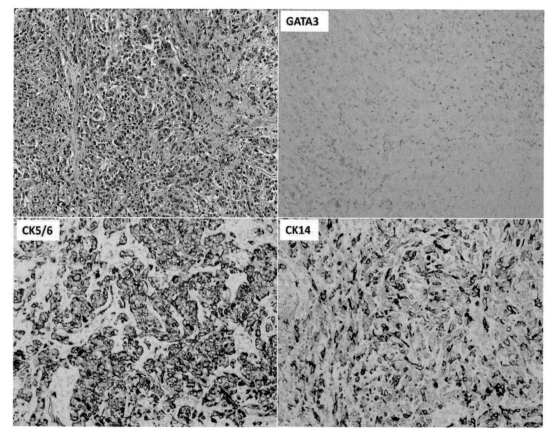

Fig. 1. Invasive urothelial carcinoma with features of basal subtype by immunohistochemistry. There is morphologic evidence of squamous differentiation in the tumor. The tumors lacks GATA3 expression and shows overexpression of basal keratins CK5/6 and CK14.

of genes involved in neuronal differentiation and development, as well as typical neuroendocrine and neural differentiation markers such as chromogranin, PEG10, PLEKHG4, and TUBB2B. In only a subset of these 20 tumors were there mutations in both *TP53* and *RB1*, which is the hallmark alteration in small cell/neuroendocrine carcinoma.[20] In contrast, the majority of tumors in this cluster (85%) had alterations in genes in the p53/cell cycle pathway and this subtype was associated with the worst clinical outcome.[1]

Applying this molecular classification to other bladder cancer cohorts resulted in patient risk stratification[1,17] and correlation with responses to chemotherapy or immunotherapy in advanced disease.[10,19,21] In other studies using RNA expression or immunohistochemical profiling, some variant histologies of urothelial carcinoma (micropapillary, nested, plasmacytoid) were found to have luminal characteristics, whereas urothelial carcinoma with squamous differentiation was found to have basal characteristics.[22,23]

Despite the important insights provided by these molecular classifications, several questions remain unanswered: Are these subtypes impacted by prior therapies for bladder cancer? Should subtyping be incorporated into clinical decision making and, if so, which disease states and/or treatments would be best applicable to such an analysis? How stable are these molecular subtypes within a given tumor and is there variation of subtyping with the same tumor (intratumoral heterogeneity)? These and several other questions are the current focus of several research groups in bladder cancer and should hopefully lead to significant insight into the biology of this disease in the near future, paving the way for novel biomarker-directed therapies.

MOLECULAR UPDATES IN SPECIFIC VARIANTS OF UROTHELIAL CARCINOMA

PLASMACYTOID UROTHELIAL CARCINOMA

Plasmacytoid urothelial carcinoma is a rare and aggressive variant of bladder cancer characterized by the presence of discohesive, individual cells with eccentrically located nuclei that resemble plasma cells as well cells with intracytoplasmic vacuoles that give the appearance of signet ring cells.[24–26] The aggressive clinical course is characterized by advanced stage at presentation, a high mortality rate, a high propensity for relapse and, frequent peritoneal carcinomatosis despite sometimes the apparent initial response to chemotherapy.[24–28] At the molecular level, it has been recently shown that the presence of *CDH1* truncating mutations (or less frequently CDH1 promoter hypermethylation) is the defining feature of plasmacytoid variant of bladder cancer.[24] Using whole exome and targeted sequencing, truncating somatic alterations in the *CDH1* gene were identified in 84% of plasmacytoid carcinomas and were specific to this histologic variant (**Fig. 2**A). Furthermore, all *CDH1* wild-type plasmacytoid carcinomas were

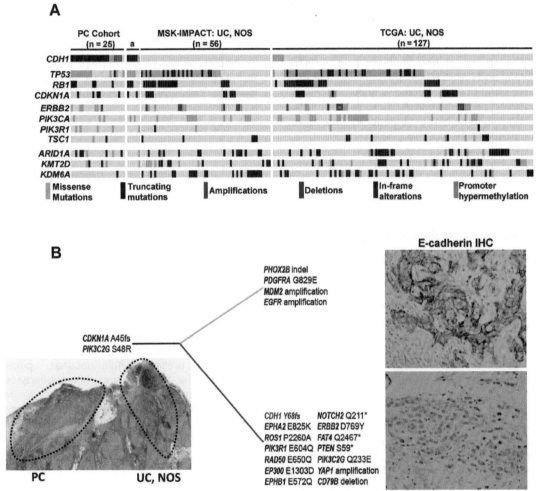

Fig. 2. Comparison of the genomic landscape of plasmacytoid urothelial carcinoma and urothelial carcinoma, not otherwise specified (NOS). (*A*) Heatmap comparing the frequency and distribution of *CDH1* alterations and select coaltered genes within 25 plasmacytoid urothelial carcinoma (PC), a prospective cohort of 62 urothelial carcinomas (including 6 with plasmacytoid histology), and 121 muscle-invasive urothelial carcinoma, NOS samples from the initial The Cancer Genome Atlas (TCGA) paper. [a] Six *CDH1* mutant plasmacytoid urothelial carcinomas from the prospective clinical cohort. (*B*) Phylogenetic tree depicting divergent evolution of plasmacytoid and urothelial NOS components within a tumor with distinct histologic regions. Exon capture and deep sequencing of macrodissected components identified shared *CDKN1A* and *PIK3C2G* mutations in both components, suggesting that these are truncal alterations occurring within a common precursor cell. However, a *CDH1* frameshift mutation was unique to plasmacytoid-variant histology, and the remaining genetic alteration profiles of the 2 histologic components were distinct. *Red* and *green lines* in the phylogenetic tree indicate plasmacytoid and urothelial NOS components, respectively. (*Reprinted* by permission from Springer Nature: Nature Publishing group, Nature Genetics. Frequent somatic CDH1 loss-of-function mutations in plasmacytoid variant bladder cancer. Al-Ahmadie HA, Iyer G, Lee BH, Scott SN, Mehra R, et al, 2016.)

associated with loss of E-cadherin expression, all but one of which were associated with CDH1 promoter hypermethylation. Aside from *CDH1* mutation, the genomic landscape of plasmacytoid carcinoma was similar to that of urothelial carcinoma, not otherwise specified, with frequent mutations in chromatin modifying genes, cell cycle regulators, and PI3 kinase pathway alterations, suggesting that plasmacytoid and classic urothelial carcinoma likely evolve from a shared cell of origin.[24] This finding was further supported by performing exon capture and deep sequencing of 2 adjacent areas of a bladder tumor that contained distinct regions of plasmacytoid and classic urothelial carcinoma (**Fig. 2**B). Both histologic regions shared mutations in *CDKN1A* (A45fs) and *PIK3C2G* (S48R), implying that these were early truncal alterations occurring within a common precursor cell. A *CDH1* Y68fs mutation, along with mutations in other genes was, however, unique to the plasmacytoid component.[24]

> ### Key Features
> #### PLASMACYTOID
> #### UROTHELIAL CARCINOMA
>
> - Rare and aggressive variant of bladder cancer.
>
> - Discohesive and infiltrating growth.
>
> - Loss of E-cadherin expression owing to truncating *CDH1* mutations or promoter hypermethylation is pathognomonic.
>
> - Genomic background otherwise similar to urothelial carcinoma.
>
> - No association with *CDH1* germline mutations.

Functional cell lines studies supported a significant role of CDH1 loss in promoting cell discohesion and stromal invasion, which could explain the higher incidence of both local recurrence and cancer-specific mortality as well as the higher rate of peritoneal spread than those with pure urothelial carcinoma. By performing clustered regularly interspersed palindromic repeat/Cas9-mediated knockout of *CDH1* in 2 CDH1 wild-type urothelial carcinoma cell lines (RT4 and MGHU4), loss of E-cadherin expression resulted in increased invasion and migratory capability of MGHU4 and RT4 cells. It was also shown that loss of E-cadherin expression was observed only in the invasive plasmacytoid carcinoma and was retained within the noninvasive component. This work and that of others reporting common E-cadherin loss by

immunohistochemistry in the majority of plasmacytoid carcinomas[25,29] indicates that E-cadherin loss, typically as a result of *CDH1* mutation and less commonly as a result of CDH1 promoter methylation, is the defining molecular event of the distinct local invasion and spread patterns observed in patients with plasmacytoid carcinoma. Notably, in contrast with the germline *CDH1* mutations typically seen in patients with diffuse hereditary gastric cancers and a subset of lobular breast cancer, no germline *CDH1* mutations were identified in plasmacytoid urothelial carcinoma.[24] These results indicate that somatic loss-of-function mutations in *CDH1*, with consequent E-cadherin loss, leads to enhanced cellular migration and invasive properties in plasmacytoid carcinoma, characterized by marked cell discohesion and single cell infiltration.

MICROPAPILLARY UROTHELIAL CARCINOMA

Micropapillary urothelial carcinoma is a rare variant of urothelial carcinoma with a reported aggressive clinical course. Although it is now increasingly recognized, it still lacks application of strict diagnostic criteria and as a result suffers from high degree of interobserver variability. This issue becomes even more problematic, particularly because many clinicians advise early cystectomy for this disease, even in the absence of invasion into the muscularis propria.[30] Morphologically, this tumor is characterized by the presence of small tight clusters of high-grade tumor cells lacking true fibrovascular cores and present within lacunar spaces (**Fig. 3**).[31] The basis behind this appearance, in the namesake entity in the breast, is the reverse orientation or polarization of the basal and luminal aspects of tumor cells resulting is the lack of cohesion between tumor and stroma.[32,33]

> ### Key Features
> #### MICROPAPILLARY
> #### UROTHELIAL CARCINOMA
>
> - Rare and aggressive variant of bladder cancer.
>
> - Characterized by small tight clusters of high-grade tumor cells lacking true fibrovascular cores and present within lacunar spaces.
>
> - Strong association with *ERBB2* gene amplification and HER2 overexpression.

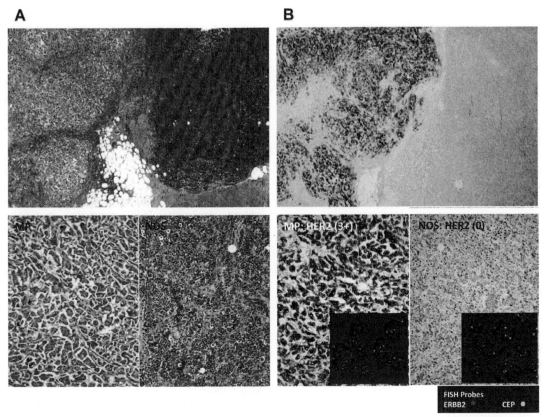

Fig. 3. An example of HER2 expression IHC score 3+ in the micropapillary component (MP) with *ERBB2* amplification. There is no HER2 expression in the not otherwise specified (NOS) component (score 0) and no *ERBB2* amplification. (*A, B*) Panoramic view of the MP and NOS components. (*From* Isharwal S, Huang H, Nanjangud G, et al. Intratumoral heterogeneity of ERBB2 amplification and HER2 expression in micropapillary urothelial carcinoma. Hum Pathol 2018;77:63–9; with permission.)

At the molecular level, higher rates of *ERBB2* amplification are reported in micropapillary urothelial carcinoma than in classic urothelial carcinoma and in some reports this amplification was additionally associated with worse cancer-specific survival after radical cystectomy.[34,35] In a recent study, we reported high rates of intratumoral heterogeneity of *ERBB2* amplification within tumor containing both micropapillary and classic urothelial components as *ERBB2* amplification was more commonly amplified in the micropapillary than the classic urothelial components.[36] Moreover, the rate of *ERBB2* in the classic urothelial components in these mixed (micropapillary + urothelial) tumors was much higher than the reported rates in pure classic urothelial carcinoma or those not mixed with micropapillary components[1,37,38] (**Fig. 4**), indicating a possible role of *ERBB2* activation in the development of this aggressive variant of urothelial carcinoma. It has been recently reported that mutations in known hotspots in *ERBB2* are common in micropapillary carcinoma of the bladder,[39] but it is likely that the frequency of

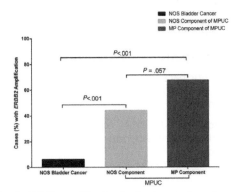

Fig. 4. *ERBB2* amplification in classic not otherwise specified (NOS) urothelial carcinoma and the NOS and micropapillary components of micropapillary urothelial carcinoma containing both components. The prevalence of *ERBB2* amplification in NOS bladder cancer is derived from The Cancer Genome Atlas dataset (6.3%). *ERBB2* amplification was significantly more common in MPUC, both within the micropapillary component and NOS components, as compared with pure NOS bladder tumors. LOH, loss of heterozygosity; N/A, not applicable. (*From* Isharwal S, Huang H, Nanjangud G, et al. Intratumoral heterogeneity of ERBB2 amplification and HER2 expression in micropapillary urothelial carcinoma. Hum Pathol 2018;77:68; with permission.)

such mutations is not higher in this variant histology than it is in classic urothelial carcinoma. In another recent study using RNA expression profiling of micropapillary bladder cancer, there was common downregulation of miR-296 and activation of chromatin-remodeling complex RUVBL1, but it remains unclear what role these alterations play and what they contribute to the development of micropapillary urothelial carcinoma.[23]

SMALL CELL/NEUROENDOCRINE CARCINOMA OF THE BLADDER

Small cell/neuroendocrine carcinoma of the bladder is a rare variant of bladder cancer that is morphologically identical to the small cell carcinoma of the lung and other organs, but may be admixed with a classic urothelial component (invasive or in situ) as well as other divergent differentiation including squamous, glandular, and sarcomatoid with or without heterologous elements in up to 50% of cases.[40]

Key Features
SMALL CELL/NEUROENDOCRINE CARCINOMA OF THE BLADDER

- Rare and aggressive variant of bladder cancer.

- Similar to small cell carcinoma in other organs.

- Strong association with *TP53/RB1* coalterations.

- Genetic background similar to bladder cancer and strongly associated with APOBEC signature.

- Aside from *TP53/RB1* coalterations, genetic background is different from lung small cell carcinoma.

The genomic landscape of small cell carcinoma of the bladder is still not fully defined, but a few recent studies provided insights into the molecular characteristics of this disease and identified some similarities and differences between small cell and urothelial components within the bladder as well as with small cell carcinoma of the lung.[20,37,41,42] A near universal finding was the presence of coalterations in *TP53* and *RB1*, resulting in a loss of function of both genes. In 1 study, *TP53* and *RB1* alterations were detected

in 90% and 87% of cases, respectively, and 80% of tumors displayed coalterations of both genes (**Fig. 5**).[20] Further, in some tumors without *RB1* loss-of-function mutations, there was loss RB expression by immunohistochemistry, suggesting an alternative mechanism, such as epigenetic silencing, that contributed to RB loss. Interestingly, and perhaps not surprisingly, unlike lung small cell carcinoma, commonly mutated genes in urothelial carcinoma were also found to be mutated in the bladder small cell carcinoma cohort, including *TERT* promoter mutations (95%) and truncating alterations within chromatin modifying genes such as *CREBBP*, *EP300*, *ARID1A*, and *KMT2D* in approximately 75% of samples.[20,42] Notable exceptions include the near absence of *KDM6A* truncating mutations, *CDKN2A* deletion, and *CCND1* amplifications in the bladder small cell carcinoma cohort, compared with urothelial carcinoma, where such alterations are common. *E2F3* amplification was found in both small cell and urothelial bladder tumors, although this event was rare in small cell lung cancer.[20]

A high level of chromosomal instability was observed in bladder small cell carcinoma, including whole genome duplication in 72% of tumors that correlated with the presence of *TP53* missense mutations, particularly those associated with biallelic silencing. The APOBEC mutation signature that was identified within muscle-invasive bladder cancer from the TCGA bladder cancer study[43] was observed in 95% of small cell bladder cancer in this cohort; notably, small cell lung cancers are typically characterized by a mutation signature associated with tobacco exposure distinct from the APOBEC signature.[20] In a subset of cases with mixed urothelial and small cell components, sequencing of the macrodissected components separately identified shared alterations between the 2 components in addition to private alterations in each of them, further supporting the concept that small cell carcinoma of the bladder develops form a precursor urothelial carcinoma. It still remains unexplained, however, how small cell carcinoma develops and what molecular mechanisms underlie its development from its urothelial precursor beyond the combined *RB1/TP53* alterations, which are co-mutated in a subset of classic urothelial carcinoma that clearly does not display small cell/neuroendocrine differentiation.[1,37,44] It also remains unclear how true small cell carcinoma, as defined histologically, is related to the neuronal/neuroendocrine subtype of bladder cancer, as defined by the TCGA and the Lund group classifications.

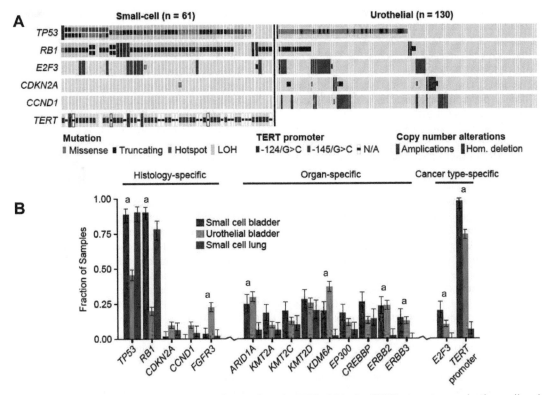

Fig. 5. (*A*) *A heatmap depicting* patterns of mutations in *TP53, RB1*, the *TERT* promoter, and other cell-cycle regulators small cell carcinoma of bladder cohort from reference[20] and urothelial carcinoma from the initial The Cancer Genome Atlas cohort. (*B*) Commonly mutated genes in small cell bladder carcinoma, urothelial carcinomas, and small-cell lung carcinoma (dark blue, light blue, and red, respectively) are grouped on the basis of their alteration frequency. [a] Nominal *P* value <.05; Fisher exact test. Hom., homozygous; LOH, loss of heterozygosity; N/A, not available. (*From* Chang MT, Penson A, Desai NB, et al. Small-cell carcinomas of the bladder and lung are characterized by a convergent but distinct pathogenesis. Clin Cancer Res 2018;24(8):1968; with permission.)

REFERENCES

1. Robertson AG, Kim J, Al-Ahmadie H, et al. Comprehensive molecular characterization of muscle-invasive bladder cancer. Cell 2017;171(3):540–56.e25.

2. Glaser AP, Fantini D, Shilatifard A, et al. The evolving genomic landscape of urothelial carcinoma. Nat Rev Urol 2017;14(4):215–29.

3. Vlachostergios PJ, Faltas BM. Treatment resistance in urothelial carcinoma: an evolutionary perspective. Nat Rev Clin Oncol 2018;15(8):495–509.

4. Teo MY, Bambury RM, Zabor EC, et al. DNA damage response and repair gene alterations are associated with improved survival in patients with platinum-treated advanced urothelial carcinoma. Clin Cancer Res 2017;23(14):3610–8.

5. Teo MY, Seier K, Ostrovnaya I, et al. Alterations in DNA damage response and repair genes as potential marker of clinical benefit from PD-1/PD-L1 blockade in advanced urothelial cancers. J Clin Oncol 2018;36(17):1685–94.

6. Desai NB, Scott SN, Zabor EC, et al. Genomic characterization of response to chemoradiation in urothelial bladder cancer. Cancer 2016;122(23):3715–23.

7. Van Allen EM, Mouw KW, Kim P, et al. Somatic ERCC2 mutations correlate with cisplatin sensitivity in muscle-invasive urothelial carcinoma. Cancer Discov 2014;4(10):1140–53.

8. Mouw KW, D'Andrea AD. DNA repair deficiency and immunotherapy response. J Clin Oncol 2018;36(17):1710–3.

9. Kim J, Mouw KW, Polak P, et al. Somatic ERCC2 mutations are associated with a distinct genomic signature in urothelial tumors. Nat Genet 2016;48(6):600–6.

10. Choi W, Porten S, Kim S, et al. Identification of distinct basal and luminal subtypes of muscle-invasive bladder cancer with different sensitivities to frontline chemotherapy. Cancer Cell 2014;25(2):152–65.

11. Damrauer JS, Hoadley KA, Chism DD, et al. Intrinsic subtypes of high-grade bladder cancer reflect the

hallmarks of breast cancer biology. Proc Natl Acad Sci U S A 2014;111(8):3110–5.

12. Sjodahl G, Lauss M, Lövgren K, et al. A molecular taxonomy for urothelial carcinoma. Clin Cancer Res 2012;18(12):3377–86.

13. Sjödahl G, Lövgren K, Lauss M, et al. Toward a molecular pathologic classification of urothelial carcinoma. Am J Pathol 2013;183(3):681–91.

14. Lerner SP, McConkey DJ, Hoadley KA, et al. Bladder cancer molecular taxonomy: summary from a consensus meeting. Bladder Cancer 2016;2(1):37–47.

15. Lindgren D, Frigyesi A, Gudjonsson S, et al. Combined gene expression and genomic profiling define two intrinsic molecular subtypes of urothelial carcinoma and gene signatures for molecular grading and outcome. Cancer Res 2010;70(9):3463–72.

16. Sjödahl G, Eriksson P, Liedberg F, et al. Molecular classification of urothelial carcinoma: global mRNA classification versus tumour-cell phenotype classification. J Pathol 2017;242(1):113–25.

17. Marzouka NA, Eriksson P, Rovira C, et al. A validation and extended description of the Lund taxonomy for urothelial carcinoma using the TCGA cohort. Sci Rep 2018;8(1):3737.

18. Kim J, Robertson G, Akbani R, et al. Genomic assessment of muscle-invasive bladder cancer: insights from The Cancer Genome Atlas (TCGA) Project. In: Hansel DE, Lerner SP, editors. Precision molecular pathology of bladder cancer. Cham (Switzerland): Springer International Publishing; 2018. p. 43–64.

19. Rosenberg JE, Hoffman-Censits J, Powles T, et al. Atezolizumab in patients with locally advanced and metastatic urothelial carcinoma who have progressed following treatment with platinum-based chemotherapy: a single-arm, multicentre, phase 2 trial. Lancet 2016;387(10031):1909–20.

20. Chang MT, Penson A, Desai NB, et al. Small-cell carcinomas of the bladder and lung are characterized by a convergent but distinct pathogenesis. Clin Cancer Res 2018;24(8):1965–73.

21. Seiler R, Ashab HAD, Erho N, et al. Impact of molecular subtypes in muscle-invasive bladder cancer on predicting response and survival after neoadjuvant chemotherapy. Eur Urol 2017;72(4):544–54.

22. Warrick JI, Kaag M, Raman JD, et al. FOXA1 and CK14 as markers of luminal and basal subtypes in histologic variants of bladder cancer and their associated conventional urothelial carcinoma. Virchows Arch 2017;471(3):337–45.

23. Guo CC, Dadhania V, Zhang L, et al. Gene expression profile of the clinically aggressive micropapillary variant of bladder cancer. Eur Urol 2016;70(4):611–20.

24. Al-Ahmadie HA, Iyer G, Lee BH, et al. Frequent somatic CDH1 loss-of-function mutations in plasmacytoid variant bladder cancer. Nat Genet 2016;48(4):356–8.

25. Keck B, Stoehr R, Wach S, et al. The plasmacytoid carcinoma of the bladder–rare variant of aggressive urothelial carcinoma. Int J Cancer 2011;129(2):346–54.

26. Nigwekar P, Tamboli P, Amin MB, et al. Plasmacytoid urothelial carcinoma: detailed analysis of morphology with clinicopathologic correlation in 17 cases. Am J Surg Pathol 2009;33(3):417–24.

27. Dayyani F, Czerniak BA, Sircar K, et al. Plasmacytoid urothelial carcinoma, a chemosensitive cancer with poor prognosis, and peritoneal carcinomatosis. J Urol 2013;189(5):1656–61.

28. Kaimakliotis HZ, Monn MF, Cheng L, et al. Plasmacytoid bladder cancer: variant histology with aggressive behavior and a new mode of invasion along fascial planes. Urology 2014;83(5):1112–6.

29. Lim MG, Adsay NV, Grignon DJ, et al. E-cadherin expression in plasmacytoid, signet ring cell and micropapillary variants of urothelial carcinoma: comparison with usual-type high-grade urothelial carcinoma. Mod Pathol 2011;24(2):241–7.

30. Sangoi AR, Beck AH, Amin MB, et al. Interobserver reproducibility in the diagnosis of invasive micropapillary carcinoma of the urinary tract among urologic pathologists. Am J Surg Pathol 2010;34(9):1367–76.

31. Amin MB, Ro JY, el-Sharkawy T, et al. Micropapillary variant of transitional cell carcinoma of the urinary bladder. Histologic pattern resembling ovarian papillary serous carcinoma. Am J Surg Pathol 1994;18(12):1224–32.

32. Nassar H, Pansare V, Zhang H, et al. Pathogenesis of invasive micropapillary carcinoma: role of MUC1 glycoprotein. Mod Pathol 2004;17(9):1045–50.

33. Luna-Moré S, Gonzalez B, Acedo C, et al. Invasive micropapillary carcinoma of the breast. A new special type of invasive mammary carcinoma. Pathol Res Pract 1994;190(7):668–74.

34. Schneider SA, Sukov WR, Frank I, et al. Outcome of patients with micropapillary urothelial carcinoma following radical cystectomy: ERBB2 (HER2) amplification identifies patients with poor outcome. Mod Pathol 2014;27(5):758–64.

35. Tschui J, Vassella E, Bandi N, et al. Morphological and molecular characteristics of HER2 amplified urothelial bladder cancer. Virchows Arch 2015;466(6):703–10.

36. Isharwal S, Huang H, Nanjangud G, et al. Intratumoral heterogeneity of ERBB2 amplification and HER2 expression in micropapillary urothelial carcinoma. Hum Pathol 2018;77:63–9.

37. Iyer G, Al-Ahmadie H, Schultz N, et al. Prevalence and co-occurrence of actionable genomic alterations in high-grade bladder cancer. J Clin Oncol 2013;31(25):3133–40.

38. Fleischmann A, Rotzer D, Seiler R, et al. Her2 amplification is significantly more frequent in lymph node

metastases from urothelial bladder cancer than in the primary tumours. Eur Urol 2011;60(2):350–7.

39. Ross JS, Wang K, Gay LM, et al. A high frequency of activating extracellular domain ERBB2 (HER2) mutation in micropapillary urothelial carcinoma. Clin Cancer Res 2014;20(1):68–75.

40. Amin MB. Histological variants of urothelial carcinoma: diagnostic, therapeutic and prognostic implications. Mod Pathol 2009;22(Suppl 2):S96–118.

41. George J, Lim JS, Jang SJ, et al. Comprehensive genomic profiles of small cell lung cancer. Nature 2015;524(7563):47–53.

42. Shen P, Jing Y, Zhang R, et al. Comprehensive genomic profiling of neuroendocrine bladder cancer pinpoints molecular origin and potential therapeutics. Oncogene 2018;37(22):3039–44.

43. Cancer Genome Atlas Research Network. Comprehensive molecular characterization of urothelial bladder carcinoma. Nature 2014;507(7492): 315–22.

44. Kim PH, Cha EK, Sfakianos JP, et al. Genomic predictors of survival in patients with high-grade urothelial carcinoma of the bladder. Eur Urol 2015;67(2): 198–201.

Recognizing Hereditary Renal Cancers Through the Microscope: A Pathology Update

Yu-Ching Peng, MD, PhD, Ying-Bei Chen, MD, PhD*

KEYWORDS

- von Hippel-Lindau • Hereditary papillary • Birt-Hogg-Dubé
- Hereditary leiomyomatosis renal cell carcinoma • Succinate dehydrogenase • Tuberous sclerosis
- Kidney cancer • Familial

Key points

- Recognize not only the histologic features of renal tumors but also the suspicious findings in the adjacent renal parenchyma and extra-renal manifestations.
- Some hereditary renal cancers (eg, VHL, HPRCC, and BHD) are often bilateral and multifocal, whereas others (eg, HLRCC and SDH-deficient RCC) are not infrequently solitary.
- Ancillary immunohistochemical markers play an important role in the diagnosis of certain hereditary renal cancers (eg, HLRCC and SDH-deficient RCC).
- Hereditary renal cancers show an expanding morphologic spectrum that overlaps with sporadic renal tumors and often require germline testing for confirmation.

ABSTRACT

A heightened understanding of hereditary renal cancer syndromes and their molecular basis has led to an increased awareness and recognition of these renal neoplasms by pathologists. Because a diagnosis of hereditary renal cell carcinoma has a profound impact on the patient and family members, when and how to raise such a suspicion via pathologic assessment has become an important yet very challenging task. This review discusses key clinicopathologic, immunohistochemical, and genetic characteristics of hereditary renal cancer syndromes, and important differential diagnostic challenges, emphasizing recent pathologic and molecular advances.

OVERVIEW

It is estimated that approximately 2% to 4% of all renal cell carcinomas (RCC) have a familial cause.[1]

Linkage studies of families with hereditary kidney cancer syndromes have provided some important insights into the oncogenic pathways of RCC, implicating genes such as *VHL*, *MET*, *FLCN*, *TSC1*, *TSC2*, *FH*, and *SDHB* in various types of familial forms of RCC (Table 1). Among these, von Hippel-Lindau (VHL) syndrome, hereditary papillary RCC (HPRC), and Birt-Hogg-Dubé syndrome are often characterized by bilateral and multifocal tumors in the kidneys, whereas the majority of reported cases of hereditary leiomyomatosis RCC (HLRCC) syndrome or succinate dehydrogenase (SDH)-deficient RCCs are unilateral and solitary renal masses. Additionally, renal lesions in patients with tuberous sclerosis complex (TSC) are mainly angiomyolipomas (AML) and cysts, but TSC-associated renal cell neoplasms can also occur and tend to be multifocal and show a wide spectrum of morphology. To recognize these hereditary renal tumors via pathologic evaluation, it is important to not only know the histologic features of the tumors, but also become familiar with the potential

Disclosure Statement: Dr. Chen was supported by the Society of Memorial Sloan Kettering research grant and NIH/NCI Cancer Center Support Grant P30 CA008748.
Department of Pathology, Memorial Sloan Kettering Cancer Center, 1275 York Avenue, New York, NY 10065, USA
* Corresponding author.
E-mail address: cheny@mskcc.org

Surgical Pathology 11 (2018) 725–737
https://doi.org/10.1016/j.path.2018.07.010
1875-9181/18/© 2018 Elsevier Inc. All rights reserved.

Table 1
Summary of clinical, genetic, and pathology of hereditary renal cancers

Syndrome	Clinical Manifestations	Gene (Chromosome) - Protein	Histologic Features of Renal Tumors
von Hippel-Lindau syndrome	Clear cell RCC, pheochromocytoma, pancreatic endocrine tumors, CNS and retinal hemangioblastomas	*VHL* (3p25) - VHL protein	Clear cell RCC
Hereditary papillary RCC	Type I papillary RCC	*MET* (7q31) - MET	Type I papillary RCC
Hereditary leiomyomatosis and RCC	RCC, Leiomyomas of skin and uterus	*FH* (1q42.1) – Fumarate hydratase	RCC with papillary/tubulocystic/other architectural patterns and, prominent nucleoli with perinucleolar halo
Birt-Hogg-Dubé syndrome	Renal tumors, fibrofolliculomas, pulmonary cysts	*BHD/FLCN* (17p11.2) – Folliculin (FLCN)	Hybrid oncocytic tumors, oncocytoma, chromophobe RCC
Tuberous sclerosis complex	Multiple renal AML, RCCs, Cardiac rhabdomyomas, Hamartomas, Neurologic disorders/seizures	*TSC1* (9q34) - Hamartin *TSC2* (16p13.3) - Tuberin	AML, renal cysts, RCC mimics clear cell RCC, TCEB1-mutated RCC, chromophobe RCC, oncocytoma, or unclassified RCC
Succinate dehydrogenase B-associated pheochromocytoma/paraganglioma syndrome Type 4	Bilateral and extraadrenal pheochromocytoma/paraganglioma, RCC and other malignancies	*SDHB* (1p36.1-p35) – Succinate dehydrogenase subunit B	Cytoplasmic inclusions containing pale eosinophilic to clear material

Abbreviations: AML, angiomyolipoma; CNS, central nervous system; RCC, renal cell carcinoma.

findings in the adjacent renal parenchyma as well as the extrarenal manifestations. Moreover, these renal tumors often show overlapping histopathologic features with sporadic tumors, in addition to morphologic features that may mimic other syndromic tumors.

VON HIPPEL-LINDAU SYNDROME

VHL syndrome is an autosomal-dominant syndrome that results from mutations in the *VHL* gene, a tumor suppressor gene on chromosome 3p25. The incidence is estimated to be 1 in 36,000 individuals. The gene product, VHL protein, plays an essential role in the degradation of hypoxia-induced factor-1α. Inactivation of the VHL protein results in the accumulation of hypoxia-induced factor-1α, leading to overexpression of multiple downstream genes including carbonic anhydrase-IX. VHL syndrome is characterized by the development of cerebellar, retinal,

and spinal hemangioblastomas, clear cell RCC (ccRCC), pheochromocytomas, pancreatic cysts and endocrine pancreatic tumors, endolymphatic sac tumors of the ear, and epididymal cystadenomas.[2,3] VHL syndrome can be divided into 2 major types depending on whether pheochromocytomas are present. Type 1 is not associated with pheochromocytomas, whereas type 2 has a high risk of pheochromocytomas. Type 2 can be further divided into 3 subtypes: type 2A has a lower risk for RCC, type 2B has a higher risk for RCC, and type 2C mainly manifests as pheochromocytomas. Although RCCs are rare in patients with VHL syndrome before the age of 20, the incidence increases thereafter, and it is estimated that 69% of patients surviving to age 60 develop RCC.[3,4]

GROSS FEATURES

The renal lesions in VHL syndrome are bilateral and multiple. The spectrum of lesions ranges from benign cysts, atypical cysts, cystic RCCs,

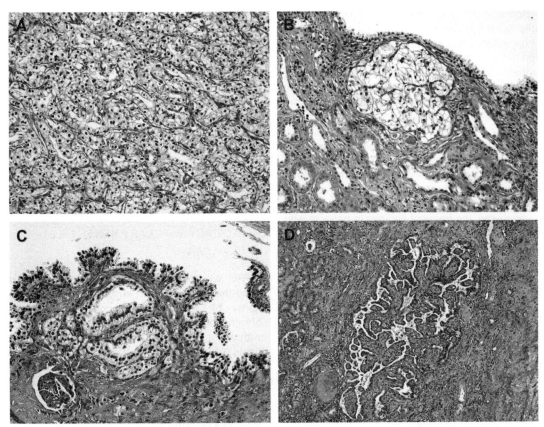

Fig. 1. (*A–C*) Von-Hippel Lindau syndrome. (*A*) Acini or nests of clear cells separated by a delicate vascular network. (*B*) Microscopic foci of clear cell nodules and clear cell-lined cysts. (*C*) Focal papillary proliferation of clear cells in the cysts. (*D*) Hereditary papillary renal cell carcinoma. Papillae are lined by low cuboidal cells with scant cytoplasm and small oval nuclei (H&E, original magnification ×20).

and solid RCCs. Grossly, the kidney may show multiple cysts and solid lesions with usually normal size and weight because most cysts and tumors are small. The number of cysts ranges from 3 to 30 (average 7.8 per kidney) and they are usually small (mean size, 0.7 cm).[5]

MICROSCOPIC FEATURES

Microscopically, renal tumors are often multifocal, tend to be low-grade, and show identical morphologic features as sporadic ccRCCs, which are characterized by acini or nests of epithelial cells with clear cytoplasm surrounded by a delicate vascular network (**Fig. 1**A). The multiple tumors in patients with VHL syndrome have been shown to develop independently.[6] Importantly, in the adjacent renal parenchyma, microscopic foci of clear cell proliferation, or aggregates and clear cell-lined cysts are typically present in patients with VHL syndrome (**Fig. 1**B). The renal cysts often manifest as unilocular, small cysts with a single layer of clear cells without cytologic atypia, but

cysts lined by multiple layers of clear cells with or without cytologic atypia or show focal papillary proliferation can also be found (**Fig. 1**C).[7]

Occasionally, VHL disease-associated RCC shows morphologic features resembling clear cell papillary RCC (ccpRCC), namely, papillary architecture with nuclei arranged away from the basement membrane, imparting a linear distribution of nuclei along the apical aspects of the tumor cells.[8,9] At this point, although it seems that these ccpRCC-like RCCs are likely molecularly distinct from sporadic ccpRCCs, which do not harbor *VHL* mutations or 3p loss, it remains unclear whether they are molecularly similar to typical ccRCCs detected in the setting of VHL syndrome.

DIFFERENTIAL DIAGNOSIS

The main differential diagnostic considerations with VHL syndrome-associated RCCs are sporadic ccRCCs, TSC-associated RCCs, and end-stage kidney disease with ccRCC.

Sporadic ccRCCs can sometimes occur at multiple foci in the kidney, prompting a consideration of hereditary predisposition. An important distinction between sporadic ccRCC and VHL syndrome is that VHL syndrome is associated with multiple renal cysts and percolating clusters of clear cells in the background kidney. In addition, the number of multiple tumors in a sporadic setting is usually small.

TSC-associated RCCs can manifest as epithelial cells with clear cytoplasm. However, the tumor cells usually have voluminous cytoplasm that either contains eosinophilic, fine granules or traversed by cobweb-like fibrillary strands. In the adjacent renal parenchyma, the frequent findings in patients with TSC are microscopic, multiple angiomyolipomas in addition to small cysts lined by cells with granular, eosinophilic cytoplasm. This distinction further emphasizes the importance of assessing the background nonneoplastic kidney.

Multiple ccRCCs can also occur in end-stage kidneys. However, the background kidney consistently shows changes in end-stage kidneys, often accompanied by acquired cystic disease. The multifocal RCCs in this setting tend to exhibit multiple tumor types, including acquired cystic disease-associated RCC, ccpRCC, papillary RCC (pRCC), and chromophobe RCC.

DIAGNOSIS

Although RCCs in VHL syndrome show similar morphologic and immunohistochemical features of sporadic ccRCCs, the constellation of pathologic features including bilateral, multifocal ccRCCs and multiple, mainly clear cell-lined cysts, as well as percolating clusters of clear cells in the adjacent kidney, should prompt one to consider a possibility of VHL syndrome. Many patients have a known family history or clinical diagnosis/suspicion of the disease, which provides a helpful clinical context for pathologists to render a correct diagnosis. The definitive diagnosis of VHL relies on genetic testing to identify germline mutations in the VHL gene.

PROGNOSIS

The management of RCCs in a patient with VHL syndrome requires a balance between excising tumors to prevent metastasis and preserving enough renal tissue to maintain renal function. In general, small tumors are managed conservatively by active surveillance and larger tumors (>3 cm) are excised by partial nephrectomy or ablation therapy. Although relatively rare, metastatic RCC is the leading cause of death in VHL.

Key Features
RENAL TUMORS IN
VON HIPPEL-LINDAU SYNDROME

1. Multifocal renal tumors morphologically identical to sporadic ccRCC.

2. Adjacent renal parenchyma shows microscopic foci of clear cell proliferation and clear cell-lined cysts.

3. Occasionally, tumors show morphologic features resembling ccpRCC.

HEREDITARY PAPILLARY RENAL CELL CARCINOMA

HPRC syndrome is an autosomal-dominant disease that results from germline activating mutations of *MET* protooncogene located at chromosome 7q31.[10,11] It is a very rare syndrome with an incidence of 1 in 10 million. Tumors in patients with HPRC often manifest at a relatively late age (50–70 years) and are highly penetrant. Unlike other hereditary RCC syndromes, no known extrarenal manifestations are associated with HPRC.

GROSS FEATURES

Grossly, the tumors are bilateral and multifocal. They are usually well-circumscribed. The number of tumors may range from dozens to hundreds.

MICROSCOPIC FEATURES

Tumors in patients with HPRC are all type 1 pRCC. These tumors show papillary or tubulopapillary architecture lined by low cuboidal cells with scant cytoplasm and small oval nuclei with inconspicuous nucleoli (Fig. 1D). Foamy macrophages and psammomatous calcifications are commonly present. Occasionally, tumor cells may focally show eosinophilic cytoplasm, mimicking the type 2 morphology of pRCC. Importantly, the adjacent renal parenchyma shows numerous papillary adenomas, which have no fibrous capsule and can measure up to 1.5 cm in size by current definition.[1]

DIFFERENTIAL DIAGNOSIS

The major differential diagnostic consideration for HPRC is multifocal, sporadic type 1 pRCC. Although it is not uncommon to have multiple type 1 pRCCs in a sporadic setting, these patients rarely have more than 10 tumors. In contrast, patients with HPRC present with numerous type 1 pRCCs, often ranging from dozens to hundreds. In addition, the background kidney in HPRC harbors innumerable microscopic papillary adenomas, which is an important clue to the hereditary condition.

DIAGNOSIS

Tumors in HPRC show similar morphologic and immunohistochemical features of sporadic type I pRCC. The presence of numerous papillary adenomas in the adjacent kidney is the most important diagnostic feature of HPRC. The definitive diagnosis of HPRC relies on genetic testing to identify germline mutations in the *MET* gene.

PROGNOSIS

Although rare, metastasis has been reported in HPRC. It is interesting to note that in a phase II and biomarker study of dual MET/VEGFR2 inhibitor foretinib, a high response rate was seen mainly in patients with germline MET mutations.[12]

HEREDITARY LEIOMYOMATOSIS RENAL CELL CARCINOMA SYNDROME

HLRCC syndrome is an autosomal dominant disorder resulting from germline mutations of *fumarate hydratase (FH)* gene, which confer an increased risk of cutaneous and uterine leiomyomatosis as well as RCC. The estimated lifetime renal cancer risk for *FH* mutation carriers is about 15%, and the mean age of presentation for cases in the literature is 41 years.[13] Most reported cases of HLRCC-associated RCCs are highly aggressive and patients often present with locally advanced disease or distant metastasis and have poor outcomes.[14–16] However, with the increased use of diagnostic biomarkers in pathologic diagnosis,[16,17] rare cases of FH-deficient RCC with low-grade morphologic features have been reported,[18,19] suggesting the HLRCC syndrome-associated RCC has a broader clinical and morphologic spectrum than previously appreciated.

Unlike the VHL or HPRC described elsewhere in this article, HLRCC-associated renal tumors can often be solitary and unilateral, and thus are difficult to distinguish from sporadic tumors clinically. Although skin or uterine leiomyomas tend to have high penetrance compared with renal tumors, the history or presence of these extrarenal manifestations can be easily missed in routine clinical encounters. Therefore, pathologic examination plays a pivotal role in facilitating the identification and clinical management of these patients and

family members.[16,20] Given a frequent lack of genetic confirmation at the time of pathologic diagnosis, the term "FH-deficient RCC" has been suggested for use in practice to encompass both HLRCC and rare cases of somatic FH-deficient RCC.

GROSS FEATURES

Tumors in HLRCC are predominantly unilateral and solitary. Grossly, they can have variable features: most of the tumors are solid and homogeneous but some are cystic or show areas of necrosis and hemorrhage. Some tumors seem to arise from the cyst wall as a distinct mural nodule. The adjacent renal parenchyma usually is unremarkable, with occasional cysts identified in some patients.

MICROSCOPIC FEATURES

Tumors show a spectrum of architectural patterns including papillary, tubular, tubulocystic, solid, cystic elements and areas closely mimicking collecting duct carcinoma or tubulocystic carcinoma. Sarcomatoid differentiation has also been reported (**Fig. 2**A–D). Mixed architectural patterns are common in a given tumor. It is worth noting that in a recent study of "tubulocystic carcinoma with poorly differentiated foci," up to 70% to 80% of cases in the multi-institution cohort are in fact FH-deficient RCC, although it is unclear how many of these were truly HLRCC with germline FH mutations.[21]

Cytologically, the most characteristic feature of HLRCC-associated RCCs as initially described by Merino and colleagues,[15] is the presence of "cherry-red," cytomegalovirus viral inclusion-like nucleoli surrounded by a perinucleolar halo (**Fig. 2**C–E). However, this feature may only be present focally in some cases[16]. In the newly identified low-grade cases of FH-deficient renal tumors (**Fig. 2**F), this feature is entirely lacking in a few instances.[18,19]

Immunohistochemically, the tumor cells show loss of FH immunoreactivity in a great majority of cases and retained immunoreactivity in endothelial or inflammatory cells within the tumor can serve as a positive internal control (see **Fig. 2**E inset). However, a small portion of confirmed HLRCC tumors shows retained weak or strong positivity, presumably owing to the retained expression of a defective FH protein. In contrast, immunohistochemical stain for S-(2-succino)-cysteine (2SC) is a highly sensitive and specific marker for the aberrant protein succination occurring in FH-deficient tumors. When showing a diffuse nuclear and

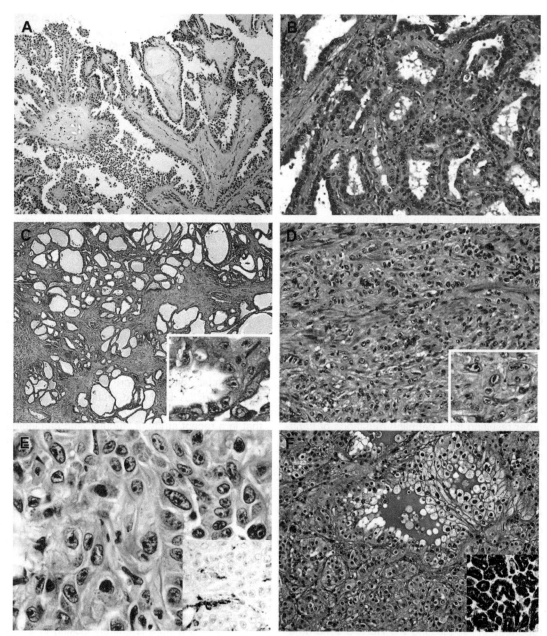

Fig. 2. Hereditary leiomyomatosis renal cell carcinoma (HLRCC) syndrome-associated RCC. Tumors demonstrate a spectrum of architectural patterns including papillary (H&E, original magnification ×10) (*A*), tubular, (H&E, original magnification × 20) (*B*), tubulocystic, (H&E, original magnification × 4) (*C*), solid, (H&E, original magnification × 20) (*D*) and sarcomatoid, (H&E, original magnification ×40) (*E*) elements. *Insets* in *C* and *D* are high-power view shows characteristic "cherry-red" nucleoli surrounded by a perinucleolar halo. *Inset* in *E* shows the loss of fumarate hydratase staining in tumor cells. Endothelial, stromal, or inflammatory cells serve as the internal positive control. (*F*) Low-grade fumarate hydratase-deficient renal tumors lack the prominent nucleoli, (H&E, original magnification ×20). *Inset* in *F*, 2SC staining confirms the status of fumarate hydratase deficiency.

cytoplasmic staining pattern, 2SC positivity highly correlates with the presence of FH mutations (see **Fig.** 2F inset). However, importantly for this marker, a cytoplasmic-only pattern (without nuclear labeling, or showing a "blue nucleus" marked only by the counterstain) should not be regarded as a positive 2SC staining for the purpose of diagnosing FH deficiency.[16]

DIFFERENTIAL DIAGNOSIS

The major differential diagnostic considerations with HLRCC-associated RCC are type 2 pRCC, collecting duct carcinoma, tubulocystic carcinoma, and other high-grade unclassified RCC. The prominent papillary structure seen in HLRCC-associated RCC may prompt one to consider a diagnosis of type 2 pRCC. In fact, many HLRCC tumors were categorized into type 2 pRCC in the literature. It is important to note that type 2 pRCC is a heterogeneous group of diseases morphologically and molecularly.[22] Because HLRCC tumors often behave more aggressively than pRCCs, it is important to properly separate this distinct entity. Tumors of type 2 pRCC are usually well-circumscribed, often with a prominent capsule. A tumor with infiltrative edges should raise the possibility of an alternative diagnosis, including HLRCC-associated RCC. The identification of the characteristic nuclear features, even only focally, may greatly aid in the diagnostic consideration of HLRCC. Finally, immunohistochemical stains for FH and 2SC can confirm the diagnosis of FH-deficient RCC (largely representing HLRCC).

Collecting duct carcinoma is a rare and very aggressive type of RCC that commonly centered in the renal medulla. The prototype is a high-grade adenocarcinoma with tubular and tubulopapillary architectural patterns in a desmoplastic stroma. However, a subset of collecting duct carcinomas may show a predominantly papillary architectural pattern. Because collecting duct carcinoma-like growth is commonly seen in HLRCC-associated RCC, rendering a diagnosis of collecting duct carcinoma typically requires excluding other possibilities in the differential diagnosis including HLRCC.

Tubulocystic carcinoma, as recommended in the current World Health Organization classification scheme, should be restricted to tumors with the classic morphology: a well-circumscribed tumor entirely composed of variably sized tubules and cysts lined by hobnail-shaped, eosinophilic cells with intermediate to large nucleoli.[23] For cases with tubulocystic carcinoma-like histology and additional poorly differentiated areas, it is very important to exclude the possibility of FH-deficient RCCs by ancillary or molecular studies.

Additional histologic features that can be seen in HLRCC-associated RCC such as cribriform pattern, sievelike prominent vacuolization, clear cell features, and sarcomatoid differentiation can also raise multiple differential diagnostic possibilities, including renal medullary carcinoma (RMC), Xp11 or t(6, 11) translocation RCC, high-grade ccRCC, and high-grade unclassified RCC. The diagnosis of RMC can be supported by the clinical features (eg, sickle cell trait) and the loss of nuclear expression of INI1 (SMARCB1/BAF47), whereas the diagnosis of *TFE3* or *TFEB* translocation tumors can be aided by TFE3/B immunohistochemistry or fluorescence in situ hybridization. The distinction of HLRCC from other high-grade RCCs with atypical features relies on finding retained FH expression and/or a negative staining result for 2SC.

DIAGNOSIS

As discussed elsewhere in this article, given the expanding clinical and pathologic spectrum of HLRCC-associated RCC, its diagnosis requires a pathologist to be vigilant about this possibility when encountering cases with unusual clinical or pathologic features. The identification of prominent nucleoli surrounded by perinucleolar haloes even focally should prompt one to perform immunohistochemical staining for FH and/or 2SC, which can help to establish or exclude the possibility of FH-deficiency. The definitive diagnosis of HLRCC relies on genetic testing to identify germline mutations in the *FH* gene.

PROGNOSIS

Among most of the reported cases in the literature, the prognosis for HLRCC-associated RCC is poor and early metastases have been described for small tumors. Common metastatic sites include the regional lymph nodes, adrenal glands, lung, liver, and bone. Currently, there is no established systemic therapy available for metastatic tumors. Clinical trials testing vascular endothelial growth factor and/or epidermal growth factor receptor inhibitors, as well as other approaches targeting the metabolic alterations, are ongoing.[24] Genetic counseling for family members and renal cancer surveillance are generally recommended, although the decision about genetic testing and surveillance should be made on an individual basis.[13]

Key Features
RENAL TUMORS IN HEREDITARY
LEIOMYOMATOSIS RENAL CELL CARCINOMA

1. Tumors show a spectrum of architectural patterns including papillary, tubular, tubulocystic, solid, and cystic areas.

2. Tumor cells are characterized by "cherry red," cytomegalovirus viral inclusion-like nucleoli surrounded by a perinucleolar halo. However, this feature may only be present focally.

3. By immunohistochemistry, tumor cells show loss of FH expression and diffuse nuclear and cytoplasmic immunoreactivity to 2SC.

⚠️ **Differential Diagnosis**
HEREDITARY LEIOMYOMATOSIS
RENAL CELL CARCINOMA

1. Type 2 pRCC

2. Tubulocystic RCC

3. Collecting duct carcinoma

4. Renal medullary carcinoma

5. Xp11 or t (6, 11) translocation RCC

6. High-grade ccRCC

7. High-grade unclassified RCC

SUCCINATE DEHYDROGENASE-DEFICIENT RENAL CELL CARCINOMA

SDH is an important component of the Krebs cycle and mitochondrial electron transport chain. Germline mutations in genes encoding its protein subunits (*SDHA*, *SDHB*, *SDHC*, and *SDHD*) or the regulatory factor *SDHAF2* have been identified as the causal aberrations in patients with familial paraganglioma-pheochromocytoma syndromes as well as other types of tumors such as gastrointestinal stromal tumors, pituitary adenomas, and RCCs. Although currently defined by the loss of immunohistochemical expression of SDHB, a marker of dysfunctional mitochondrial complex II, SDH-deficient RCC is strongly hereditary, and most commonly involving *SDHB* gene.[25,26] The overall incidence of RCC is estimated to be 0.05% to 0.1% of all resected renal cell tumors.[25]

GROSS FEATURES

SDH-deficient RCCs are often solitary and unilateral. Bilateral tumors were observed in 26% of reported cases. Grossly, tumors are mostly well-circumscribed, often with a pushing border and sometimes associated with a pseudocapsule. However, tumors rarely can show an infiltrative border and exhibit high-grade histology. Cut surfaces of the tumors are often solid, variegated, tan-brown, or red-brown.

MICROSCOPIC FEATURES

These tumors often show a predominantly solid architecture with cystic change. The tumor cells have characteristic intracytoplasmic vacuolations and inclusions, flocculated eosinophilic cytoplasm and uniform low-grade nuclei (**Fig. 3**A, B). These inclusions are shown to be giant mitochondria on ultrastructural examination. Intratumoral mast cells can often be identified. High-grade features, including sarcomatoid change, coagulative necrosis, and high nuclear grade are uncommon and are associated aggressive biology. By immunohistochemistry, the loss of SDHB staining is a sensitive and specific marker for these tumors (**Fig. 3**C). Of note, a lack of SDHB staining can be seen in tumors with mutations in *SDHA*, *SDHC*, *SDHD*, or *SDHAF2*, owing to protein destabilization. The tumors are typically negative for CK7 or CD117, but the latter stain often highlights the intratumoral mast cells.

DIFFERENTIAL DIAGNOSIS

The major differential diagnostic considerations with SDH-deficient RCC are renal oncocytoma, eosinophilic variant of chromophobe RCC, TSC-associated RCC, recently described eosinophilic solid and cystic (ESC) RCC,[27] rare low-grade HLRCC-associated RCC described elsewhere in this article, rare *TFEB*-translocation tumors, and other unclassified RCC with oncocytic features.

Renal oncocytoma has uniform, round nuclei with abundant granular eosinophilic cytoplasm

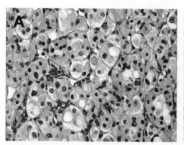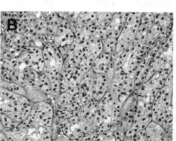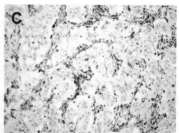

Fig. 3. Succinate dehydrogenase (SDH)-deficient renal cell carcinoma. (*A, B*) Tumors often comprise solid nests of cells. Tumor cells have intracytoplasmic vacuolations and inclusions, flocculated eosinophilic cytoplasm, and uniform low-grade nuclei (H&E, original magnification *A* ×40; *B* ×20). (*C*) Tumor cells demonstrate a loss of SDHB staining. Staining in the blood vessels serve as a positive internal control (SDHB staining, original magnification × 20).

arranged in solid nests or microcysts in a background of loose stroma. Although architecturally similar to SDH-deficient RCC, it lacks intracytoplasmic vacuolations and inclusions. Nuclear pleomorphism can be seen in cells with degenerative changes, but true high-grade nuclear features are lacking in oncocytoma. Additionally, renal oncocytoma is usually positive for CD117 and shows retention of SDHB staining.

The eosinophilic variant of chromophobe RCC shows dense granular eosinophilic cytoplasm with irregular, wrinkled nuclei and perinuclear halos, and lacks intracytoplasmic inclusions. They have retained SDHB and usually are positive for CD117 staining. CK7 is also positive in a portion of cases.

The distinction of SDH-deficient RCC from other rare subtypes of RCC typically requires ancillary studies such SDHB, FH, or TFE3/TFEB.

DIAGNOSIS

The diagnosis of SDH-deficient RCC can be rendered when the tumor shows at least focal histology features of intracytoplasmic inclusions and absence of immunohistochemical staining for SDHB. The definitive diagnosis of SDH complex deficiency syndrome relies on genetic testing to identify germline mutations in the *SDHA-D* or *SDHAF2* gene.

PROGNOSIS

Most SDH-deficient RCC demonstrates an indolent clinical behavior. However, up to 33% of these tumors show metastasis and an aggressive clinical course. Most cases with metastasis exhibit high-grade features, such as high-grade nuclear atypia and coagulative necrosis. Thus, a careful histologic examination of the tumor is important in determining the prognosis of these tumors.

Key Features
SUCCINATE DEHYDROGENASE-DEFICIENT RENAL CELL CARCINOMA

1. Tumors often show a solid growth pattern with cystic change.

2. Tumor cells have intracytoplasmic vacuolations and inclusions that are shown to be giant mitochondria. Tumor cells usually have low-grade nuclei.

3. Loss of SDHB staining is a sensitive and specific marker for these tumors.

⚠️ Differential Diagnosis
SUCCINATE DEHYDROGENASE-DEFICIENT RENAL CELL CARCINOMA

1. Renal oncocytoma

2. Eosinophilic variant of chromophobe RCC

3. TSC-associated RCC

4. ESC RCC

5. Low-grade HLRCC-associated RCC

6. TFEB-translocation tumors

7. Unclassified RCC with oncocytic features

BIRT-HOGG-DUBÉ SYNDROME

BHD syndrome is an autosomal-dominant syndrome that results from mutations in *FLCN* gene, located on chromosome 17p11.2. BHD syndrome is characterized by the development of cutaneous hamartomas, kidney tumors, lung cysts, and spontaneous pneumothorax. Among these, pulmonary findings are most common features. More than 80% of patients with BHD syndrome have lung cysts on CT imaging and about 40% of BHD have a history of spontaneous pneumothorax. Skin lesions usually appear before renal manifestations. Renal tumors occur in 15% to 30% of patients with a mean age of onset of 46 to 52 years and are usually bilateral and multifocal. The most common tumor histology is hybrid oncocytic tumors (50%) with features of chromophobe RCC, and renal oncocytoma, and other histologies include chromophobe RCC, ccRCC, and renal oncocytoma.[28,29] The function of folliculin, the gene product, has not been clearly delineated, but it is believed to be a tumor suppressor gene and plays a role in modulating AKT-mammalian target of rapamycin pathway.[30]

GROSS FEATURES

Approximately 50% of patients with BHD syndrome present with bilateral and multifocal renal tumors. Tumors usually have homogeneous, brown cut surface without hemorrhage or necrosis. A central scar may be present. Ample sampling of the available adjacent renal parenchyma, which may or may not contain grossly visible small nodules, is recommended for recognizing the presence of renal oncocytosis.

MICROSCOPIC FEATURES

The most commonly encountered histologic subtype is hybrid oncocytic tumors, in which there are admixed areas reminiscent of chromophobe

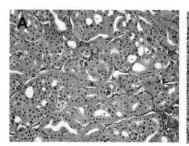
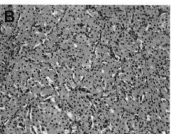
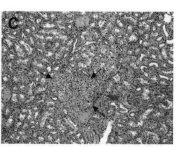

Fig. 4. Birt-Hogg-Dubé syndrome. (*A*) Representative hybrid oncocytic tumor with admixed features of chromophobe renal cell carcinoma and oncocytoma. (*B*) Representative hybrid oncocytic tumor shows nuclear contour irregularities but lacks the perinuclear halos. (*C*) Clusters of oncocytic cells (*arrows*) percolating between native renal parenchyma (H&E, original magnification *A, B* ×20; *C* ×10).

RCC or oncocytoma, or tumor cells displaying nuclear contour irregularities but lacking the perinuclear halos (**Fig. 4**). Characteristically, oncocytic tumors in BHD syndrome can contain clusters of clear cells in an otherwise oncocytic tumor. Tumors with the histology of chromophobe, clear cell, or pRCC, as well as renal oncocytoma, have also been described; however, the underlying molecular alterations in these tumors may differ from their sporadic counterparts.[31]

To raise a suspicion of BHD based on pathologic review, it is essential to evaluate the surrounding renal parenchyma for features of oncocytosis, such as numerous microscopic oncocytic nodules with features of oncocytoma, chromophobe RCC or hybrid tumors, cysts lined by oncocytic cells, or clusters of oncocytic cells percolating between native renal parenchyma, and oncocytic changes in nonneoplastic renal tubules.[32]

DIFFERENTIAL DIAGNOSIS

The major differential diagnostic considerations with BHD syndrome-associated renal tumors are sporadic renal oncocytoma and chromophobe RCC. Currently, there are no specific ancillary tools to support the diagnosis. A history of bilateral and multifocal renal tumors should prompt one to consider a possibility of the syndromic condition. Examination of the adjacent renal parenchyma is crucial.

Sporadic renal oncocytoma lacks the focal nuclear atypia resembling chromophobe RCC and the scattered clusters of cells with clear cytoplasm. Sporadic chromophobe RCC has the characteristic hyperchromatic, raisinoid nuclei with perinuclear haloes, whereas this feature in the hybrid oncocytic tumors of BHD patients is less convincing or only focally present.

DIAGNOSIS

Multiple oncocytic neoplasms and features of oncocytosis in the background kidney should raise

a possibility of BHD or renal oncocytosis. The definitive diagnosis of BHD relies on the presence of extrarenal and renal manifestations and confirmed by a genetic test that is positive for a germline *FLCN* mutation.

PROGNOSIS

Tumors are usually small at the time of presentation and have minimal metastatic potential. Patients with BHD with renal manifestations commonly develop chronic kidney disease.

Key Features
RENAL TUMORS IN
BIRT-HOGG-DUBÉ SYNDROME

1. In hybrid oncocytic tumors, there are admixed areas reminiscent of chromophobe RCC or oncocytoma; tumor cells often display nuclear contour irregularities but lack perinuclear halos.

2. The surrounding renal parenchyma shows features of oncocytosis.

TUBEROUS SCLEROSIS COMPLEX

TSC is an autosomal-dominant genetic disorder that results from germline mutations in either *TSC1* (9q34), encoding the protein harmatin, or in *TSC2* (16p13), encoding the protein tuberin. These 2 proteins are components of the mammalian target of rapamycin signaling pathway. Up to 50% of cases have no family history and represent either new mutations or a variation of disease penetrance. TSC can affect nearly every organ system to varying degrees. Renal involvement occurs in approximately 80% of individuals with TSC and is the leading cause of death in patients with TSC. Renal manifestations commonly observed in patients with TSC include angiomyolipoma and renal epithelial cysts, affecting up to 50% to 80% and 40% of patients, respectively. In comparison, RCCs or renal epithelial neoplasia are much less common, with an estimated incidence of 2% to 4%, which is slightly higher than the estimated incidence in the general population.[33,34]

GROSS FEATURES

Multiple tan-yellow nodules, which represent angiomyolipomas, and simple or multiple cysts are frequent features in the kidney of patients with TSC. Diffuse cystic formation similar to autosomal-dominant polycystic kidney disease develops in 5% of TSC2 patients owing to dual deletion of 2 genes located contiguously on chromosome 16, TSC2 and PKD1.[35,36]

MICROSCOPIC FEATURES

TSC-associated RCCs are often multifocal and present in association with multiple angiomyolipomas and renal cysts. Microscopically, TSC-associated RCCs demonstrate a wide spectrum of cytologic features and architectural patterns.[37,38] A subset of tumors predominantly show clear and voluminous cytoplasm arranged in papillary, acinar, tubular, or alveolar architectural patterns (Fig. 5A), closely mimicking ccRCC or the recently described TCEB1-mutated RCC.[39] These tumors frequently have prominent fibromuscular stroma, a feature also seen in TCEB1-mutated RCC and renal angiomyoadenomatous tumor–like tumors. The second group of tumors comprises nests or sheets of cells with eosinophilic or onco-cytic cytoplasm, resembling chromophobe RCC, oncocytoma, or hybrid oncocytic tumors (Fig. 5B). The remaining TSC-associated tumors may have more unclassifiable features and mainly consist of eosinophilic cells with variable architectures and can focally display high-grade nuclear features (Fig. 5C). The recently described ESC

RCC can be morphologically indistinguishable from some tumors in the 2 latter categories.[17] Although 1 architectural pattern may be dominant in a tumor, mixed growth patterns were not uncommon. The cytoplasm of TSC-associated tumors often contains eosinophilic, finely granular stippling or fibrillary material, and sometimes displaying aggregated eosinophilic globules.

Given the wide morphologic spectrum, the immunohistochemical features of TSC-associated RCC also vary. Tumors with clear cells are often at least focally positive for carbonic anhydrase-IX and show variable positivity for CD10 and CK7, and are negative for AMACR. Tumors resembling chromophobe, oncocytoma, or hybrid oncocytic tumor may be positive for CD117. Overall, the tumors are positive for PAX8 and show a strong expression of markers of mammalian target of rapamycin pathway, such as p-4EBP1 and p-S6.[40]

DIFFERENTIAL DIAGNOSIS

Depending on the histologic features, the major differential diagnostic considerations for TSC-associated RCC differ. In tumors with predominantly clear cytoplasm, the main differentials are TCEB1-mutated RCC, ccRCC, or TFE3 translocation RCC. In tumors with eosinophilic cytoplasm, the differential often includes ESC RCC, eosinophilic chromophobe, hybrid oncocytic tumor, TFE3/TFEB translocation RCC, and other unclassified RCC. Because there are currently no specific markers developed for TSC-associated RCC, their distinction from other RCCs with morphologic similarity depends on a careful examination of the adjacent renal parenchyma for the presence of angiomyolipomas (often are microscopic) and renal cysts. A clinical history of extrarenal manifestations can also be helpful in considering a syndromic association.

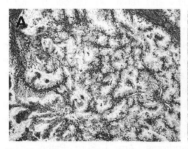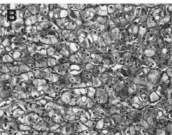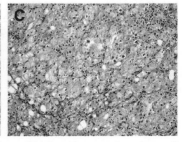

Fig. 5. Tuberous sclerosis complex-associated renal tumors. (*A*) The tumor predominantly comprises clear cells with voluminous cytoplasm and shows papillary and alveolar architectural patterns. (*B*) Tumor composed of nests of cells with pale to eosinophilic or oncocytic cytoplasm, mimicking chromophobe renal cell carcinoma or hybrid oncocytic tumors. (*C*) Some tuberous sclerosis complex-associated tumors consist of eosinophilic cells with variable architectures and can focally display high-grade nuclear features (H&E, original magnification ×20).

TCEB1-mutated RCC is characterized by thick fibromuscular bands traversing tumor parenchyma, imparting a multinodular appearance on low-power view. Tumor cells have clear and voluminous cytoplasm and form solid acinar and papillary architecture. By immunohistochemistry, tumor cells are positive for carbonic anhydrase-IX (diffuse box-like membranous staining) and CK7. These morphologic and immunohistochemical features can be virtually identical to some of the tumors seen in TSC. Identifying *TCEB1* (*ELOC*) hotspot mutation and concurrent 8/8q loss confirms the diagnosis.

DIAGNOSIS

The presence of multifocal angiomyolipomas should strongly suggest the possibility of TSC. The possibility of TSC-associated RCC should be raised when a patient has multifocal renal tumors exhibiting morphologies resembling *TCEB1*-mutated RCC, ESC RCC, hybrid oncocytoma, or chromophobe-like features in a background kidney with multiple angiomyolipomas and renal cysts. The definitive diagnosis of TSC relies on genetic testing to identify germline mutations in the *TSC1 or TSC2* gene.

PROGNOSIS

Renal tumors in patients with TSC generally follow an indolent clinical course. They rarely metastasize. Deaths owing to RCC in patients with TSC are uncommon.

Key Features
RENAL TUMORS IN
TUBEROUS SCLEROSIS COMPLEX

1. Clear and voluminous cytoplasm arranged in papillary, acinar, tubular, or alveolar architectural patterns.

2. Nests or sheets of tumor cells with oncocytic cytoplasm.

3. Eosinophilic cells with variable architectures and can focally display high-grade nuclear features.

4. Associated with multiple angiomyolipomas and renal cysts.

REFERENCES

1. Moch H, Humphrey PA, Ulbright TM, et al, editors. WHO classification of tumours of the urinary system and male genital organs. 4th edition. Lyon (France): IARC; 2016.

2. Gossage L, Eisen T, Maher ER. VHL the story of a tumour suppressor gene. Nat Rev Cancer 2015; 15(1):55–64.

3. Lonser RR, Glenn GM, Walther M, et al. von Hippel-Lindau disease. Lancet 2003;361(9374):2059–67.

4. Chauveau D, Duvic C, Chretien Y, et al. Renal involvement in von Hippel-Lindau disease. Kidney Int 1996;50(3):944–51.

5. Solomon D, Schwartz A. Renal pathology in von Hippel-Lindau disease. Hum Pathol 1988;19(9): 1072–9.

6. Beroukhim R, Brunet JP, Di Napoli A, et al. Patterns of gene expression and copy-number alterations in von-Hippel Lindau disease-associated and sporadic clear cell carcinoma of the kidney. Cancer Res 2009; 69(11):4674–81.

7. Chen YB, Tickoo SK. Spectrum of preneoplastic and neoplastic cystic lesions of the kidney. Arch Pathol Lab Med 2012;136(4):400–9.

8. Williamson SR, Zhang S, Eble JN, et al. Clear cell papillary renal cell carcinoma-like tumors in patients with von Hippel-Lindau disease are unrelated to sporadic clear cell papillary renal cell carcinoma. Am J Surg Pathol 2013;37(8):1131–9.

9. Rao P, Monzon F, Jonasch E, et al. Clear cell papillary renal cell carcinoma in patients with von Hippel-Lindau syndrome–clinicopathological features and comparative genomic analysis of 3 cases. Hum Pathol 2014;45(9):1966–72.

10. Schmidt L, Duh FM, Chen F, et al. Germline and somatic mutations in the tyrosine kinase domain of the MET proto-oncogene in papillary renal carcinomas. Nat Genet 1997;16(1):68–73.

11. Lubensky IA, Schmidt L, Zhuang Z, et al. Hereditary and sporadic papillary renal carcinomas with c-met mutations share a distinct morphological phenotype. Am J Pathol 1999;155(2):517–26.

12. Choueiri TK, Vaishampayan U, Rosenberg JE, et al. Phase II and biomarker study of the dual MET/VEGFR2 inhibitor foretinib in patients with papillary renal cell carcinoma. J Clin Oncol 2013;31(2):181–6.

13. Menko FH, Maher ER, Schmidt LS, et al. Hereditary leiomyomatosis and renal cell cancer (HLRCC): renal cancer risk, surveillance and treatment. Fam Cancer 2014;13(4):637–44.

14. Toro JR, Nickerson ML, Wei MH, et al. Mutations in the fumarate hydratase gene cause hereditary leiomyomatosis and renal cell cancer in families in North America. Am J Hum Genet 2003;73(1):95–106.

15. Merino MJ, Torres-Cabala C, Pinto P, et al. The morphologic spectrum of kidney tumors in hereditary leiomyomatosis and renal cell carcinoma (HLRCC) syndrome. Am J Surg Pathol 2007; 31(10):1578–85.

16. Chen YB, Brannon AR, Toubaji A, et al. Hereditary leiomyomatosis and renal cell carcinoma syndrome-associated renal cancer: recognition of

the syndrome by pathologic features and the utility of detecting aberrant succination by immunohistochemistry. Am J Surg Pathol 2014;38(5):627–37.

17. Trpkov K, Hes O, Agaimy A, et al. Fumarate Hydratase-deficient renal cell carcinoma is strongly correlated with Fumarate Hydratase mutation and hereditary Leiomyomatosis and renal cell carcinoma syndrome. Am J Surg Pathol 2016;40(7):865–75.

18. Smith SC, Sirohi D, Ohe C, et al. A distinctive, low-grade oncocytic fumarate hydratase-deficient renal cell carcinoma, morphologically reminiscent of succinate dehydrogenase-deficient renal cell carcinoma. Histopathology 2017;71(1):42–52.

19. Li Y, Reuter VE, Matoso A, et al. Re-evaluation of 33 'unclassified' eosinophilic renal cell carcinomas in young patients. Histopathology 2018;72(4):588–600.

20. Kopp RP, Stratton KL, Glogowski E, et al. Utility of prospective pathologic evaluation to inform clinical genetic testing for hereditary leiomyomatosis and renal cell carcinoma. Cancer 2017;123(13):2452–8.

21. Smith SC, Trpkov K, Chen YB, et al. Tubulocystic carcinoma of the kidney with poorly differentiated foci: a frequent morphologic pattern of Fumarate Hydratase-deficient renal cell carcinoma. Am J Surg Pathol 2016;40(11):1457–72.

22. Cancer Genome Atlas Research Network, Linehan WM, Spellman PT, et al. Comprehensive molecular characterization of papillary renal-cell carcinoma. N Engl J Med 2016;374(2):135–45.

23. Srigley JR, Delahunt B, Eble JN, et al. The International Society of Urological Pathology (ISUP) Vancouver Classification of Renal Neoplasia. Am J Surg Pathol 2013;37(10):1469–89.

24. Linehan WM, Rouault TA. Molecular pathways: fumarate hydratase-deficient kidney cancer–targeting the Warburg effect in cancer. Clin Cancer Res 2013;19(13):3345–52.

25. Gill AJ, Hes O, Papathomas T, et al. Succinate dehydrogenase (SDH)-deficient renal carcinoma: a morphologically distinct entity: a clinicopathologic series of 36 tumors from 27 patients. Am J Surg Pathol 2014;38(12):1588–602.

26. Gill AJ. Succinate dehydrogenase (SDH) and mitochondrial driven neoplasia. Pathology 2012;44(4):285–92.

27. Trpkov K, Hes O, Bonert M, et al. Eosinophilic, solid, and cystic renal cell carcinoma: clinicopathologic study of 16 unique, sporadic neoplasms occurring in women. Am J Surg Pathol 2016;40(1):60–71.

28. Pavlovich CP, Walther MM, Eyler RA, et al. Renal tumors in the Birt-Hogg-Dube syndrome. Am J Surg Pathol 2002;26(12):1542–52.

29. Furuya M, Yao M, Tanaka R, et al. Genetic, epidemiologic and clinicopathologic studies of Japanese Asian patients with Birt-Hogg-Dube syndrome. Clin Genet 2016;90(5):403–12.

30. Schmidt LS, Linehan WM. Molecular genetics and clinical features of Birt-Hogg-Dube syndrome. Nat Rev Urol 2015;12(10):558–69.

31. Iribe Y, Yao M, Tanaka R, et al. Genome-wide uniparental disomy and copy number variations in renal cell carcinomas associated with Birt-Hogg-Dube syndrome. Am J Pathol 2016;186(2):337–46.

32. Tickoo SK, Reuter VE, Amin MB, et al. Renal oncocytosis: a morphologic study of fourteen cases. Am J Surg Pathol 1999;23(9):1094–101.

33. Crino PB, Nathanson KL, Henske EP. The tuberous sclerosis complex. N Engl J Med 2006;355(13):1345–56.

34. Rakowski SK, Winterkorn EB, Paul E, et al. Renal manifestations of tuberous sclerosis complex: incidence, prognosis, and predictive factors. Kidney Int 2006;70(10):1777–82.

35. Brook-Carter PT, Peral B, Ward CJ, et al. Deletion of the TSC2 and PKD1 genes associated with severe infantile polycystic kidney disease–a contiguous gene syndrome. Nat Genet 1994;8(4):328–32.

36. Martignoni G, Bonetti F, Pea M, et al. Renal disease in adults with TSC2/PKD1 contiguous gene syndrome. Am J Surg Pathol 2002;26(2):198–205.

37. Guo J, Tretiakova MS, Troxell ML, et al. Tuberous sclerosis-associated renal cell carcinoma: a clinicopathologic study of 57 separate carcinomas in 18 patients. Am J Surg Pathol 2014;38(11):1457–67.

38. Yang P, Cornejo KM, Sadow PM, et al. Renal cell carcinoma in tuberous sclerosis complex. Am J Surg Pathol 2014;38(7):895–909.

39. Hakimi AA, Tickoo SK, Jacobsen A, et al. TCEB1-mutated renal cell carcinoma: a distinct genomic and morphological subtype. Mod Pathol 2015;28(6):845–53.

40. Chen YB, Gopalan A, Al-Ahmadie H, et al. Tuberous sclerosis-associated renal cell carcinoma: morphologic spectrum and molecular characterization. Mod Pathol 2013;26:201A.

A Contemporary Review of Common Adult Non–germ Cell Tumors of the Testis and Paratestis

Kelly L. Mooney, MD, Chia-Sui Kao, MD*

KEYWORDS

- Testis • Non–germ cell tumor • Sex cord–stromal tumor • Paratesticular tumor • Leydig cell tumor
- Sertoli cell tumor • Immunohistochemistry

Key points

- Sex cord–stromal tumors comprise a majority of non–germ cell tumors of the testis.

- Features suggestive of malignancy in sex cord–stromal tumors are the following: large size, infiltrative borders, severe cytologic atypia, increased mitoses, necrosis, and lymphovascular invasion.

- Lymphoma and metastasis, although rare, remain important differential diagnoses of testicular neoplasia, especially in elderly men.

ABSTRACT

This article provides a comprehensive review of non–germ cell tumors of the testis and paratestis in adults, incorporating the latest 2016 World Health Organization updates. Clinical features, gross pathologic findings, key morphologic details, immunohistochemical profiles, and differential diagnoses are covered, with an emphasis on how to resolve commonly encountered, and sometimes difficult, differential diagnoses.

germ cell tumors. Similarly, paratesticular tumors remain important differential diagnoses when encountering a tumor in the testis, given the possibility of secondary involvement. This article focuses on tumors seen more commonly in adults, and interested readers are referred to a previous excellent comprehensive review of testicular tumors of the young by Ulbright and Young.[1] The important clinicopathologic features of non–germ cell testicular and paratesticular tumors of adult men, including recent World Health Organization (WHO) updates and how to resolve difficult differential diagnosis in this category of tumors, are discussed.

OVERVIEW

Sex cord–stromal tumors comprise the second largest tumor category of testicular tumors; nonetheless, their rarity may result in diagnostic difficulty and confusion with the more common

SEX CORD–STROMAL TUMORS

INTRODUCTION

Sex cord–stromal tumors make up 2% to 5% of adult testicular tumors and approximately 25%

Disclosure Statement: The authors have nothing to disclose.
Department of Pathology, Stanford University School of Medicine, 300 Pasteur Drive, L235, Stanford, CA 94305, USA
* Corresponding author.
E-mail address: ckao2@stanford.edu

1875-9181/18/© 2018 Elsevier Inc. All rights reserved.

of pediatric testicular tumors, due to the relatively lower incidence of germ cell tumors in the pediatric population.[2–4] In contrast to germ cell tumors, sex cord–stromal tumors are seen more commonly in younger patients (particularly in the setting of genetic syndromes) and are mostly benign, with an approximately 5% to 10% chance of malignant behavior. Also, unlike germ cell tumors, sex cord–stromal tumors are not pathologically staged unless deemed malignant, although malignant behavior of sex cord–stromal tumors is often not predictable based on morphology alone. Because the gross appearance of sex cord–stromal tumors is often indistinguishable from germ cell tumors, the grossing protocol of any testicular tumor remains the same, and such protocol has been detailed in a prior publication (see Howitt and Berney[5]).

Recent work on testicular sex cord–stromal tumors was reflected in the latest WHO classification of urologic tumors (2016) with several key changes to the framework set forth in the 2004 version.[6] First, there are no separate categories of benign and malignant sex cord–stromal tumors, because malignant behavior is not uniformly predictable based on morphology. Second, sclerosing and lipid cell variants of Sertoli cell tumor (SCT) are now considered morphologic variants of SCT, not otherwise specified (NOS), because CTNNB1 gene mutations have been identified in both the NOS and sclerosing SCTs.[7,8] Although no specific study of CTNNB1 gene mutations in lipid cell variant of SCT is available, it is now known that many SCT NOS contain variable amounts of lipid, and, therefore, lipid-rich SCTs are considered within the morphologic spectrum of SCT NOS. Third, large cell calcifying SCT (LCCSCT) and intratubular large cell hyalinizing Sertoli cell neoplasia (ILHSCN) are considered separate entities, with key differences in clinical presentation, pathologic features, and specific germline mutations (discussed later). Fourth, a "mixed and unclassified sex cord–stromal tumor" category replaces the previously separate categories of "mixed" and "incompletely differentiated" forms of sex cord–gonadal stromal tumors. Fifth, the entity "germ cell–sex cord/gonadal stromal tumor, unclassified" has been removed from the WHO classification due to its debatable existence,[9] and a new classification has been introduced: "tumor containing both germ cell and sex cord stromal elements" with only 1 entity—gonadoblastoma. Lastly, "undifferentiated gonadal tissue" is introduced as a precursor lesion of gonadoblastoma, and myoid gonadal

stromal tumor (MGST) is introduced as an emerging entity.

Although each tumor within the testicular sex cord–stromal tumor category is distinct, a few generalizations can be made. The morphologic features are similar to those seen in their ovarian counterparts, if applicable, with similar immunohistochemical reactivity. The role of immunohistochemistry is limited, given the overlapping immunoreactivity within the sex cord–stromal tumor family. Inhibin and calretinin have been the more commonly used confirmatory marker for sex cord–stromal tumors of the testis, but recent work suggests that steroidogenic factor 1 (SF1) is overall more sensitive and specific, whereas SOX9 and FOXL2, although not lineage specific, may provide additional evidence of Sertoli and granulosa/stromal differentiation, respectively.[10,11] Short of metastasis to confirm malignant behavior of a sex cord–stromal tumor, morphologic features that are suggestive of malignancy are, in general, a combination of large tumor size, infiltrative boarders, necrosis, lymphovascular invasion, cytologic atypia, and high mitotic activity. Radical orchiectomy is curative for clinically benign sex cord–stromal tumors, and malignant tumors are resistant to chemotherapy and radiation.

LEYDIG CELL TUMOR

Clinical Features

Leydig cell tumors (LCTs) account for 1% to 2% of all testicular tumors and are the most common neoplasia in the testicular sex cord–stromal tumor category.[12] They can occur at all ages with 2 peaks, one at 5 years to 10 years and a second at 30 years to 35 years.[12] Reported clinical features include painless testicular enlargement, elevated serum testosterone, and estrogen levels resulting in hormonal manifestations, such as gynecomastia (up to 15%) or, rarely, precocious puberty and Cushing syndrome.[12–15] Rare associations with Klinefelter syndrome, hereditary leiomyomatosis, and renal cell cancer syndromes have been described.[16,17] A minority are clinically malignant and present with metastases (most commonly in retroperitoneal lymph nodes).[14,18,19] Orchiectomy alone is generally curative for nonmetastasizing LCTs, with testis-sparing surgery as a safe alternative in patients with tumors smaller than 2.5 cm.[15,20–22] Malignant LCTs are treated by orchiectomy with retroperitoneal lymph node dissection, with no significant response to chemotherapy.[23] The cancer-specific mortality for LCTs is 2%, with an overall 5-year survival of greater than 90% after orchiectomy.[4,24] Although most

LCTs are benign, it is important to highlight that their early detection and removal are imperative due to the infertility risk of long-term excess estrogen.[25]

Pathologic Features

Macroscopically, LCTs are usually small (<5 cm in diameter), well circumscribed, and solid with golden brown cut surfaces. Low-power histology reveals diffuse sheets or large nodules of eosinophilic tumors cells (Fig. 1A); less common patterns include insular, trabecular, pseudotubular, ribbon-like, spindled, and microcystic.[14,26,27] The cells are characterized by uniform round nuclei, prominent central nucleoli, and abundant eosinophilic cytoplasm. Ground-glass nuclear change is distinct when present (Fig. 1B). The cytoplasm may contain Reinke crystals (up to 30% of cases; Fig. 1C), with variations showing scant or foamy cytoplasm.[27] Calcification, ossification, and adipocytic metaplasia may be seen. Malignant tumors have more than 2 of the following features: greater than 5 cm in diameter, infiltrative borders, cytologic atypia (Fig. 1D), mitoses (>3/10 high-power fields [HPFs]), vascular invasion, and/or necrosis.[14] Using immunohistochemistry, LCTs are typically positive for inhibin (95%), calretinin (90%), and melan-A.[13]

△△ **Differential Diagnosis**
   LEYDIG CELL TUMOR

- Leydig cell hyperplasia (usually microscopic, <0.5 cm; when macroscopic, remain small and multifocal)

- Benign ectopic Leydig cells (do not confuse with invasive nests)

- Testicular tumor of adrenogenital syndrome (bilateral, multifocal, cytoplasmic lipofuscin, spotty atypia, and thick dissecting fibrous bands)

- Granular cell tumor (melan-A negative in granular cell tumor and positive in LCT)

- Malakoplakia (involves tubules and interstitium, with xanthogranulomatous inflammation and Michaelis-Gutmann bodies)

- Lymphomas (more frequently bilateral, intertubular effacement with intratubular growth, and distinct cytologic features)

- Yolk sac tumor (presence of germ cell neoplasia in situ in background tubules and SALL4/GPC3/AFP positive)

SERTOLI CELL TUMOR, NOT OTHERWISE SPECIFIED

Clinical Features

Sertoli cell tumor, not otherwise specified (SCT NOS) is the second most common testicular sex cord–stromal tumor and accounts for approximately 1% of all testicular tumors. They generally present in adults over 30 years old as unilateral, slow-growing, possibly painful testicular masses, with or without hormonal manifestations,[28] but rare cases have been reported in infants.[29] Mutations in the CTNNB1 gene (encoding β-catenin protein) are found in a portion of SCT NOS, including the sclerosing type.[7,8] Although most patients follow benign clinical courses after surgical excision (in particular, those with tumors showing extensive sclerotic change—sclerosing type), metastases, including late metastases, develop in a minority of patients, with a risk of mortality in the setting of malignant tumors.[28]

Pathologic Features

Histologically, the morphology is variable, depending on the extent and type of tubular differentiation. Tubular and/or corded architecture with a nodular growth is the hallmark of SCT; however, other patterns, such as nests, sheets, and, rarely, single cells in a fibrous stroma may be the predominant pattern with only focal tubular differentiation, if at all recognizable. Tubules may be in different forms, such as elongated (Fig. 2A), solid, hollow (Fig. 2B), irregular, or, rarely, retiform (Fig. 2C). Unusual patterns include focal dilatation of tubules, resulting in a cystic morphology, prominent palisading simulating Verocay bodies of a schwannoma, and hyaline bodies.[28] The cells are often pale and cytoplasm may contain lipid or vacuolization (Fig. 2D). The background is usually fibrous or myxoid; when the stroma is more than 50% fibrotic, the tumor may be placed in the sclerosing subtype of SCT NOS (Fig. 2E, F), which has an excellent prognosis. Malignant criteria for SCT NOS include the following: large size (≥5 cm), increased mitotic activity (>5 mitotic figures per HPFs), tumor necrosis, moderate to severe nuclear atypia, lymphovascular invasion, and infiltrative growth pattern.[28,30] CTNNB1 gene mutations are found in 60% to 70% of these tumors, resulting in a characteristic nuclear accumulation of β-catenin by immunohistochemistry (Fig. 2G).[8] Additional immunohistochemical reactivity includes pancytokeratin, epithelial membrane antigen (EMA), inhibin, melan-A, WT1, SF1, CD99, calretinin, synaptophysin, chromogranin, and SOX9 (Fig. 2H).[11,28,31,32]

△△ **Differential Diagnosis**
SERTOLI CELL TUMOR

- LCT (more frequently positive for inhibin; negative for nuclear β-catenin)

- Adenomatoid tumors (paratesticular location)

- Seminoma (tubular type, in particular, may be confused with SCT, but seminoma expresses OCT3/4 and exhibits nuclei with squared-off edges and prominent nucleoli)

- Carcinoid tumors (negative for SF1/inhibin/calretinin)

- Metastases (exclude with history and immunohistochemistry)

LARGE CELL CALCIFYING SERTOLI CELL TUMOR

Clinical Features

Large cell calcifying Sertoli cell tumors (LCCSCTs) are exceptionally rare.[33,34] They are a feature of autosomal dominant Carney complex (characterized by a germline *PRKAR1A* gene mutation) but more commonly occur sporadically (60%).[34] When these are syndromic, they are usually bilateral and multifocal, whereas sporadic tumors are almost always unifocal and unilateral. Increased aromatase expression in LCCSCTs, possibly secondary to increased cyclic adenosine monophosphate signaling, may lead to endocrine symptoms clinically.[35] Most benign cases present in younger patients (mean 17 years, range 2–38 years) whereas malignant cases typically present in older patients (mean 39 years, rage 28–51 years) without associated syndromes.[34,36,37] In the setting of Carney complex or other genetic neoplasia syndrome, surgery may not be indicated due to effective treatment with aromatase inhibitors.[37,38]

Pathologic Features

Histologically, LCCSCTs are characterized by large Sertoli cells with abundant eosinophilic cytoplasm organized in sheets, nests, and solid tubules and cords with focal to massive calcifications (**Fig. 3**A) and an often substantial

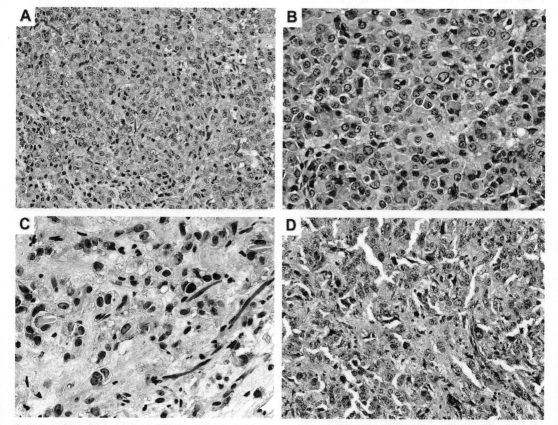

Fig. 1. Leydig cell tumor. (*A*) Diffuse growth with uniform eosinophilic cells containing round nuclei and conspicuous nuclei. (*B*) Some nuclei have a ground-glass appearance. (*C*) Multiple rod-shaped Reinke crystals are seen in the cytoplasm. (*D*) Severe nuclear atypia in this tumor is manifest as pleomorphism and hyperchromasia.

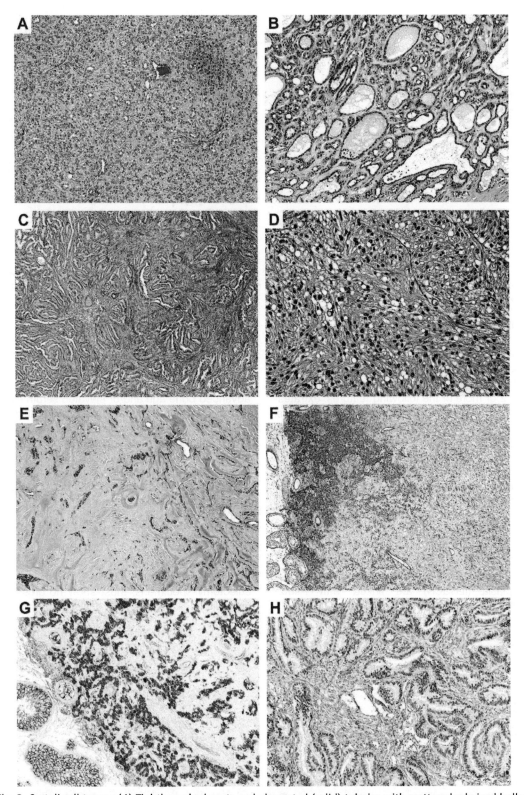

Fig. 2. Sertoli cell tumor. (*A*) Tightly packed nests and elongated (solid) tubules with scattered admixed hollow tubules. (*B*) A mixture of solid and hollow tubules in a fibromyxoid background. The hollow tubules contain luminal fluid and some with irregular shape (*bottom right*). (*C*) Retiform tubules. (*D*) Diffuse type with eosinophilic cytoplasm mimicking LCT with cytoplasmic vacuoles and intranuclear inclusions. (*E*) Sclerosing-type SCT with dense fibrotic background separating the tumor cells into thin cords, resembling the appearance of a carcinoid tumor. (*F*) Another sclerosing-type tumor with less conspicuous tubular differentiation. (*G*) Same case as (*F*) with immunostain demonstrating β-catenin nuclear accumulation. Normal Sertoli cells in the background seminiferous tubules show membranous β-catenin reactivity. (*H*) SOX9 positive (nuclear) reactivity.

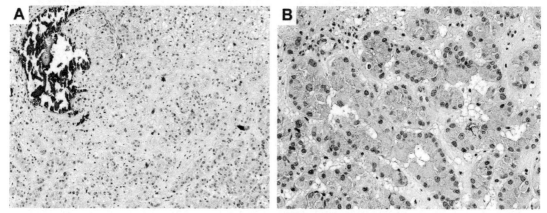

Fig. 3. Large cell calcifying Sertoli cell tumor. (*A*) Coarse calcifications associated with large Sertoli cells growing in cords and small clusters. (*B*) The tumor cells are large, round and cuboidal with eosinophilic cytoplasm and are associated with a neutrophilic infiltrate.

neutrophilic infiltrate (**Fig. 3**B); an intratubular component may be present.[34] In one study, malignant tumors were all unilateral and unifocal, ranged in size from 2 cm to 15 cm in dimension (mean 5.4 cm), and were strongly associated with 2 or more of the following features: extratesticular growth, size greater than 4 cm, necrosis, high-grade cytologic atypia, lymphovascular invasion, and increased mitoses (over 3 per 10 HPFs).[34] Variable S100 positivity is seen in LCCSCTs on immunohistochemistry, in addition to positive inhibin, vimentin, and CK (focal).[34]

INTRATUBULAR LARGE CELL HYALINIZING SERTOLI CELL NEOPLASIA

Clinical Features

Intratubular large cell hyalinizing Sertoli cell neoplasia (ILHSCN) are linked with Peutz-Jeghers syndrome, with a characteristic *STK11*

gene mutation.[6,39] These tumors are seen in boys of mean age 6.5 years (range 4–13 years) presenting with bilateral testicular enlargement usually in the absence of a discrete mass and often associated with gynecomastia. In some cases, advanced bone age and/or elevated serum estradiol may be seen.[39,40] This tumor is bilateral, multifocal, and benign. Conservative therapy with an aromatase inhibitor is the treatment of choice to reduce the estrogen effects and orchiectomy is reserved for cases when it is necessary to control hormonal manifestations refractory to estrogen-receptor modulating agents or aromatase inhibitors.[39–41]

Pathologic Features

Although small white foci have been described in biopsy specimens and ill-defined nodularity in orchiectomy specimens, most show no gross abnormality.[39,40] ILHSCN consists of patchy

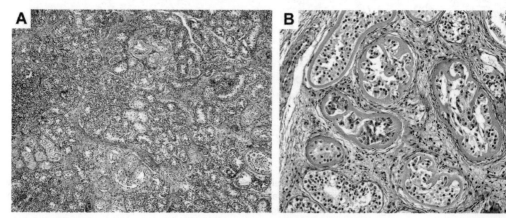

Fig. 4. Intratubular large cell hyalinizing Sertoli cell neoplasia. (*A*) Multifocal clusters of abnormal seminiferous tubules showing thickened peritubular basement membranes. (*B*) The abnormal seminiferous tubules are lined by large Sertoli cells with eosinophilic cytoplasm and prominent hyalinization of basement membranes that frequently extend into the tubular lumens. (*Courtesy of* Dr Thomas M. Ulbright, Indianapolis, IN with permission.)

clusters of expanded seminiferous tubules with petal-like arrays of large Sertoli cells with eosinophilic to vacuolated cytoplasm admixed with globoid basement membrane deposits extending from a thickened peritubular basement membrane (**Fig. 4**).[39–42] The lesion, to an extent, resembles LCCSCT, but the clinical presentation of gynecomastia, almost always present intratubular growth, and genetic alterations (*STK11* vs *PRKAR1A* gene mutation) are different.[40] A minority of cases show calcification within the basement membrane material, and stromal invasion is uncommon as well as atypia.[39,42]

> ### *Key Points*
> ### VARIOUS TESTICULAR SERTOLI CELL TUMORS
>
> - SCT NOS
>   - No syndromic associations
>   - Presence of tubular differentiation with various morphology, including sclerosing and lipid rich
>   - β-catenin mutation (nuclear accumulation of β-catenin on immunohistochemistry in approximately 60% of cases)
>   - SOX9 positive
>   - Features of malignancy: large size (≥5 cm), increased mitotic activity (>5 mitotic figures per 10 HPFs), tumor necrosis, moderate to severe nuclear atypia, lymphovascular invasion, and infiltrative growth pattern
> - Sclerosing SCT (now considered in the same category as SCT NOS; shares same *CTNNB1* gene mutation)
>   - Dense fibrotic stroma (at least 50% of tumor)
>   - Significantly reduced risk of malignancy compared with SCT NOS
> - LCCSCT
>   - Carney complex (*PRKAR1A* gene mutation)
>   - Large cells with abundant eosinophilic cytoplasm
>   - Prominent calcifications
>   - Substantial neutrophilic infiltrate
>   - More robust staining for S100 and inhibin compared with SCT NOS
>   - Higher risk of malignancy in nonsyndromic cases (older men)

- ILHSCN
  - Peutz-Jeghers syndrome (*STK11* gene mutation)
  - Expanded seminiferous tubules with petal-like arrays of large Sertoli cells with eosinophilic to vacuolated cytoplasm
  - Round basement membrane deposits extending from a thickened peritubular basement membrane
  - Benign

ADULT GRANULOSA CELL TUMOR

Clinical Features

Adult granulosa cell tumors (AGCTs) of the testis are rare and are seen in men of a broad age range (16–83 years, average 42 years), usually as an isolated unilateral testicular mass and occasionally (approximately 20%) with gynecomastia.[43,44] Juvenile granulosa cell tumors are more common than the adult form and occur almost exclusively in infants under 6 months of age. AGCTs of the testis are generally cured by surgical resection with an overall indolent clinical course; however, metastases have been reported to retroperitoneal lymph nodes (retroperitoneal lymph node dissection is indicated in this situation), with rare case reports of metastases to the liver, lungs, and bone.[43,45] Consequently, long-term follow-up is recommended for all patients, with special attention to cases with pathologic features worrisome for aggressive behavior.

Pathologic Features

The histologic findings match those of the ovarian counterpart, including diffuse, or less commonly, trabecular, insular, microfollicular or macrofollicular, or cystic growth patterns of round to ovoid (carrot-shaped) cells with elongated grooved nuclei, 1 to 2 eccentrically placed nucleoli, and scant pale cytoplasm (**Fig. 5**A). Granulosa cells may be seen palisading around Call-Exner bodies (**Fig. 5**B), and focal smooth muscle or osteoid differentiation may be identified.[2,6,43,46] Although nuclear grooves are characteristic of AGCT, they are not exclusive to this entity and can be seen in other sex cord–stromal tumors as well; therefore, if architectural patterns are typical, the lack of apparent nuclear grooves is not a contradicting feature for the diagnosis of AGCT. Malignant tumors are usually larger (over 4 cm), with mitoses, necrosis, and lymphovascular invasion.[43,47]

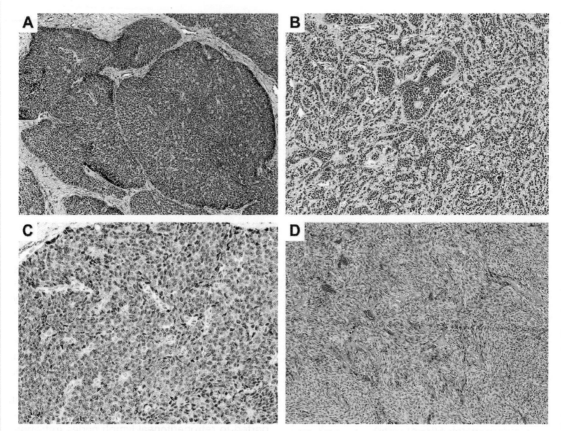

Fig. 5. Adult granulosa cell tumor (*A–C*) and fibrothecoma (*D*). (*A*) Insular pattern. (*B*) Tumor cells arranged predominantly in cords with Call-Exner bodies. (*C*) FOXL2 positive (nuclear) reactivity. (*D*) Storiform arrangement of thin spindled tumor cells in a collagenous background.

Recently, a somatic mutation in the *FOXL2* gene was reported in adult granulosa tumors in men, and this is reflected in the immunoreactivity with FOXL2 (**Fig. 5**C).[11,48]

Key Features
ADULT GRANULOSA CELL TUMOR

- Composed of round to ovoid cells with elongated grooved nuclei (which may or may not be conspicuous) and scant cytoplasm

- May see Call-Exner bodies

- Less common than juvenile granulosa cell tumor (in men)

- Somatic *FOXL2* gene mutation seen in testicular AGCTs; positive for FOXL2 immunostain

- Features of malignancy: large size (over 4 cm in span), lymphovascular invasion, necrosis, infiltrative growth pattern, and moderate to severe cytologic atypia

---

FIBROTHECOMA

Clinical Features

Reported in patients in their second to eighth decades presenting with a testicular mass, fibrothecomas are also exceedingly rare. The tumor has also been called "fibroma of gonadal stromal origin," "sex cord stromal tumor of the testis with a predominance of spindle cells," "fibroma," "thecoma," and "thecal cell tumor."[49,50] Historically, efforts were made to differentiate fibroma from thecoma using inhibin and oil red O fat staining, which are more likely positive in thecomas; however, the 2 processes are closely related and often merge, so the term *fibrothecoma* is preferred.[49] Fibrothecomas, even those with increased mitoses and cellularity, appear uniformly benign and are cured by excision with no evidence of disease on follow-up.[49,50]

Pathologic Features

On histology, tumor cells are spindle-shaped and arranged in short fascicles or a storiform pattern (**Fig. 5**D). Increased mitoses (up to 10 per 10

HPFs), minimal invasion into the surrounding testis, and hypercellularity may be seen but are not features of malignancy. The background may contain collagen deposition in bands or investing single cells, and seminiferous tubule entrapment.[49] Diagnosis is predominantly based on morphology, with a varying immunoprofile, including possible positivity for inhibin, calretinin, melan-A, pancytokeratin, BCL2, CD34, S100, smooth muscle actin, and desmin.[49] Fibrothecomas exhibit a pericellular reticulin staining pattern.

MYOID GONADAL STROMAL TUMOR

Clinical Features

Myoid gonadal stromal tumor (MGST) is currently categorized as an "emerging entity" with rare reports in the literature describing such tumors mostly in adult men (median age 41, range 4–49).[51,52] Although a deeper clinical understanding of this rare emerging entity relies on additional experience, MGSTs demonstrate favorable outcomes after orchiectomy.[6,51,52]

Pathologic Features

MGSTs are small (under 4 cm in span) and often located adjacent to the rete testis.[51] Microscopy reveals tumor cells arranged in tightly packed short fascicles. The cells are fusiform and cytologically bland with tapered nuclei, inconspicuous to small nucleoli, and scant to moderate eosinophilic cytoplasm. Mitoses may be present (up to 5 per 10 HPFs). The background is heterogeneously collagenous with scattered small thin-walled vessels and peripherally entrapped normal tubules. No sex cord component is present.[51] Tumor cells show features of both smooth muscle and gonadal stroma differentiation and their nature is reflected in the strong and diffuse coexpression of smooth muscle actin and S100 protein. Additional immunohistochemical features include positivity for FOXL2 and SF1 and negative staining for caldesmon, calretinin, and SOX9; inhibin and calponin may be focally positive.[51,52]

MIXED AND UNCLASSIFIED SEX CORD–STROMAL TUMORS

Clinical Features

Mixed sex cord–stromal tumors may behave in a malignant fashion and the morphologic criteria used to assess malignancy in SCTs and LCTs may be used.[6] Currently, extended follow-up with serial abdominal/pelvic imaging is recommended given the possibility of late progression and malignancy of gonadal sex cord–stromal tumors.[53]

Pathologic Features

Mixed sex cord–stromal tumors demonstrate morphologic and immunophenotypic findings consistent with 2 or more distinct sex cord–stromal tumor elements. Unclassified sex cord–stromal tumors, on the other hand, are mostly composed of nests and/or sheets of indeterminate or poorly differentiated cells that do not fit into any of the established entities.

NON–GERM CELL, NON–SEX CORD–STROMAL TUMORS

HEMANGIOMA

Clinical Features

Intratesticular vascular neoplasms are extremely rare and can be seen in a wide age range, from infants to adults.[54,55] They may present as a painless or rapidly enlarging mass, mimicking a malignant neoplasm of the testis clinically and on imaging, with ultrasound hypervascularity but with negative preoperative tumor markers.[55] Due to the benign nature of hemangiomas (no recurrences after excision), tumor enucleation is the recommended therapy.[54,56] To avoid unnecessary orchiectomy, intraoperative frozen section may be performed in the setting of clinical concern for hemangioma or a small testicular mass without serum tumor marker elevation and vascularity on Doppler sonography.[57,58]

Pathologic Features

Hemangiomas of the testis are generally small in size (under 1 cm) and circumscribed, with red nodular cut surfaces.[59] On histology, cavernous, epithelioid, capillary, and anastomosing types of morphology have been described.[59–61] The vascular lesion may exhibit an infiltrative pattern, entrapping benign seminiferous tubules and invading the tunica albuginea (Fig. 6A).[54] Immunohistochemical staining shows typical positive reactivity with endothelial markers of CD31, CD34, Expanded Factor VIII-related protein, FLI-1, and ERG.[54,58]

HEMATOLOGIC NEOPLASMS

Malignant lymphomas of the testis account for 2% to 5% of all primary testicular tumors, and approximately half of those are seen in men over age 60.[62] Testicular lymphoma may be primary and confined to the testis (rare) but is more often a manifestation of widespread disease.[40,63,64] The most common testicular hematologic neoplasm is diffuse large B-cell

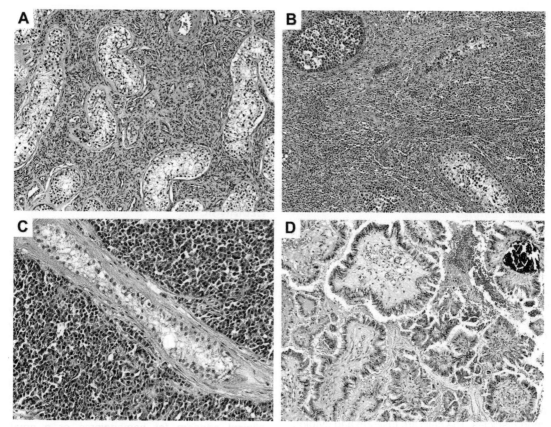

Fig. 6. (*A*) Hemangioma of testis infiltrating in between the seminiferous tubules. (*B*) Diffuse large B-cell lymphoma showing effacement of testicular parenchyma with focal intratubular growth (*top left*). (*C*) Plasmacytoma with prominent intertubular growth with entrapped seminiferous tubule. (*D*) Serous borderline tumor with tall ciliated columnar cells with nuclear stratification and epithelial budding lining fibrovascular cores and focal psammomatous calcification.

lymphoma (**Fig. 6**B), with other tumors including but not limited to mucosa-associated lymphoid tissue lymphomas, follicular lymphomas, extranodal natural killer/T-cell lymphomas, Burkitt lymphoma, and plasmacytoma (**Fig. 6**C).[65–67] On gross evaluation, testicular lymphomas usually consist of partial or complete organ effacement by a firm to fleshy homogenous mass with tan cut surfaces resembling a seminoma. Microscopic evaluation reveals conspicuous involvement of the testis interstitium with frequent invasion of the seminiferous tubules (see **Fig. 6**B). Intratubular growth is not specific and may be seen in other types of tumors that are important differential diagnostic considerations for elderly men, such as spermatocytic tumors and metastases. Adult testicular lymphoma treatment generally includes orchiectomy and chemotherapy, with or without iliac and/or para-aortic lymph node radiation therapy in addition to intrathecal chemotherapy to prevent central nervous system relapse, with molecular approaches in

exploration.[64] Discussion of each hematologic neoplasm is beyond the scope of this article, but it is important to be aware of its occurrence as a testicular tumor and consider it as a differential diagnosis, especially in older men.

METASTASES TO THE TESTIS (SECONDARY TUMORS)

Common sources of metastases to the testis include prostate, kidney, colon, bladder or renal pelvis, lung, stomach, pancreas, and cutaneous malignant melanoma.[40,68,69] Each of these entities can be correctly identified with appropriate clinical history (if available) and careful morphologic examination paying special attention to the nuclear features (shape and nucleolar appearance), cellular architecture (round, cuboidal, or columnar), and growth pattern (single cells, gland formation, and solid sheets) with the appropriate use of adjunct immunostains.

OVARIAN EPITHELIAL–TYPE TUMORS (MOSTLY PARATESTICULAR)

This group of tumors, mostly paratesticular with some intratesticular, is morphologically identical to ovarian surface epithelial tumors, including serous cystadenoma, serous tumor of borderline malignancy, serous cystadenocarcinoma, mucinous cystadenoma, mucinous borderline tumor, mucinous cystadenocarcinoma, endometrioid adenocarcinoma, clear cell adenocarcinoma, and Brenner tumor.[6] The histogenesis of Müllerian neoplasms in men is unclear, and possible etiologies include Müllerian duct remnants (ie, appendix testis), Müllerian neometaplasia of mesothelium, or from the mucinous epithelium of a teratoma.[70–72] This section focuses on the most frequent tumor seen in this category: serous borderline tumor (SBT).[73–77]

Clinical Features

Ovarian epithelial–type tumors of the testis have been reported in patients in their second to the eighth decades (mean age 50), presenting with a testicular or paratesticular mass.[71,75,78] The most common among all, SBTs, have been shown to be benign with no recurrence after excision on clinical follow-up.[71,75,78]

Pathologic Features

SBTs are also histologically identical to their female counterparts, composed of fibrovascular cores lined by stratified columnar epithelium that may have atypia or mitosis and psammoma bodies (Fig. 6D). In general, testicular Müllerian neoplasms stain with cytokeratin (CK) AE1/AE3 and BerEP4.[70,71,75,78] SBTs are also positive for estrogen receptor (ER), progesterone receptor (PR), WT1, PAX8, and MOC-31, while negative for CK20, carcinoembryonic antigen (CEA), calretinin, and HER2/neu stains.[78,79]

PARATESTICULAR TUMORS

ADENOMATOID TUMOR

Clinical Features

Adenomatoid tumors are the most common paratesticular tumor and present in infants and adults but predominantly in patients 30 years of age to 50 years of age, in the setting of asymptomatic, slow-growing masses.[80–85] These tumors are found in the epididymis most commonly but also in the tunica albuginea, spermatic cord, and, very rarely, isolated within the testis.[80,84] Negative tumor markers and sonographic findings (hypoechoic and homogenous) may prompt frozen

section evaluation to avoid unnecessary orchiectomy.[81,86] Excision is curative because it is benign.

Pathologic Features

At gross examination, these tumors usually consist of well-circumscribed 2 cm to 3 cm nodules with white to pink cut surfaces.[40,84] Histologic findings classically include a solid pattern with conspicuous lymphoid aggregates on low-power view (Fig. 7A) and acinar or tubular/gland-like structures composed of flattened to cuboidal cells with vacuolated cytoplasm on high-power examination (Fig. 7B).[40,81,84,85] Thin, bridging strands of cytoplasm across the lumen (so called thread-like bridging strands) are common (see Fig. 7B).[85] In the setting of infarct, recognition of ghost outlines of associated adenomatoid tumor is critical in the setting of surrounding reactive change that raises concern for a malignant infiltrating neoplasm.[87] Using immunohistochemistry, adenomatoid tumors express mesothelial markers including WT1, calretinin (Fig. 7C), and podoplanin as well as pancytokeratin (Fig. 7D) and CK7.[81,84,88]

MESOTHELIOMA

Clinical Features

Mesothelioma arises from the tunica vaginalis of the testis and is a rare entity that tends to occur at an older age.[89] Asbestos exposure is a known risk factor; however, many cases are sporadic.[90,91] The diagnosis should be considered in the setting of scrotal swelling with an atypical/recurrent hydrocele.[92–94] On clinical staging, lymphadenopathy may be identified and scrotal skin involvement is possible.[90,92] Mesothelioma of the paratestis carries a high recurrence risk and is usually fatal.[95] With no official treatment guidelines due to disease rarity, therapy usually involves radial inguinal orchiectomy with or without retroperitoneal or inguinal lymph node dissection, and chemoradiation therapy for advanced or recurrent disease, usually with poor response.[89,90,92,96]

Pathologic Features

Gross examination reveals thickening of the tunica vaginalis with multiple tan-white papillary excrescences (0.5–1 cm in diameter) on the parietal and visceral sides of the tunica vaginalis and/or tunica albuginea.[96] Microscopy shows tunica vaginalis involvement by solid, clefted, tubular, and/or micropapillary patterns of epithelioid cells with pleomorphic hyperchromatic nuclei, large nucleoli, eosinophilic cytoplasm, and multiple mitoses (Fig. 7E).[90,96] Although a well-differentiated papillary variant of mesothelioma exists and is

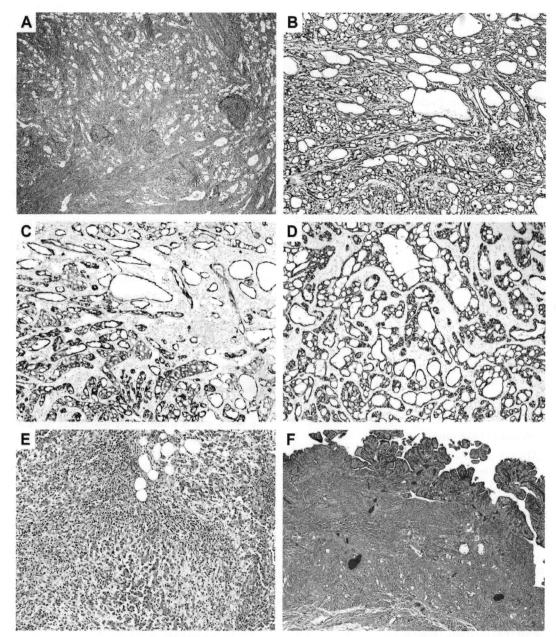

Fig. 7. Adenomatoid tumor (*A–D*) and mesothelioma (*E, F*). (*A*) Low-power view of adenomatoid tumor with prominent admixed lymphoid aggregates. (*B*) Gland-like tubules with vacuoles in a fibrotic background. Many of the tubules have thread-like bridging strands of cytoplasm across the lumens. (*C*) Calretinin and (*D*) cytokeratin AE1/AE3 positivity in adenomatoid tumor. (*E*) Mesothelioma with epithelioid morphology invading paratesticular soft tissue. (*F*) Mesothelioma with prominent papillary architecture at the surface with underlying deep stromal invasion.

similar to that seen in the abdominal cavity in women, any evidence of stromal invasion excludes this diagnosis and qualifies as malignant mesothelioma (**Fig.** 7F). Papillary architecture may be present in malignant mesothelioma and can be indistinguishable from well-differentiated papillary mesothelioma. Therefore, when considering a diagnosis of well-differentiated papillary mesothelioma, the entire specimen must be submitted for histologic evaluation to exclude an invasive component. On immunohistochemistry, the cells express typical mesothelial markers, including calretinin, EMA, CK7, WT1, and CK5/6.[90,96]

SOFT TISSUE TUMORS

Essentially any soft tissue tumor can be seen in the paratesticular soft tissue region, including the spermatic cord, but rarely in the testis itself, which is usually secondary involvement by direct extension. This section discusses the most common paratesticular soft tissue tumors in adult men.

Lipoma and Liposarcoma

Adipocytic tumors may involve the spermatic cord, testicular tunics, and epididymis of patients approximately 40 years old to 90 years old (mean age approximately 60 years old) and range in size from 3 cm to 30 cm (mean 12 cm).[97,98] A majority are well-differentiated liposarcomas, with a smaller proportion of dedifferentiated liposarcomas (both low-grade and high-grade dedifferentiation) and rare cases of lipomas. Cytogenetic alterations of ring chromosomes containing amplified sequences from 12q14-15 are present.[99] Well-differentiated liposarcomas can locally recur but have no metastatic potential in the absence of dedifferentiation. Dedifferentiated liposarcomas, on the other hand, have the potential to metastasize and carry mortality risk.[100,101]

Leiomyoma and Leiomyosarcoma

Leiomyomas are rare and usually present as slow-growing masses in patients 30 years old to 60 years old. The tumors are circumscribed and hypoechoic on sonography, with histology showing bland spindle cells in interlacing fascicles that stain with desmin, caldesmon, and smooth muscle actin.[102] In contrast, leiomyosarcomas exhibit atypia, mitoses, and necrosis and have been reported in the testis, spermatic cord, epididymis, and scrotal skin of adults.[103,104] Leiomyomas are benign and do not recur. Leiomyosarcomas may recur locally but have low metastatic potential if low grade (predominant); however, if high grade, metastasis is often and may lead to patient death.[105]

Fibroblastic and Myofibroblastic Tumors

Nodular periorchitis (fibrous pseudotumor)

A common non-neoplastic paratesticular entity is nodular periorchitis, a reactive fibrotic process that can produce a mass (or masses) growing between the testicular tunica layers, which can be associated with hydrocele, infection, or trauma.[106] Cases have been reported in the setting of IgG4-associated sclerosing disease.[107] On histology, the entity is characterized by dense fibrous tissue and inflammation (Fig. 8A) with inconspicuous atypia and mitoses.[106] Nodular periorchitis is negative for anaplastic lymphoma kinase-1 (ALK1) and

β-catenin, providing no support for inflammatory myofibroblastic tumor or fibromatosis. Although non-neoplastic, it deserves mention because it may be mass-producing and its awareness is required for recognition of this benign and reactive process.

Fibroma of tunica albuginea

Fibroma of the tunica albuginea is an exceedingly rare benign entity, with cases reported in patients in their second to eighth decades.[108] The lesions are well-circumscribed, white-tan whorled nodules on the tunica albuginea (Fig. 8B), which may be pedunculated. On histology, these fibromas are mildly to moderately cellular, composed of bland spindled/stellate cells organized in whorls, similar to fibromas elsewhere (Fig. 8C). Compared with nodular periorchitis, which may be morphologically similar, this entity lacks the association with hydrocele, trauma, or inflammation that is often present in non-neoplastic, reactive proliferations.

Cellular angiofibroma

Cellular angiofibromas are slow-growing and painless tumors that are seen in middle-aged or elderly men.[109] Most tumors are well-circumscribed, composed of hypercellular bland spindle cells with prominent thick-walled blood vessels with hyalinization or fibroid change, scattered mast cells, and collagenized stroma (Fig. 8D).[109,110] On immunohistochemistry, the tumor cells are positive for ER, PR, with variable smooth muscle actin and CD34 reactivity, and less commonly express desmin. Long-term follow-up is recommended for these lesions, which have a risk of local recurrence (albeit rare).[110]

Mammary-type myofibroblastoma

Mammary-type myofibroblastomas are rare indolent mesenchymal tumors that grow in the superficial soft tissues of the groin/perineal region, including cases that present as a paratesticular mass, even within the seminal vesicle.[111–114] Histologically, the tumors consist of a well-circumscribed proliferation of fascicles of myofibroblastic cells within coarse collagenous stroma, which express desmin, CD34, ER, and androgen receptor.[111–113] The differential diagnosis includes solitary fibrous tumor, cellular angiofibroma, and spindle cell lipoma, all of which are probably related entities due to shared 13q rearrangement with RB1 deletion/loss.[111,112] Surgical excision is curative and local recurrence is very rare.[113]

Deep (aggressive) angiomyxoma

In men, the deep (aggressive) angiomyxoma tumor is seen mostly in adults and occurs in the spermatic cord or scrotum.[115–118] Histologically, it is

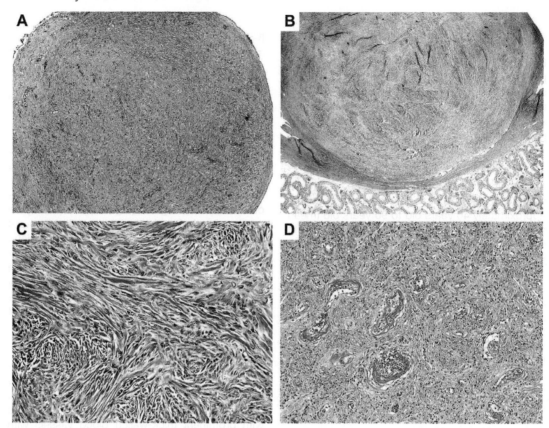

Fig. 8. (*A*) Nodular periorchitis. This tumor is mass-forming composed of fibroblasts with admixed chronic inflammation. (*B*) Fibroma of tunica albuginea. The tumor is seen originating from the tunica and the underlying testis is uninvolved. (*C*) Fibroma of tunica albuginea. High-power view shows similar morphology to that observed in the testicular fibrothecoma. (*D*) Cellular angiofibroma. Stellate fibroblastic cells are seen in the stroma with intervening thick-walled vessels demonstrating fibrinoid change.

characterized by an infiltrative lesion with monotonous bland small spindled and stellate fibroblasts set within myxoid hypocellular stroma with prominent dilated thick-walled vessels. On immunohistochemistry, the tumors are positive for androgen receptor with patchy ER positivity.[117] Most cases tested show involvement of *HMGA2* gene at 12q14.3, resulting in positive immunostaining for HMGA2,[119] which may be helping in differential diagnosis.[120] There is a potential for recurrence but metastasis is rare; wide local excision, when feasible, is the treatment of choice.

COMMON DIFFERENTIAL DIAGNOSES IN TESTICULAR NON–GERM CELL TUMORS AND PARATESTICULAR TUMORS

TESTICULAR TUMOR OF ADRENOGENITAL SYNDROME VERSUS LEYDIG CELL TUMOR

It is important to differentiate between a testicular tumor of the adrenogenital syndrome (TTAGS) and an LCT because the former regresses with corticosteroid therapy and does not typically require

surgery.[121] Key histologic and clinical features of TTAGS include bilaterality, prominent fibrous bands between tumor nests, abundant cytoplasmic lipofuscin pigment, spotty cytologic atypia, mitotic activity, and an abnormal hormone profile with elevated 17-hydroxyprogesterone and adrenal androgen levels.[122] In contrast to LCTs, TTAGS do not express androgen receptor, and more commonly express neuroendocrine markers.[123–125]

SERTOLI CELL NODULE VERSUS SERTOLI CELL TUMOR

Sertoli cell nodules (Pick adenomas or Sertoli cell adenomas) often occur in undescended testes and are non-neoplastic aggregates of seminiferous tubules containing immature Sertoli cells.[28] Sertoli cell nodules are usually microscopic but mass-producing (macroscopic) nodules have been reported.[126] Microscopic findings supportive of a Sertoli cell nodule include conspicuous basement membrane deposits, association with spermatogonia, and, perhaps the most important feature, lack of stromal invasion.

SERTOLI CELL TUMOR VERSUS LEYDIG CELL TUMOR

Some SCT NOS may resemble LCT if the growth pattern is predominantly diffuse with larger eosinophilic tumor cells. The most helpful histologic feature is the presence of tubular differentiation in most SCTs, although pseudotubular morphology may be seen in LCTs. Presence of Reinke crystals is pathognomonic for LCTs but it occurs only in approximately one-third of LCTs. Compared with LCTs, SCTs are less frequently reactive with inhibin, have stronger cytokeratin staining, and show characteristic nuclear accumulation of β-catenin (~60%)[31]; therefore, a negative inhibin stain is more consistent with SCT than LCT.

SERTOLI CELL TUMOR VERSUS SEMINOMA

Because clinical management for SCT versus seminoma differs drastically, distinguishing these two tumors from one another has been discussed extensively in other reviews.[5,40,127] Briefly, a diffuse pattern of SCT can mimic seminoma, and a tubular seminoma can resemble SCT. Seminomas in general have a consistent admixture of lymphocytes, frequent mitotic figures, and characteristic nuclear features (squared-off nuclear edges with conspicuous nucleoli). The presence of granulomatous inflammation and/or background germ cell neoplasia in situ are also supportive of seminoma. Immunostains for OCT3/4, SALL4, SF1, inhibin, and calretinin are helpful in making a correct diagnosis because seminoma is positive for the former two stains whereas SCT is positive for the latter three.[30,128,129] The use of SALL4 and 1 of the general sex cord–stromal tumor markers—SF1, calretinin, and inhibin—is the recommended immunostaining panel for differentiating a germ cell tumor from a sex cord–stromal tumor.[10]

> **Differential Diagnosis**
> SEX CORD–STROMAL TUMORS
> VERSUS GERM CELL TUMORS
>
> - Morphology on light microscopy is usually sufficient.
>
> - SCT may be confused with seminoma (particularly in the setting of a solid pattern of SCT or a tubular pattern of seminoma) or solid yolk sac tumor.
>
> - Perform appropriate germ cell markers (SALL4/OCT3/4/GPC3) and sex cord–stromal tumor markers (SF1/inhibin/calretinin).

SERTOLI CELL TUMOR VERSUS ADENOMATOID TUMOR

The tubular appearance of an SCT may be mistaken for an adenomatoid tumor. SCT is intratesticular whereas adenomatoid tumor is almost always paratesticular. Rare cases of intratesticular adenomatoid tumors, however, have been reported.[130] The tubules of adenomatoid tumor are usually lined by flattened cells that form thread-like bridging strands across lumens and stain with cytokeratins.[81,83] Both SCTs and adenomatoid tumors can stain with WT1 and calretinin as well as various keratins; however, negativity for these markers is supportive of SCT. Furthermore, inhibin may be positive in SCTs and is negative in adenomatoid tumors.

ADENOMATOID TUMOR VERSUS HEMANGIOMA VERSUS METASTATIC ADENOCARCINOMA

The small tubules of an adenomatoid tumor may resemble vascular spaces of a hemangioma or epithelial glands of a metastatic adenocarcinoma (in particular signet ring cell carcinoma). Immunohistochemistry is especially useful in this context. Adenomatoid tumors are positive for calretinin, podoplanin, and WT1. Hemangiomas are reactive for vascular markers, and although both adenomatoid tumors and metastatic signet ring cell carcinomas are positive for cytokeratins, the positive staining with mesothelial markers in the former resolves this differential diagnosis.

VARIOUS SPINDLED NON–GERM CELL TUMORS

The differential diagnosis for the category, various spindled non–germ cell tumors, includes sex cord–stromal tumors with spindled morphology and paratesticular soft tissue tumors. LCT with pure spindled morphology is extremely rare, and additional sampling almost always reveals associated more characteristic patterns of LCT. Myoid gonadal stromal tumor (MGST) shows its distinct dual expression of immunohistochemical profile smooth muscle actin and S100. Fibrothecoma and MGST both show individual pericellular staining with reticulin, whereas a mixed or undifferentiated sex cord–stromal tumor shows nests of sex–cord elements highlighted by the reticulin stain that were not otherwise obvious on routine hematoxylin-eosin stains.[127] It is important to distinguish fibrothecoma and MGST (benign entities) from unclassified sex cord–stromal tumor (malignant potential). Finally, considerations for paratesticular soft tissue tumors include liposarcoma (in particular dedifferentiated), leiomyosarcoma, fibromatosis, and others, which can be distinguished using appropriate immunohistochemical stains and/or molecular studies.

Differential Diagnosis
SPINDLED TESTICULAR (NON–GERM CELL) TUMORS

- Leydig cell tumor (spindled or sarcomatoid)
- Fibrothecoma
- Myoid gonadal stromal tumor
- Unclassified sex cord–stromal tumor
- Secondary involvement by paratesticular soft tissue tumors

SEROUS BORDERLINE TUMOR VERSUS MESOTHELIOMA

SBTs may be indistinguishable from mesotheliomas grossly, but on histology, SBT papillae have a more pronounced budding appearance, with cellular stratification and frequent psammoma bodies. SBTs are also positive for CD15 and CEA and negative for calretinin, whereas mesotheliomas demonstrate the opposite immunoprofile.

MESOTHELIAL HYPERPLASIA VERSUS MESOTHELIOMA

Mesothelioma is more commonly seen in the setting of a mass or visible nodularity in a hydrocele sac, whereas mesothelial hyperplasia is more commonly a microscopic finding in a hernia sac. Mesothelial hyperplasia is predominantly tubular with associated inflammation, with cell clusters confined above a well-delineated linear interface within the hydrocele sac and no invasion of the fibrous stroma. On the other hand, mesotheliomas often show irregular downward infiltration into the fibrous stroma.

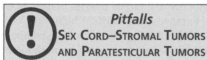

Pitfalls
SEX CORD–STROMAL TUMORS AND PARATESTICULAR TUMORS

! Benign ectopic Leydig cells are seen in the paratestis adjacent to small neurovascular bundles and can be mistaken for perineural or lymphovascular invasion.

! LCTs are positive for S100 and melan-A; these stains have limited value when the differential diagnosis is melanoma.

! LCTs and SCTs are positive for synaptophysin and chromogranin, so these stains are not useful when carcinoid tumor (well-differentiated neuroendocrine tumor) is in the differential

! Adenomatoid tumor and SCT are both positive for WT1 and calretinin.

! Smooth muscle actin is not reliable in distinguishing fibromatous tumors from myogenic ones because both can show positive staining- desmin is a better stain for this purpose

---

REFERENCES

1. Ulbright TM, Young RH. Testicular and paratesticular tumors and tumor-like lesions in the first 2 decades. Semin Diagn Pathol 2014;31(5):323–81.
2. Young RH. Sex cord-stromal tumors of the ovary and testis: their similarities and differences with consideration of selected problems. Mod Pathol 2005;18(Suppl 2):S81–98.
3. Moch H, Cubilla AL, Humphrey PA, et al. The 2016 WHO classification of tumours of the urinary system and male genital organs-part a: renal, penile, and testicular tumours. Eur Urol 2016;70(1):93–105.
4. Osbun N, Winters B, Holt SK, et al. Characteristics of patients with sertoli and leydig cell testis neoplasms from a national population-based registry. Clin Genitourin Cancer 2017;15(2):e263–6.
5. Howitt BE, Berney DM. Tumors of the testis: morphologic features and molecular alterations. Surg Pathol Clin 2015;8(4):687–716.
6. Idrees MT, Ulbright TM, Oliva E, et al. The World Health Organization 2016 classification of testicular non-germ cell tumours: a review and update from the International Society of Urological Pathology Testis Consultation Panel. Histopathology 2017; 70(4):513–21.
7. Verdorfer I, Horst D, Höllrigl A, et al. Leydig cell tumors of the testis: a molecular-cytogenetic study based on a large series of patients. Oncol Rep 2007;17(3):585–9.
8. Perrone F, Bertolotti A, Montemurro G, et al. Frequent mutation and nuclear localization of β-catenin in sertoli cell tumors of the testis. Am J Surg Pathol 2014;38(1):66–71.
9. Ulbright TM, Srigley JR, Reuter VE, et al. Sex cord-stromal tumors of the testis with entrapped germ cells: a lesion mimicking unclassified mixed germ cell sex cord-stromal tumors. Am J Surg Pathol 2000;24(4):535–42.
10. Ulbright TM, Tickoo SK, Berney DM, et al, Members of the ISUP Immunohistochemistry in Diagnostic Urologic Pathology Group. Best practices recommendations in the application of immunohistochemistry in

testicular tumors: report from the International Society of Urological Pathology consensus conference. Am J Surg Pathol 2014;38(8):e50–9.

11. Kao CS, Cheng L, Ulbright TM, et al. The utility of SOX9, FOXL2, and SF1 immunohistochemical (IHC) stains in the diagnosis of testicular sex cord-stromal tumors (SCST) compared to other commonly used markers (abstract). Mod Pathol 2015;28:233A.

12. Jou P, MacLennan GT. Leydig cell tumor of the testis. J Urol 2009;181(5):2299–300.

13. Al-Agha OM, Axiotis CA. An in-depth look at Leydig cell tumor of the testis. Arch Pathol Lab Med 2007; 131(2):311–7.

14. Kim I, Young RH, Scully RE. Leydig cell tumors of the testis. A clinicopathological analysis of 40 cases and review of the literature. Am J Surg Pathol 1985;9(3):177–92.

15. Suardi N, Strada E, Colombo R, et al. Leydig cell tumour of the testis: presentation, therapy, long-term follow-up and the role of organ-sparing surgery in a single-institution experience. BJU Int 2009;103(2):197–200.

16. Soria JC, Durdux C, Chrétien Y, et al. Malignant Leydig cell tumor of the testis associated with Klinefelter's syndrome. Anticancer Res 1999;19(5C):4491–4.

17. Carvajal-Carmona LG, Alam NA, Pollard PJ, et al. Adult leydig cell tumors of the testis caused by germline fumarate hydratase mutations. J Clin Endocrinol Metab 2006;91(8):3071–5.

18. Bokemeyer C, Harstrick A, Gonnermann O, et al. Metastatic leydig-cell tumors of the testis - report of 4 cases and review of the literature. Int J Oncol 1993;2(2):241–4.

19. Mati W, Lam G, Dahl C, et al. Leydig cell tumour–a rare testicular tumour. Int Urol Nephrol 2002;33(1): 103–5.

20. Heer R, Jackson MJ, El-Sherif A, et al. Twenty-nine Leydig cell tumors: histological features, outcomes and implications for management. Int J Urol 2010; 17(10):886–9.

21. Loeser A, Vergho DC, Katzenberger T, et al. Testis-sparing surgery versus radical orchiectomy in patients with Leydig cell tumors. Urology 2009;74(2): 370–2.

22. Giannarini G, Mogorovich A, Menchini Fabris F, et al. Long-term followup after elective testis sparing surgery for Leydig cell tumors: a single center experience. J Urol 2007;178(3 Pt 1):872–6, [quiz: 1129].

23. Cost NG, Maroni P, Flaig TW. Metastatic relapse after initial clinical stage I testicular Leydig cell tumor. Oncology (Williston Park) 2014;28(3):211–4.

24. Banerji JS, Odem-Davis K, Wolff EM, et al. Patterns of care and survival outcomes for malignant sex cord stromal testicular cancer: results from the national cancer data base. J Urol 2016;196(4): 1117–22.

25. Mineur P, De Cooman S, Hustin J, et al. Feminizing testicular Leydig cell tumor: hormonal profile before and after unilateral orchidectomy. J Clin Endocrinol Metab 1987;64(4):686–91.

26. Billings SD, Roth LM, Ulbright TM. Microcystic Leydig cell tumors mimicking yolk sac tumor: a report of four cases. Am J Surg Pathol 1999;23(5):546–51.

27. Ulbright TM, Srigley JR, Hatzianastassiou DK, et al. Leydig cell tumors of the testis with unusual features: adipose differentiation, calcification with ossification, and spindle-shaped tumor cells. Am J Surg Pathol 2002;26(11):1424–33.

28. Young RH, Koelliker DD, Scully RE. Sertoli cell tumors of the testis, not otherwise specified: a clinicopathologic analysis of 60 cases. Am J Surg Pathol 1998;22(6):709–21.

29. Talon I, Moog R, Kauffmann I, et al. Sertoli cell tumor of the testis in children: reevaluation of a rarely encountered tumor. J Pediatr Hematol Oncol 2005; 27(9):491–4.

30. Henley JD, Young RH, Ulbright TM. Malignant Sertoli cell tumors of the testis: a study of 13 examples of a neoplasm frequently misinterpreted as seminoma. Am J Surg Pathol 2002;26(5):541–50.

31. Zhang C, Ulbright TM. Nuclear localization of β-Catenin in sertoli cell tumors and other sex cord-stromal tumors of the testis: an immunohistochemical study of 87 cases. Am J Surg Pathol 2015;39(10):1390–4.

32. Mesa H, Gilles S, Datta MW, et al. Comparative immunomorphology of testicular Sertoli and sertoliform tumors. Hum Pathol 2017;61:181–9.

33. Proppe KH, Scully RE. Large-cell calcifying Sertoli cell tumor of the testis. Am J Clin Pathol 1980; 74(5):607–19.

34. Kratzer SS, Ulbright TM, Talerman A, et al. Large cell calcifying Sertoli cell tumor of the testis: contrasting features of six malignant and six benign tumors and a review of the literature. Am J Surg Pathol 1997;21(11):1271–80.

35. Forlino A, Vetro A, Garavelli L, et al. PRKACB and carney complex. N Engl J Med 2014;370(11): 1065–7.

36. Giglio M, Medica M, De Rose AF, et al. Testicular sertoli cell tumours and relative sub-types. Analysis of clinical and prognostic features. Urol Int 2003; 70(3):205–10.

37. Gourgari E, Saloustros E, Stratakis CA. Large-cell calcifying Sertoli cell tumors of the testes in pediatrics. Curr Opin Pediatr 2012;24(4):518–22.

38. Crocker MK, Gourgari E, Lodish M, et al. Use of aromatase inhibitors in large cell calcifying sertoli cell tumors: effects on gynecomastia, growth velocity, and bone age. J Clin Endocrinol Metab 2014; 99(12):E2673–80.

39. Ulbright TM, Amin MB, Young RH. Intratubular large cell hyalinizing sertoli cell neoplasia of the

testis: a report of 8 cases of a distinctive lesion of the Peutz-Jeghers syndrome. Am J Surg Pathol 2007;31(6):827–35.

40. Young RH. Testicular tumors—some new and a few perennial problems. Arch Pathol Lab Med 2008; 132(4):548–64.

41. Armijo B, Bocklage T, Heideman R. Intratubular large cell hyalinizing sertoli cell tumor of the testes in a 4-year-old male with peutz-jeghers syndrome. J Pediatr Hematol Oncol 2015;37(3):e184–7.

42. Venara M, Rey R, Bergadá I, et al. Sertoli cell proliferations of the infantile testis: an intratubular form of Sertoli cell tumor? Am J Surg Pathol 2001;25(10): 1237–44.

43. Cornejo KM, Young RH. Adult granulosa cell tumors of the testis: a report of 32 cases. Am J Surg Pathol 2014;38(9):1242–50.

44. Hammerich KH, Hille S, Ayala GE, et al. Malignant advanced granulosa cell tumor of the adult testis: case report and review of the literature. Hum Pathol 2008;39(5):701–9.

45. Jimenez-Quintero LP, Ro JY, Zavala-Pompa A, et al. Granulosa cell tumor of the adult testis: a clinicopathologic study of seven cases and a review of the literature. Hum Pathol 1993;24(10):1120–5.

46. Al-Bozom IA, El-Faqih SR, Hassan SH, et al. Granulosa cell tumor of the adult type: a case report and review of the literature of a very rare testicular tumor. Arch Pathol Lab Med 2000;124(10):1525–8.

47. Hanson JA, Ambaye AB. Adult testicular granulosa cell tumor. Arch Pathol Lab Med 2011;135:4.

48. Lima JF, Jin L, de Araujo ARC, et al. FOXL2 mutations in granulosa cell tumors occurring in males. Arch Pathol Lab Med 2012;136(7):825–8.

49. Zhang M, Kao C-S, Ulbright TM, et al. Testicular fibrothecoma: a morphologic and immunohistochemical study of 16 cases. Am J Surg Pathol 2013;37(8):1208–14.

50. Sourial M-W, Sabbagh R, Doueik A, et al. A 17 year old male with a testicular fibrothecoma: a case report. Diagn Pathol 2013;8:152.

51. Kao C-S, Ulbright TM. Myoid gonadal stromal tumor: a clinicopathologic study of three cases of a distinctive testicular tumor. Am J Clin Pathol 2014; 142(5):675–82.

52. Du S, Powell J, Hii A, et al. Myoid gonadal stromal tumor: a distinct testicular tumor with peritubular myoid cell differentiation. Hum Pathol 2012;43(1):144–9.

53. Brekelbaum CE, Abreo F, Fowler M, et al. Undifferentiated sex cord/stromal testis tumor. Urology 2000;55(3):436.

54. Kryvenko ON, Epstein JI. Testicular hemangioma: a series of 8 cases. Am J Surg Pathol 2013;37(6): 860–6.

55. Ben Abda R, Bess D, Nieves-Robbins N. Testicular hemangioma mimicking a malignant neoplasm. Radiol Case Rep 2016;11(2):121–3.

56. Gołąbek T, Chłosta PL. How to manage testicular capillary haemangioma. J Ultrason 2016;16(64): 97–8.

57. Mungan S, Turgutalp H, Ersöz S, et al. A rare neoplasm of the testis: capillary hemangioma. Turk Patoloji Derg 2011;27(1):80–3.

58. Zaidi SN, Fathaddin AA. Testicular capillary hemangioma–a case report of a rare tumor. Indian J Pathol Microbiol 2012;55(4):557–9.

59. Xu R, Shi T-M, Liu S-J, et al. Neonatal testicular hemangiolymphangioma: a case report. Arch Iran Med 2015;18(6):386–8.

60. Takaoka E-I, Yamaguchi K, Tominaga T. Cavernous hemangioma of the testis: a case report and review of the literature. Hinyokika Kiyo 2007;53(6):405–7.

61. Erdag G, Kwon EO, Lizza EF, et al. Cavernous hemangioma of tunica albuginea testis manifesting as testicular pain. Urology 2006;68(3):673.e13-15.

62. Al-Abbadi MA, Hattab EM, Tarawneh M, et al. Primary testicular and paratesticular lymphoma: a retrospective clinicopathologic study of 34 cases with emphasis on differential diagnosis. Arch Pathol Lab Med 2007;131(7):1040–6.

63. Schniederjan SD, Osunkoya AO. Lymphoid neoplasms of the urinary tract and male genital organs: a clinicopathological study of 40 cases. Mod Pathol 2009;22(8):1057–65.

64. Zouhair A, Herrmann E, Ugurluer G, et al. Primary testicular lymphoma. Swiss Med Wkly 2010;140: w13076.

65. Froberg MK, Hamati H, Kant JA, et al. Primary low-grade T-helper cell testicular lymphoma. Arch Pathol Lab Med 1997;121(10):1096–9.

66. Akhtar M, al-Dayel F, Siegrist K, et al. Neutrophil-rich Ki-1-positive anaplastic large cell lymphoma presenting as a testicular mass. Mod Pathol 1996; 9(8):812–5.

67. Seliem RM, Chikwava K, Swerdlow SH, et al. Classical Hodgkin's lymphoma presenting as a testicular mass: report of a case. Int J Surg Pathol 2007;15(2):207–12.

68. Datta MW, Young RH. Malignant melanoma metastatic to the testis: a report of three cases with clinically significant manifestations. Int J Surg Pathol 2000;8(1):49–57.

69. Ulbright TM, Young RH. Metastatic carcinoma to the testis: a clinicopathologic analysis of 26 nonincidental cases with emphasis on deceptive features. Am J Surg Pathol 2008;32(11): 1683–93.

70. Jones MA, Young RH, Srigley JR, et al. Paratesticular serous papillary carcinoma. A report of six cases. Am J Surg Pathol 1995;19(12):1359–65.

71. Ulbright TM, Young RH. Primary mucinous tumors of the testis and paratestis: a report of nine cases. Am J Surg Pathol 2003;27(9):1221–8.

72. Sundarasivarao D. The Müllerian vestiges and benign epithelial tumours of the epididymis. J Pathol Bacteriol 1953;66(2):417–32.

73. Kosmehl H, Langbein L, Kiss F. Papillary serous cystadenoma of the testis. Int Urol Nephrol 1989; 21(2):169–74.

74. Olla L, Di Naro N, Puliga G, et al. Intraparenchymal serous papillary cystadenoma of the testis: a case report. Pathologica 2013;105(1):15–7.

75. Young RH, Scully RE. Testicular and paratesticular tumors and tumor-like lesions of ovarian common epithelial and müllerian types. A report of four cases and review of the literature. Am J Clin Pathol 1986;86(2):146–52.

76. Guarch R, Rivas A, Puras A, et al. Papillary serous carcinoma of ovarian type of the testis with borderline differentiation. Histopathology 2005;46(5): 588–90.

77. Ibrahim AS, Li C, Al-Jafari MS. Borderline serous papillary tumour of the testis: a case report and review of the literature. Anticancer Res 2012;32(11): 5011–3.

78. McClure RF, Keeney GL, Sebo TJ, et al. Serous borderline tumor of the paratestis: a report of seven cases. Am J Surg Pathol 2001;25(3):373–8.

79. Bürger T, Schildhaus H-U, Inniger R, et al. Ovarian-type epithelial tumours of the testis: immunohistochemical and molecular analysis of two serous borderline tumours of the testis. Diagn Pathol 2015;10:118.

80. Sun AY, Polackwich AS, Sabanegh ES. Adenomatoid tumor of the testis arising from the tunica albuginea. Rev Urol 2016;18(1):51–3.

81. Amin W, Parwani AV. Adenomatoid tumor of testis. Clin Med Pathol 2009;2:17–22.

82. Liu W, Wu R, Yu Q. Adenomatoid tumor of the testis in a child. J Pediatr Surg 2011;46(10):E15–7.

83. Alam K, Maheshwari V, Varshney M, et al. Adenomatoid tumour of testis. BMJ Case Rep 2011;1–3.

84. Sheng B, Zhang Y-P, Wei H-H, et al. Primary adenomatoid tumor of the testis: report of a case and review of literature. Int J Clin Exp Pathol 2015;8(5): 5914–8.

85. Chen D, Yu Z, Ni L, et al. Adenomatoid tumors of the testis: a report of two cases and review of the literature. Oncol Lett 2014;7(5):1718–20.

86. Aganovic L, Cassidy F. Imaging of the scrotum. Radiol Clin North Am 2012;50(6):1145–65.

87. Skinnider BF, Young RH. Infarcted adenomatoid tumor: a report of five cases of a facet of a benign neoplasm that may cause diagnostic difficulty. Am J Surg Pathol 2004;28(1):77–83.

88. Sangoi AR, McKenney JK, Schwartz EJ, et al. Adenomatoid tumors of the female and male genital tracts: a clinicopathological and immunohistochemical study of 44 cases. Mod Pathol 2009; 22(9):1228–35.

89. Zhang N, Fu N, Peng S, et al. Malignant mesothelioma of the tunica vaginalis testis: a case report and literature review. Mol Clin Oncol 2017;7(6):1053–6.

90. Hispán P, Pascual JC, González I, et al. Cutaneous metastases from malignant mesothelioma of the tunica vaginalis testis. Am J Dermatopathol 2016; 38(3):222–5.

91. Attanoos RL, Gibbs AR. Primary malignant gonadal mesotheliomas and asbestos. Histopathology 2000;37(2):150–9.

92. Recabal P, Rosenzweig B, Bazzi WM, et al. Malignant mesothelioma of the tunica vaginalis testis: outcomes following surgical management beyond radical orchiectomy. Urology 2017;107:166–70.

93. Tan WK, Tan M-Y, Tan HM, et al. Well-differentiated papillary mesothelioma of the tunica vaginalis. Urology 2016;90:e7–8.

94. Bertolotto M, Boulay-Coletta I, Butini R, et al. Imaging of mesothelioma of tunica vaginalis testis. Eur Radiol 2016;26(3):631–8.

95. Hai B, Yang Y, Xiao Y, et al. Diagnosis and prognosis of malignant mesothelioma of the tunica vaginalis testis. Can Urol Assoc J 2012;6(6):E238–41.

96. Arda E, Arıkan MG, Cetin G, et al. Malignant mesothelioma of tunica vaginalis testis: macroscopic and microscopic features of a very rare malignancy. Cureus 2017;9(11):e1860.

97. Kodzo-Grey Venyo A, Deoleker M. Paratesticular liposarcoma of the spermatic cord: a case report and a review of the literature. West Afr J Med 2011;30(6):447–52.

98. Raza M, Vinay HG, Ali M, et al. Bilateral paratesticular liposarcoma - a rare case report. J Surg Tech Case Rep 2014;6(1):15–7.

99. Jour G, Gullet A, Liu M, et al. Prognostic relevance of Fédération Nationale des Centres de Lutte Contre le Cancer grade and MDM2 amplification levels in dedifferentiated liposarcoma: a study of 50 cases. Mod Pathol 2015;28(1):37–47.

100. Montgomery E, Fisher C. Paratesticular liposarcoma: a clinicopathologic study. Am J Surg Pathol 2003;27(1):40–7.

101. Fabre-Guillevin E, Coindre J-M, Somerhausen Nde SA, et al. Retroperitoneal liposarcomas: follow-up analysis of dedifferentiation after clinicopathologic reexamination of 86 liposarcomas and malignant fibrous histiocytomas. Cancer 2006; 106(12):2725–33.

102. Frias-Kletecka MC, MacLennan GT. Benign soft tissue tumors of the testis. J Urol 2009;182(1):312–3.

103. Agrawal R, Gupta M, Mohan N, et al. Recurrent leiomyosarcoma scrotum: an important differential in scrotal masses. Indian J Pathol Microbiol 2017; 60(4):581–3.

104. Ali Y, Kehinde EO, Makar R, et al. Leiomyosarcoma complicating chronic inflammation of the testis. Med Princ Pract 2002;11(3):157–60.

105. Fisher C, Goldblum JR, Epstein JI, et al. Leiomyosarcoma of the paratesticular region: a clinicopathologic study. Am J Surg Pathol 2001;25(9):1143–9.

106. Miyamoto H, Montgomery EA, Epstein JI. Paratesticular fibrous pseudotumor: a morphologic and immunohistochemical study of 13 cases. Am J Surg Pathol 2010;34(4):569–74.

107. Bösmüller H, von Weyhern CH, Adam P, et al. Paratesticular fibrous pseudotumor–an IgG4-related disorder? Virchows Arch 2011;458(1):109–13.

108. Jones MA, Young RH, Scully RE. Benign fibromatous tumors of the testis and paratesticular region: a report of 9 cases with a proposed classification of fibromatous tumors and tumor-like lesions. Am J Surg Pathol 1997;21(3):296–305.

109. Iwasa Y, Fletcher CDM. Cellular angiofibroma: clinicopathologic and immunohistochemical analysis of 51 cases. Am J Surg Pathol 2004;28(11):1426–35.

110. Aydin M, Uzuner H, Akgunes E, et al. Cellular angiofibroma of the spermatic cord. Aktuelle Urol 2017;48(2):159–60.

111. Mukonoweshuro P, McCormick F, Rachapalli V, et al. Paratesticular mammary-type myofibroblastoma. Histopathology 2007;50(3):396–7.

112. Kojima F, Ishida M, Takikita-Suzuki M, et al. Mammary-type myofibroblastoma of seminal vesicle. Histopathology 2012;60(3):524–7.

113. Flucke U, van Krieken JHJM, Mentzel T. Cellular angiofibroma: analysis of 25 cases emphasizing its relationship to spindle cell lipoma and mammary-type myofibroblastoma. Mod Pathol 2011;24(1):82–9.

114. McMenamin ME, Fletcher CD. Mammary-type myofibroblastoma of soft tissue: a tumor closely related to spindle cell lipoma. Am J Surg Pathol 2001;25(8):1022–9.

115. Ismail MI, Wong YP, Tan GH, et al. Paratesticular aggressive angiomyxoma: a rare case. Urol Ann 2017;9(2):197–9.

116. Morag R, Fridman E, Mor Y. Aggressive angiomyxoma of the scrotum mimicking huge hydrocele: case report and literature review. Case Rep Med 2009;2009:157624.

117. Chihara Y, Fujimoto K, Takada S, et al. Aggressive angiomyxoma in the scrotum expressing androgen and progesterone receptors. Int J Urol 2003;10(12):672–5.

118. Kim H-S, Park S-H, Chi JG. Aggressive angiomyxoma of childhood: two unusual cases developed in the scrotum. Pediatr Dev Pathol 2003;6(2):187–91.

119. Dreux N, Marty M, Chibon F, et al. Value and limitation of immunohistochemical expression of HMGA2 in mesenchymal tumors: about a series of 1052 cases. Mod Pathol 2010;23(12):1657–66.

120. Micci F, Panagopoulos I, Bjerkehagen B, et al. Deregulation of HMGA2 in an aggressive angiomyxoma with t(11;12)(q23;q15). Virchows Arch Int J Pathol 2006;448(6):838–42.

121. Naouar S, Braiek S, El Kamel R. Testicular tumors of adrenogenital syndrome: From physiopathology to therapy. Presse Med 2017;46(6 Pt 1):572–8.

122. Vukina J, Chism DD, Sharpless JL, et al. Metachronous bilateral testicular leydig-like tumors leading to the diagnosis of congenital adrenal hyperplasia (Adrenogenital Syndrome). Case Rep Pathol 2015;2015:459318.

123. Ashley RA, McGee SM, Isotaolo PA, et al. Clinical and pathological features associated with the testicular tumor of the adrenogenital syndrome. J Urol 2007;177(2):546–9, [discussion: 549].

124. Wang Z, Yang S, Shi H, et al. Histopathological and immunophenotypic features of testicular tumour of the adrenogenital syndrome. Histopathology 2011;58(7):1013–8.

125. Rutgers JL, Young RH, Scully RE. The testicular "tumor" of the adrenogenital syndrome. A report of six cases and review of the literature on testicular masses in patients with adrenocortical disorders. Am J Surg Pathol 1988;12(7):503–13.

126. Vallangeon BD, Eble JN, Ulbright TM. Macroscopic sertoli cell nodule: a study of 6 cases that presented as testicular masses. Am J Surg Pathol 2010;34(12):1874–80.

127. Renshaw AA, Gordon M, Corless CL. Immunohistochemistry of unclassified sex cord-stromal tumors of the testis with a predominance of spindle cells. Mod Pathol 1997;10(7):693–700.

128. Ye H, Ulbright TM. Difficult differential diagnoses in testicular pathology. Arch Pathol Lab Med 2012;136(4):435–46.

129. Ulbright TM. The most common, clinically significant misdiagnoses in testicular tumor pathology, and how to avoid them. Adv Anat Pathol 2008;15(1):18–27.

130. Delahunt B, Kenwright DN. Benign solid and acinar mesothelioma (Adenomatoid Tumor). AJSP Rev Rep 2005;10(4):206.

Updates on Grading and Staging of Prostate Cancer

Beth L. Braunhut, MD[a], Sanoj Punnen, MD[b,c], Oleksandr N. Kryvenko, MD[a,b,c],*

KEYWORDS

- Prostate cancer • Gleason grading system • Grade Groups • Staging

---

Key points

- The Gleason grading system has evolved since its introduction more than 50 years ago but it remains critically important for clinical management and determining the prognosis of men with prostate cancer.

- With the 2005 and 2014 revisions, grading of Gleason patterns 3 and 4 has been revised substantially and reporting has become more standardized. The transition to the Grade Group system provides a more simplified and intuitive grading system for counseling patients, in particular those with low-risk, indolent cancers that may be well-managed with active surveillance.

- The new grading system has been validated to predict risk of recurrence and death from prostate cancer.

- Genomic tests predicting the behavior of prostate cancer are now commercially available and gaining in their role as an ancillary test in prostate cancer management.

ABSTRACT

Since its development between 1966 and 1977, the Gleason grading system has remained one of the most important prognostic indicators in prostatic acinar adenocarcinoma. The grading system was first majorly revised in 2005 and again in 2014. With the publication of the 8th edition of the American Joint Committee on Cancer TNM staging manual in 2018, the classification of prostate cancer and its reporting have further evolved and are now included as part of staging criteria. This article reflects the aspects that are most influential on daily practice. A brief summary of 3 ancillary commercially available genomic tests is also provided.

GLEASON GRADING: OVERVIEW

The Gleason grading system is a 5-tier system that was developed and validated by Dr Donald Gleason from 1960 to 1975 as part of the Veterans Administration Cooperative Urological Research Group.[1–4] Unlike grading systems in many other organs, the Gleason grading system for prostatic adenocarcinoma is based solely on the architectural features of the neoplastic glands. Individual histologic patterns are assigned scores ranging from 1 to 5, reflecting the degree of differentiation of the cancerous glands and their associated prognosis. Other characteristics, such as the degree of nuclear pleomorphism and mitotic frequency, are not included in consideration when assigning a Gleason grade. Also, unique among

---

[a] Department of Pathology and Laboratory Medicine, University of Miami Miller School of Medicine, 1400 North West 12th Avenue, Miami, FL, 33136 USA; [b] Department of Urology, University of Miami Miller School of Medicine, 1150 North West 14th Street, Miami, FL 33136, USA; [c] Sylvester Comprehensive Cancer Center, University of Miami Miller School of Medicine, 1475 North West 12th Ave, Miami, FL 33136, USA
* Corresponding author. Department of Pathology and Laboratory Medicine, University of Miami Miller School of Medicine, 1400 Northwest 12th Avenue, Room 4076, Miami, FL 33136.
E-mail address: o.kryvenko@med.miami.edu

Surgical Pathology 11 (2018) 759–774
https://doi.org/10.1016/j.path.2018.07.003
1875-9181/18/© 2018 Elsevier Inc. All rights reserved.

cancer grading systems, the Gleason grade represents a summed score based on the 2 most prevalent patterns of carcinoma (prostatectomy) or a sum of the most prevalent pattern and the highest-grade pattern (prostate biopsy). This helps address the issue of tumor heterogeneity that is characteristic of prostate cancer.

The Gleason grading system represents a continuum with low-grade tumors assigned the lowest score and high-grade tumors assigned the highest score. In general, low-grade tumors demonstrate well-formed individual glands to high-grade tumors demonstrating no gland formation whatsoever. Historically, Gleason scores ranged from 2 (1 + 1) with the best prognosis to 10 (5 + 5) with the worst prognosis. Increasing Gleason grade is strongly correlated with tumor size, more advanced clinical stage, metastatic disease, and decreased survival.[3,5] Therefore, Gleason grade is a critical piece of information that is incorporated into National Comprehensive Cancer Network guidelines for risk stratification and the treatment guidelines in prostate cancer patients.[6]

The Gleason grading system has evolved from its original form over the years after the 2005 and 2014 consensus conferences of the International Society of Urological Pathology (ISUP).[7,8] These consensus conferences addressed the classification of architectural patterns in Gleason 3 and Gleason 4 cancer, grading of variants of prostatic acinar carcinoma, and reporting issues. With the most recent consensus conference in 2014, a new classification system was reviewed and endorsed, known as Grade Goups.[9] This new 5-tiered grading system is a simplified and intuitive system for the counseling of patients and it has been validated in multiple studies and shown to have improved prognostic significance compared with conventional Gleason grading.[10–16] The Grade Groups were then adopted for use by the 8th edition of the World Health Organization Classification of Tumours of the Urinary System and Male Genital Organs, College of American Pathologists (CAP), and American Joint Committee on Cancer (AJCC) TNM staging manual.[17]

OVERVIEW OF GLEASON PATTERNS

GLEASON PATTERN 1 AND PATTERN 2

In the original Gleason grading system, grade 1 and grade 2 prostate cancers both represented well-circumscribed nodules with small, uniform, well-formed, back-to-back round glands separated by delicate stroma without an infiltrative

pattern (grade 1) or only focal peripheral infiltration between or around benign glands (grade 2). Since the advent of immunohistochemistry; however, it is now recognized that many of lesions that would previously have been classified as Gleason pattern 1 or pattern 2 prostate cancer actually represent benign mimickers of prostate cancer, such as adenosis. In an editorial from 2000, Epstein[18] argued that a Gleason score of 2 to 4 prostatic adenocarcinoma is "a diagnosis that should not be made" on needle biopsy because there is poor reproducibility in diagnosing these patterns even among expert genitourinary pathologists, and often patients are upgraded in subsequent radical prostatectomy specimens. Also, assigning a Gleason score of less than 6 on biopsy can give a false sense of reassurance to clinicians and patients and result in under-treatment.[18] The 2005 ISUP consensus conference recommended that a diagnosis of Gleason score cancer less than 6 should never be made on core biopsy and the 2014 consensus maintained this position.[19] Although a modified Gleason grading diagram after the 2014 ISUP consensus conference retained these patterns, for practical purposes they need to be considered vanished and not used even in radical prostatectomy specimens.[9,17,19,20] The incidence of diagnosis of Gleason scores 2 to 4 prostatic adenocarcinoma has decreased precipitously after the 2005 ISUP consensus meeting.[21–23] With the implementation of Grade Groups, all cancers with a summed Gleason scores of less than or equal to 6 have been consolidated into Grade Group 1. Thus, with the transition to using Grade Groups as a stand-alone grade without an accompanying Gleason score, it is no longer necessary to discriminate between patterns 1 to 3.

GLEASON PATTERN 3

Gleason grade 3 carcinoma is the most commonly encountered pattern in most settings. It is assigned to cancers composed only of well-formed individual glands that demonstrate an infiltrative growth pattern between benign glands. The glands are often small but larger glands are also allowable. According to the 2014 ISUP consensus, well-formed glands that demonstrate branching without cribriform gland formation are still considered to represent pattern 3 (Fig. 1A).[9] A few poorly formed glands or seemingly fused glands among other well-formed glands are allowable, because these may represent tangential sectioning of Gleason 3 glands. In cases of morphology that is borderline between Gleason pattern 3 and pattern 4, it is advised to err on the side of the

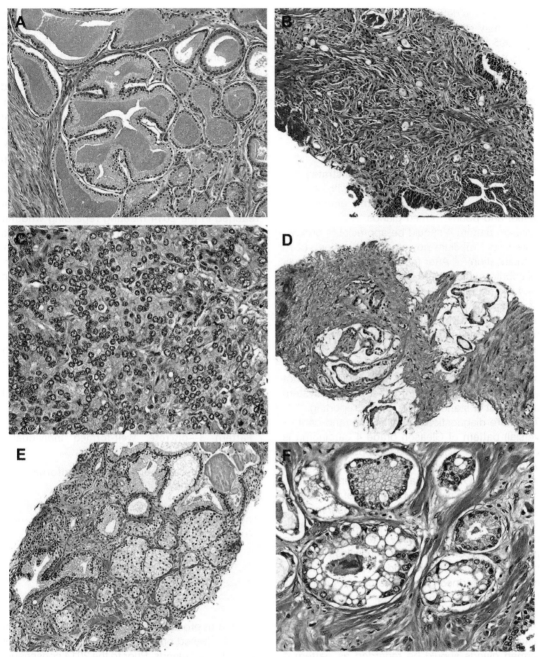

Fig. 1. (*A*) Well-formed branching gland representing a variant of Gleason pattern 3. (*B*) A cluster of poorly formed glands where this finding may not be explained by a tangential cutting and enough to diagnose as Gleason pattern 4 in limited prostatic adenocarcinoma. (*C*) Solid sheet of tumor cells with rosette-like structures without lumina formation representing Gleason pattern 5 prostate cancer. (*D*) Mucinous prostatic adenocarcinoma in a limited biopsy composed of individual well-formed glands representing Gleason pattern 3. (*E*) Foamy gland prostatic adenocarcinoma in a biopsy specimen forming nests of solid sheets of cells sufficient to grade it as Gleason pattern 5. (*F*) Individual well-formed glands of Gleason pattern 3 prostate cancer with signet ring cell–like features.

lower-grade/better prognosis for the patient.[24] A diagnosis of even a minor component of Gleason pattern 4 could potentially change patient management but under-calling a minor percentage of pattern 4 would most likely not harm a patient if put on active surveillance.

The original Gleason grading system included large and small cribriform glands as pattern 3.

Although some debate remained if small cribriform glands may still be considered as pattern 3 after the 2005 ISUP consensus conference, since the ISUP consensus conference in 2014, this is no longer acceptable in modern practice; 100% of participants at the 2014 consensus conference agreed that all cribriform glands should be considered Gleason pattern 4.[9]

GLEASON PATTERN 4

Gleason grade 4 carcinoma demonstrates the greatest variability in morphology, with 4 main architectural patterns: cribriform, glomeruloid, fused, and poorly formed glands. A diagnosis of Gleason pattern 4 should be appreciable on low-power or medium-power magnification ($\times$10 magnification).[8,9] After the 2014 ISUP consensus, all cribriform glands are now considered to represent Gleason grade 4. Glomeruloid glands consist of malignant glands within a dilated gland only focally attached to it, thus resembling a glomerulus. The presence of cribriform pattern 4 carcinoma has been associated with an adverse prognosis compared with other patterns of Gleason 4 prostate cancer, but this finding has not yet been incorporated into the grading system and is not a standard part of the reporting.[25–29] The more diagnostically challenging (and controversial) pattern of Gleason grade 4 carcinoma is poorly formed glands. These appear ill defined with poorly visualized lumina and they were included in Gleason pattern 4 after the 2005 ISUP consensus meeting. Diagnosis of this pattern of Gleason 4 has the highest interobserver variability, particularly in limited prostatic adenocarcinoma. A recent survey among urologic pathologists concluded that regardless of their number, poorly formed glands immediately adjacent to well-formed glands and clusters of poorly formed glands of 5 or fewer should not be regarded as pattern 4. The consensus was reached that clusters of 10 or more poorly formed glands that are not immediately adjacent to well-formed glands should be regarded as pattern 4 (**Fig. 1**B).[30] The presence of discrete foci of pattern 4 as opposed to scattered glands among pattern 3 glands is associated with higher interobserver reproducibility in Gleason scoring.[31]

GLEASON PATTERN 5

Gleason grade 5 prostate adenocarcinoma is the most aggressive pattern and demonstrates no glandular formation. This pattern has undergone the least revisions compared with the original description by Gleason and may take the form of solid sheets of tumor cells, single infiltrative tumor cells, or cords of infiltrating tumor cells. Gleason pattern 5 with signet ring cell–like change forming solid sheets can be a mimicker of Gleason pattern 4 (cribriform) carcinoma. Comedonecrosis is always considered Gleason pattern 5, even if the necrosis involves cribriform glands or glomeruloid structures that otherwise would be considered to represent Gleason pattern 4. According to the 2014 ISUP consensus conference, nests of cells with rosette-like structures but no definitive lumina also should be considered to represent Gleason pattern 5 (**Fig. 1**C).[9,17] A consensus was not reached in the 2014 meeting regarding whether to assign Gleason pattern 5 to discrete glands containing necrotic debris that architecturally otherwise are considered pattern 3 (49% of participants voted yes). The authors do not assign pattern 5 to this finding.

> ### Key Features
> OF GLEASON PATTERNS
>
> Patterns 1 and 2—vanished; consider pattern 3 as the lowest possible grade.
>
> Pattern 3—discrete, well-formed individual glands
>
> Pattern 4—fused/poorly formed/cribriform/glomeruloid glands
>
> Pattern 5—comedonecrosis or no gland formation (solid sheets, single infiltrative cells, or cords of cells)

GRADING OF VARIANTS OF PROSTATIC ADENOCARCINOMA

Grading of prostatic cancer with variant histology is largely based on the underlying architecture of the malignant glands. Prior to the 2014 consensus, mucinous carcinoma of the prostate was regarded as Gleason 4. After the 2014 ISUP consensus, prostatic mucinous adenocarcinoma is graded by assessing the underlying architecture of the glands and the presence of necrosis as if the extracellular mucin were not present. Thus, there are occasional cases graded as Gleason score 3 + 3 = 6 (Grade Group 1) mucinous prostatic adenocarcinoma (**Fig. 1**D). Mucinous carcinomas have a behavior comparable to grade-matched conventional acinar prostatic adenocarcinoma.[29,32] It is rarely seen in its pure form and most of the time represents a component admixed with acinar prostatic adenocarcinoma. Such cases can be reported as prostatic adenocarcinoma with mucinous features. Similarly, when grading foamy gland carcinoma, the foamy cytoplasm should be ignored and the grade should be assigned based on the underlying architecture of the glands (Fig. 1E). Not infrequently prostate cancer has large clear intracytoplasmic vacuoles that do not contain mucin and thus are referred to as signet ring cell–like features. Similar to other variants, prostatic cancer with signet ring cell–like morphology is graded based on the underlying architecture (Fig. 1F; Fig. 2A). Conversely, basal cell carcinoma of the prostate should not be assigned a Gleason grade because these may display a variety of morphologic patterns that do not necessarily correlate with the behavior and, therefore, the prognosis of typical prostatic acinar carcinoma.[33]

Prostatic ductal carcinoma is, by convention, graded as Grade 4. This consists of papillary or cribriform glands with pseudostratified high-grade epithelium (Fig. 2B). Prostatic duct adenocarcinomas with necrosis are assigned Gleason pattern 5. Occasional basal cells may be present in prostatic duct carcinomas. High-grade prostatic intraepithelial neoplasia–like ductal adenocarcinoma has a favorable prognosis and is graded as Gleason pattern 3.[34,35]

Key Features
GRADING OF PROSTATIC ADENOCARCINOMA VARIANTS

No Gleason grade is assigned

   Intraductal prostatic adenocarcinoma

   Prostatic basal cell carcinoma

   Small cell carcinoma

   Large cell carcinoma

Gleason grade based on underlying architecture

   Mucinous adenocarcinoma

   Foamy gland carcinoma

   Carcinomas with signet ring cell–like features

Gleason grade 3

   High-grade prostatic intraepithelial neoplasia–like ductal carcinoma

Gleason grade 4

   Conventional prostatic ductal carcinoma

PROSTATIC CARCINOMAS WITH NEUROENDOCRINE DIFFERENTIATION

A recent review suggested classifying prostate cancers with neuroendocrine differentiation into (1) usual prostatic adenocarcinoma with neuroendocrine differentiation, (2) adenocarcinoma with Paneth cell–like neuroendocrine differentiation, (3) low-grade neuroendocrine carcinoma/carcinoid tumor, (4) small cell carcinoma, and (5) large cell carcinoma.[36] Usual prostatic acinar adenocarcinoma with neuroendocrine differentiation represents the most frequent scenario, and the frequency of neuroendocrine differentiation increases with higher grades. The expression of neuroendocrine markers by conventional carcinoma has not shown an effect on survival, and routine staining of usual-appearing prostatic adenocarcinoma for neuroendocrine markers is not recommended.[37] Reporting stains on cancers in the absence of architectural and cytologic evidence of neuroendocrine differentiation (ie, small cells cell or Paneth cell–like carcinoma) may be misleading to clinicians and patients because of uncertainty if these cases represent a small cell carcinoma. In the authors' practice, conventional prostatic adenocarcinoma with neuroendocrine differentiation is seen in cases submitted in consultation when the stains were performed elsewhere. The authors routinely comment that these cancers are not small cell carcinomas and the presence of neuroendocrine differentiation does not have a proved clinical significance. Paneth cell–like differentiation is not infrequent and may be seen in benign glands, high-grade prostatic intraepithelial neoplasia, and cancers with different grades. In most cases, these findings are focal and the cancers with Paneth cell–like changes are graded based on the underlying architecture (Fig. 2C). The exception may represent cases with extensive Paneth cell–like changes, particularly those with paucity of eosinophilic neuroendocrine granules, which may mimic Gleason pattern 5 architecturally.[38] In such cases, it is suggested to comment on the extensive Paneth cell–like differentiation and not grade these tumors but to acknowledge that these tumors seem to have a favorable prognosis. Small cell carcinomas and large cell carcinomas have a distinctly aggressive behavior and are not assigned a Gleason grade. Most small cell prostatic carcinomas develop in patients with prior androgen deprivation therapy.[39]

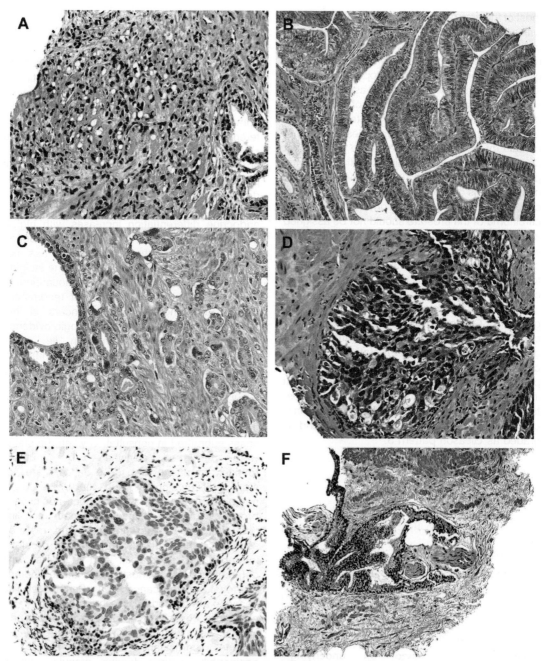

Fig. 2. (*A*) Single tumor cells of Gleason pattern 5 prostate cancer with signet ring cell–like feature. (*B*) Prostatic duct adenocarcinoma forming papillae with fibrovascular cores lined by cells with high-grade pseudostratified columnar nuclei. (*C*) Prostate cancer with Paneth cell–like differentiation. Based on underlying architecture this cancer is Gleason pattern 3. (*D*) Intraductal carcinoma of the prostate demonstrating solid growth pattern with marked cytologic atypia. (*E*) GATA-3 immunostain performed to rule out intraductal spread of high-grade urothelial carcinoma demonstrates the presence of basal cells in intraductal prostatic carcinoma (same case as [*D*]). (*F*) A focus of perineural invasion where despite the architectural complexity the cancer should be graded Gleason pattern 3.

INTRADUCTAL CARCINOMA OF THE PROSTATE

Prostatic intraductal carcinoma is defined as an intraglandular proliferation of malignant cells within acini or prostatic ducts with preserved basal cells. This may take the form of solid or dense cribriform growth (lamina constitute <30% of tumor), loose cribriform or micropapillary proliferations with marked nuclear atypia (nuclei 6-times larger than normal), or presence of comedonecrosis (**Fig.** 2D, E).[40] In most cases, intraductal carcinoma is associated with high-grade cancer elsewhere in the gland, higher pathologic stage, and adverse prognosis.[41] In approximately 10% of radical prostatectomies, however, the intraductal carcinoma is not associated with high-grade cancer and has been suggested to be considered a precursor-like lesion that primarily developed in the ducts and had not yet developed into an invasive cancer.[41] A similar finding of 10% favorable outcomes was demonstrated by a prior study with intraductal prostatic adenocarcinoma on biopsy without invasive cancer.[42] The presence of intraductal carcinoma in a biopsy without invasive cancer or with Gleason score 3 + 3 = 6 (Grade Group 1) prostatic carcinoma may be considered sufficient evidence to advocate for definitive therapy and the authors regularly comment on that in such cases.[42] In the 2014 ISUP consensus, 82% of participants agreed that intraductal carcinoma in absence of invasion should not be assigned a Gleason grade.[9] There is controversy regarding whether intraductal prostatic carcinoma that is present alongside an invasive component should be incorporated into the grade. The 2014 consensus article provides multiple arguments for and against doing so.[9] Currently, if intraductal carcinoma is present along with an invasive component, it is recommended that the intraductal component should be ignored and the Gleason grade should be assigned based on the architecture of the invasive component alone. The presence of intraductal carcinoma has also been validated as an adverse prognostic factor.

SPECIAL CONSIDERATIONS: PERINEURAL INVASION AND MUCINOUS FIBROPLASIA

Both findings, perineural invasion and mucinous fibroplasia, represent unequivocal features of prostatic adenocarcinoma and allow a definitive diagnosis even when infiltrative pattern may not be assessed. Perineural invasion and mucinous fibroplasia (formerly collagenous micronodules) often alter the architecture of the glands and impart a more complex appearance, resembling Gleason pattern 4 carcinoma. By convention, however, s vast majority of such invasive foci are considered Gleason pattern 3 (**Fig.** 2F). In rare instances, upgrading of prostatic adenocarcinoma in these areas should be done only if there is a large cribriform structure and the degree of architectural complexity cannot be explained by the adjacent nerve or mucinous fibroplasia alone (**Fig.** 3A). Upgrading may also occur if necrosis is present.

Pitfalls
PERINEURAL INVASION AND
MUCINOUS FIBROPLASIA

! Perineural invasion and mucinous fibroplasia impart architectural complexity mimicking higher-grade carcinoma (Gleason pattern 4).

! By convention, prostate cancer in areas of perineural invasion or mucinous fibroplasia is considered Gleason pattern 3.

! In rare instances, the degree of complexity cannot be explained by the adjacent structure and upgrading to Gleason pattern 4 is appropriate.

SPECIAL CONSIDERATIONS: GLEASON GRADING POST-THERAPY

Radiation therapy, hormonal therapy, and other treatment modalities, such as high-intensity focused ultrasound (HIFU), may induce significant cytologic and architectural changes in the prostatic glands and stroma, both within the cancerous and the noncancerous components. With the 2 former modalities, residual cancer tends to appear as small poorly formed glands with cytoplasmic vacuolization or as single infiltrating cells which, in absence of a known history of prior therapy, could easily be categorized as Gleason pattern 4 or pattern 5 (**Fig.** 3B, C). The cancers, however, have a favorable prognosis.[43] Therefore, cancers exhibiting hormonal or radiation treatment effect should not be assigned a grade and reported as prostatic adenocarcinoma with hormonal or radiation therapy effect.[17] If cancer in a treated gland

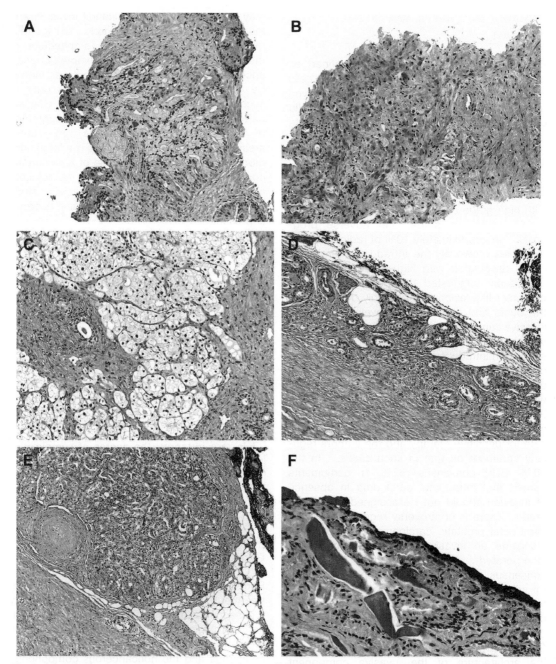

Fig. 3. (*A*) Cribriform prostate cancer gland with a small focus of mucinous fibroplasia where the latter cannot explain the extent of architectural complexity and the cancer should be graded as Gleason pattern 4. (*B*) Irradiated prostate cancer in a core biopsy presenting as single cells with foamy cytoplasm. No grade is assigned. (*C*) Hormonally treated prostate presenting as sheets of vacuolated cells with pyknotic nuclei. No grade is assigned. (*D*) Focal extraprostatic extension where the glands just barely infiltrate the fat. (*E*) Nonfocal extraprostatic extension with a substantial amount of cancer outside the prostate boundary. (*F*) The presence of any intervening tissue between the prostatic glands and cauterized inked margin should be interpreted as negative margin.

demonstrates no treatment effect, however, then it should be graded and the report should specifically state that treatment effect is not identified. HIFU therapy usually causes coagulative necrosis without inflammation and in the areas that did not undergo ablation the carcinoma does not change the histologic appearance.[44]

Pitfalls
GRADING PROSTATE CANCER POST-THERAPY

! Radiation therapy/hormonal therapy may induce cytologic and architectural changes mimicking high-grade prostate cancer.

! Cancers exhibiting hormonal or radiation treatment effect should not be assigned a Gleason grade. The case should be reported as "prostatic adenocarcinoma with treatment effect."

! If cancer in a post-therapy gland does not exhibit treatment effect, then a Gleason grade should be assigned. The case should be reported as "prostatic adenocarcinoma without treatment effect, Gleason score ___ (Grade Group ___)."

A NEW GRADING SYSTEM FOR PROSTATE CANCER: GRADE GROUPS

In the original Gleason grading system of prostatic adenocarcinoma, summed scores assigned at the time of biopsy ranged from 2 to 10 and the combination of 2 patterns from 1 to 5 allowed 25 variations of grade. In modern practice, however, the lowest score is 6. This shift led to some confusion and increased anxiety among patients in particular who associated a score of 6/10 with moderate risk more than average prostate cancer when, in fact, most of these patients have indolent disease and excellent prognosis. This shift likely contributed to overtreatment of patients who otherwise could have been managed with active surveillance. In response to this problem and in an effort to further improve prognostication of prostate cancer, a new 5-tier grading system was developed by the Hopkins group and formally adopted by the ISUP 2014 consensus conference.[9] The nomenclature for this new grading system has been agreed on as in the original publication and referred to it as Grade Groups.[11,45] This terminology was subsequently adopted by the 2016 edition of the World Health Organization *Classification of Tumours of the Urinary System and Male Genital Organs*, the 8th edition of the AJCC, and the CAP.[46] For the foreseeable future, the 2014 modified Gleason score should be reported alongside the Grade Group. The Grade Groups range from 1 to 5, with Grade Group 1 having the most favorable prognosis and Grade Group 5 having the least favorable prognosis.[10,11,16,47] The Grade Groups are designed to be patient centric and to allocate the lowest grade 1 of 5 to the most favorable cancer.[48] Grade Group 1 cases have a Gleason score of less than or equal to 6. Cancers with a Gleason score of 7 are separated into 2 distinct groups, reflecting their

different prognoses; Grade Group 2 consists of cases with Gleason score 3 + 4 = 7 whereas Grade Group 3 cases are Gleason score 4 + 3 = 7.[10] Grade Group 4 is the most heterogeneous and consists of all cases, with a Gleason score of 8 (3 + 5 = 8, 5 + 3 = 8, or 4 + 4 = 8). Finally, Grade Group 5 consists of cases with a Gleason score of greater than or equal to 9 (4 + 5 = 9, 5 + 4 = 9, or 5 + 5 = 10).

The original Gleason grading system correlated Gleason grades with clinical outcomes in prospective studies at the Veterans Administration.[2] Gleason grade has reliably been an independent prognostic indicator for risk of mortality and disease recurrence. The new Grade Group grading system has been validated and shown superior to conventional Gleason grading.[11-16,49,50] Although tertiary pattern 5 is not currently incorporated into the Grade Group system, this could change in the future, because it has been shown to have independent prognostic value.[8]

Some controversy exists regarding Grade Group 4, which currently includes all cancers with a Gleason score of 8 (3 + 5 = 8, 4 + 4 = 8, and 5 + 3 = 8). Some investigators argue that these Gleason grades behave differently, and it is therefore misleading to lump them all together as a single Grade Group 4.[51-54] The authors have demonstrated that contemporary graded cancers with Gleason score 3 + 5 = 8 and 4 + 4 = 8 have comparable clinical behavior.[52] Consequently, it has been suggested that Gleason score 5 + 3 = 8 cancer is more appropriately classified as Grade Group 5.[54] This is an ongoing discussion requiring additional evidence with contemporarily graded cases. As more evidence is accumulated, the Gleason score makeup of the various Grade Groups may be altered to better reflect their prognostic meaning.

> ## Key Features
> ### DEFINITIONS OF GRADE GROUPS
>
> Grade Group 1 (any Gleason score ≤6)—only discrete well-formed glands
>
> Grade Group 2 (3 + 4 = 7)—predominantly discrete well-formed glands with less than 50% fused/poorly formed/cribriform/glomeruloid glands
>
> Grade Group 3 (4 + 3 = 7)—predominantly fused/poorly formed/cribriform/glomeruloid glands with less than 50% discrete well-formed glands
>
> Grade Group 4 (any Gleason score 8: 4 + 4 = 8, 3 + 5 = 8, or 5 + 3 = 8)
>
> - Only fused/poorly formed/cribriform/glomeruloid glands or
> - Predominantly well-formed glands with less than 50% lacking glands or
> - Predominantly lacking glands and less than 50% well-formed glands
>
> Grade Group 5 (any Gleason score 9 or 10: 4 + 5 = 9, 5 + 4 = 9, or 5 + 5 = 10)—comedonecrosis or absence of gland formation with or without fused/poorly formed/cribriform/glomeruloid glands

REPORTING OF BIOPSY SPECIMENS

In the prostate biopsy, the Gleason score is composed of the most dominant (primary) pattern and the highest-grade (secondary) pattern. Although in the past, an individual Gleason score was advocated to be assigned to each needle core with cancer, a recent expert review suggested that when the cores are submitted in a specific anatomic manner (eg, sextant site putting 2 cores in the container rather than splitting separate medial and lateral specimens), the grade of the cores in the same container should be averaged together given they are taken from the same location in the prostate.[8] At the University of Miami, the authors submit a single core per container, which is not an infrequent practice for large prostate cancer centers.[55] For the confirming reads and consults from outside institutions, the authors still report grade per core according to the criteria of the Miami Active Surveillance Trial (MAST- ClinicalTrials.gov identifier NCT02242773), which allows inclusion of men with up to 4 positive biopsy cores, 2 of which may contain Gleason score 3 + 4 = 7 (Grade Group 2) prostate cancer. Averaging containers with 2 separate cores of Gleason score 3 + 3 = 6 (Grade Group 1) and 3 + 4 = 7 (Grade Group 2) cancers may incorrectly disqualify patients from being considered for active surveillance at the authors' institution. In cases of fragmented specimens, a global score is assigned even if the record indicates that more than 1 biopsy was submitted in the jar.[17,55] It is recommended that in

Grade Groups 2 and 3 prostate cancers the percentage of pattern 4 should always be reported. Large studies have demonstrated an incremental increase in biochemical recurrence on the basis of increasing percentages of Gleason pattern 4.[25,56] As an example, Grade Group 2 cancers with less than 5% pattern 4 and those approaching 50% might have a different prognosis and management approach.

Tertiary patterns are not reported in needle core biopsy specimens. Instead, in needle biopsies, if 3 patterns are present, then the higher grade (worst) should always be reported instead of the secondary pattern, even if it comprises less than 5% of the cancer. For example, if a biopsy core shows cancer with pattern 3 (70%), pattern 4 (25%), and the smallest amount of pattern 5 (5%), the reported Gleason score is 3 + 5 = 8 (Grade Group 4). If a minor component (<5%) of a lower pattern is present, then the lower pattern should be ignored (eg, report 4 + 4 = 8 [Grade Group 4] if less than 5% of pattern 3 is present). The overarching approach is that the higher grade should always be reported in biopsy. For example, if a core contains 97% pattern 3% and 3% pattern 4, the core should be assigned a Gleason score 3 + 4 = 7 (Grade Group 2) and the percentage of pattern 4 should be reported as less than 5%.

The extent of cancer is reported by percent of biopsy core involvement with optional inclusion of cancer length. In cases of a discontinuous involvement, the percent of core estimated from one end of the cancer to another with inclusion of the skip lesion.[17,55,57]

Key Features
REPORTING OF BIOPSY SPECIMENS

1. No tertiary pattern

2. The Gleason score is composed of the most dominant and highest grade.

3. If the highest grade is dominant and lower grade is less than 5%—ignore lower grade.

4. Cores taken from the same anatomic location may be lumped together for grading.

REPORTING OF RADICAL PROSTATECTOMY SPECIMENS

The 2005 and 2014 consensus conferences both recommend assigning individual Gleason scores and Grade Groups to each tumor nodule present in the prostatectomy specimen.[8,19] This is accomplished at the authors' institution by submitting radical prostatectomy specimens in their entirety and mapping the locations of the tumor nodules on the slides enabling the discrimination between the different nodules. Each tumor nodule is then assigned its own Gleason score (Grade Group). The Gleason score (Grade Group) assigned to the case is based on the tumor nodule with the highest grade. The dominant tumor nodule tends to be the largest and has the highest grade and stage. Infrequently, a smaller dominant tumor nodule with higher grade may be present along with a larger secondary tumor nodule of lower grade. It is virtually not seen in practice for the larger-volume lower-grade secondary tumor nodule to be of a higher stage than smaller-volume higher-grade dominant tumor nodule. The authors report the Gleason score (Grade Group) of the dominant tumor nodule and its location, followed by the percentage of pattern 4 (if applicable) and grade of any secondary nodules with their locations.

In radical prostatectomy specimens, the Gleason score is reported as the primary (most prevalent) pattern, followed by the secondary (second most common) pattern. The tertiary pattern is reported only in cases of Gleason score 3 + 4 = 7 (Grade Group 2) and 4 + 3 = 7 (Grade Group 3), with pattern 5 representing less than 5% of the tumor nodule. Even a minor component of pattern 5 can negatively affect prognosis.[58,59] In cases of only 2 patterns, the second higher grade pattern is always reported. Thus, a radical prostatectomy cannot be interpreted as Gleason score 3 + 3 = 6 (Grade Group 1) with tertiary pattern 4 (<5%), because such cases are capable of metastasis and need to be regarded as Gleason score 3 + 4 = 7 (Grade Group 2) with low-volume pattern 4.[60] The possible terminology when Grade Groups replace Gleason grade for tertiary pattern 5 is Grade Group 2 or Grade Group 3 with a minor higher-grade component.

The CAP and AJCC staging protocols require indication of the extent of the cancer in radical prostatectomy. Reporting the percent of gland involvement is among the most common methods. There is no provision if the dominant tumor nodule or overall carcinoma should be reported. Although the volume of prostate cancer has been validated as a prognostic factor for extraprostatic extension, seminal vesicle invasion, and positive surgical margin, its independent effect on long-term outcome has not been effectively assessed yet. For the purpose of defining the insignificant prostate cancer, the volume of the dominant tumor nodule is used.[61,62] The authors report the percent of gland involved by entire cancer with increments of 1% up to 10%.

The 8th edition of the AJCC staging manual eliminated reporting a, b, and c substaging of organ-confined prostate cancer (pT2). Although not reflected in the staging, extraprostatic extension should be classified into focal and nonfocal (**Fig. 3**D, E). The latter has a significant negative impact on the likelihood of biochemical recurrence.[63] Although the nomenclature may be somewhat confusing, it does not reflect the number of foci where the extraprostatic extension is seen but rather the amount of cancer that has spread outside the prostatic boundaries (the prostate does not have a true capsule).[64] Bladder neck invasion is considered a nonfocal extraprostatic extension. There is no clear separation between the prostatic stroma and bladder neck. At the authors' institutions, perpendicular sections of the prostate base are submitted and a diagnosis of microscopic bladder neck invasion rendered when the cancer glands are present at the surgical resection margin. In the radical prostatectomy specimen, the positive margin is only reported when the glands are transected at the margin with the overlying ink. The presence of any amount of intervening tissue should be interpreted as negative margin (**Fig. 3**F). The distance of carcinoma to the surgical resection margin is not used in clinical practice, although some reports indicated that this may be an important measure in anteriorly located tumors.[65] The length of positive margin and the grade at the margin are expected to be included in the surgical pathology report and clinically important for adjuvant radiation therapy.

Key Features
REPORTING OF RADICAL
PROSTATECTOMY SPECIMENS

1. Grade each tumor nodule separately.

2. The Gleason score is composed of the most dominant and highest-grade patterns.

3. Tertiary component reported in cases of Gleason score 3 + 4 = 7 (Grade Group 2) or 4 + 3 = 7 (Grade Group 3), with pattern 5 representing less than 5% of the tumor nodule.

4. In tumor nodules with 2 patterns and higher-grade pattern less than 5%—report the higher grade as secondary.

5. Categorize extraprostatic extension into focal and nonfocal.

6. Report the length of positive margin and Gleason score present at the margin.

COMPOSITE (TOTAL) GLEASON SCORE

In the United States, urologists manage patients with a biopsy-proved prostate cancer based on the core with the highest Gleason score (Grade Group), and the reporting of a composite (total) Gleason score is generally not practiced.[17] The development of the Grade Groups was also performed based on the highest grade of the biopsy core and/or tumor nodules with the highest grade. This significantly differs from the practice in Europe and Australia, where the composite (total) grade is assigned to both biopsies and radical prostatectomies. Occasional works indicated a marginal superiority of reporting composite Gleason score.[66] The CAP staging protocol offers inclusion of a composite (total) Gleason score (Grade Group) for both biopsy and radical prostatectomy but no provisions are provided regarding how to assess such a score.[67] In the authors' practice, a composite (total) score for the prostate cancer cases is not provided.

ANCILLARY GENOMIC STUDIES

In the past, treatment decision making was based only on the Gleason grade and extent of prostate cancer found within the gland. Although this is still mostly true today, other tests that provide independent but complementary information have emerged as popular tools to enhance risk stratification.[68] For example, 3 commercial genomic signatures that can be run on prostate biopsy tissue

have emerged and have been validated to help in deciding on the need for treatment versus observation in prostate cancer. The Genomic Health Oncotype test (Redwood City, CA, USA) is a 17-gene signature that was specifically selected to address the tumor heterogeneity issue and multifocality issue.[69] It was validated in 395 men with matched biopsy and radical prostatectomy pathology, where it was found to predict the likelihood of adverse pathology at radical prostatectomy (stage T3+, primary pattern 4). Similarly, the Myriad Polaris (Salt Lake City, UT, USA) has a 31–gene cell cycle progression (CCP) signature that was validated in a 413-men radical prostatectomy cohort, where the investors found the CCP scores from the biopsy were highly correlated with the likelihood of recurrence.[70] Finally, GenomeDx has the Decipher test (Vancouver, BC, Canada), which is a 22-gene panel signature that was previously validated to predict prostate cancer metastasis.[71] It was recently assessed in 57 men who had a biopsy and underwent radical prostatectomy, and the Decipher score was found an independent predictor of metastasis. Therefore, each of these signatures has good data validating itself as an independent predictor of prostate cancer outcomes and can provide helpful information in addition to the histopathology to better risk-stratify patients with prostate cancer. Although the Oncotype test is only available on biopsy tissue, the Decipher and Prolaris tests were originally meant to be conducted on radical prostatectomy tissue to predict more relevant long-term endpoints, such as metastasis and death.[72] As a result, these biomarkers were originally validated in deciding on the need for adjuvant or salvage radiotherapy and androgen deprivation therapy after surgery.

While performing tests on radical prostatectomy tissue, the entire prostate is available and the tumor with the highest grade is often selected for genomic analysis. When the test is performed on biopsy tissue, however, it is uncertain how vulnerable it is to the tumor heterogeneity and multifocality issues that limit proper risk stratification. A recent study by Wei and colleagues[73] looked at 4 radical prostatectomy specimens and sequence biopsy cores from various areas. They found that the expression levels of the genes that were involved in each of these tests were variably expressed throughout the different biopsy cores, suggesting the tumor heterogeneity is an issue not only for pathology but also for genomics.

Similarly, studies looking at random and MRI-targeted biopsy cores, with comparison to the radical prostatectomy specimen, have suggested that both the histology and the genomics from the targeted biopsy cores were more similar to that from the radical prostatectomy compared with the random cores.[74] This provides more data to suggest that although genomic signatures may help address the tumor heterogeneity issues, they certainly do not overcome the problem.

At the University of Miami, the authors are currently conducting a prospective trial for men who are interested in active surveillance (Miami Active Surveillance [MAST] Trial), with the goal of integrating novel imaging and genomic markers to enhance prostate cancer risk stratification and the selection of appropriate men for prospective conservative management. The trial allows men with up to 4 cores of cancer to be enrolled, allowing up to 2 of those cores to be Gleason 3 + 4 = 7. There are no exclusions based on the volume of cancer seen within the core. Men who enroll on the trial have an MRI and template and MRI-targeted biopsy within 3 months of enrollment and every year thereafter for 3 years. The authors will also collect blood and urine on men every year, and biopsy tissue from various biopsy cores are being sequenced and tested for the genomic signatures (discussed previously). The authors believe this trial will answer many important questions, such as how to best integrate novel imaging and genomic markers and how much these markers do and do not address the tumor heterogeneity problem. It is only by answering these questions that how to best use these novel markers will be learned.

SUMMARY

The Gleason grading system has evolved since its introduction more than 50 years ago but it remains critically important for clinical management and determining the prognosis of men with prostate cancer. With the 2005 and 2014 revisions, grading of Gleason patterns 3 and 4 has been revised substantially and reporting has become more standardized. The transition to the Grade Group system provides a more simplified and intuitive grading system for counseling patients, in particular those with low-risk, indolent cancers that may be well-managed with active surveillance. The new grading system has been validated to predict risk of recurrence and death from prostate cancer. Genomic tests predicting the behavior of prostate cancer are now commercially available and gaining in their role as an ancillary test in prostate cancer management.

REFERENCES

1. Bailar JC 3rd, Mellinger GT, Gleason DF. Survival rates of patients with prostatic cancer, tumor stage, and differentiation–preliminary report. Cancer Chemother Rep 1966;50(3):129–36.
2. Gleason DF, Mellinger GT. Prediction of prognosis for prostatic adenocarcinoma by combined histological grading and clinical staging. J Urol 1974;111(1): 58–64.
3. Gleason DF. Histologic grading of prostate cancer: a perspective. Hum Pathol 1992;23(3):273–9.
4. Gleason DF. Classification of prostatic carcinomas. Cancer Chemother Rep 1966;50(3):125–8.
5. Humphrey PA. Gleason grading and prognostic factors in carcinoma of the prostate. Mod Pathol 2004; 17(3):292–306.
6. Mohler JL, A.E., Armstrong AJ, et al. Prostate Cancer, Version 1.2016. J Natl Compr Canc Netw 2016 Jan;14(1):19–30.
7. Zareba P, Zhang J, Yilmaz A, et al. The impact of the 2005 International Society of Urological Pathology (ISUP) consensus on Gleason grading in contemporary practice. Histopathology 2009;55(4):384–91.
8. Epstein JI, Amin MB, Reuter VE, et al. Contemporary Gleason grading of prostatic carcinoma: an update with discussion on practical issues to implement the 2014 international society of urological pathology (ISUP) consensus conference on Gleason grading of prostatic carcinoma. Am J Surg Pathol 2017; 41(4):e1–7.
9. Epstein JI, Egevad L, Amin MB, et al. The 2014 international society of urological pathology (ISUP) consensus conference on Gleason grading of prostatic carcinoma: definition of grading patterns and proposal for a new grading system. Am J Surg Pathol 2016;40(2):244–52.
10. Epstein JI, Zelefsky MJ, Sjoberg DD, et al. A contemporary prostate cancer grading system: a validated alternative to the Gleason score. Eur Urol 2016;69(3):428–35.
11. Pierorazio PM, Walsh PC, Partin AW, et al. Prognostic Gleason grade grouping: data based on the modified Gleason scoring system. BJU Int 2013; 111(5):753–60.
12. Spratt DE, Jackson WC, Abugharib A, et al. Independent validation of the prognostic capacity of the ISUP prostate cancer grade grouping system for radiation treated patients with long-term follow-up. Prostate Cancer Prostatic Dis 2016; 19(3):292–7.
13. Grogan J, Gupta R, Mahon KL, et al. Predictive value of the 2014 International Society of Urological Pathology grading system for prostate cancer in patients undergoing radical prostatectomy with long-term follow-up. BJU Int 2017;120(5):651–8.
14. Vollmer RT. Gleason grading, biochemical failure, and prostate cancer-specific death. Am J Clin Pathol 2017;147(3):273–7.
15. Mathieu R, Moschini M, Beyer B, et al. Prognostic value of the new Grade Groups in Prostate

Cancer: a multi-institutional European validation study. Prostate Cancer Prostatic Dis 2017;20(2): 197–202.

16. Samaratunga H, Delahunt B, Gianduzzo T, et al. The prognostic significance of the 2014 International Society of Urological Pathology (ISUP) grading system for prostate cancer. Pathology 2015;47(6):515–9.

17. Kryvenko ON, Epstein JI. Prostate cancer grading: a decade after the 2005 modified Gleason grading system. Arch Pathol Lab Med 2016;140(10): 1140–52.

18. Epstein JI. Gleason score 2-4 adenocarcinoma of the prostate on needle biopsy: a diagnosis that should not be made. Am J Surg Pathol 2000;24(4): 477–8.

19. Epstein JI, Allsbrook WC Jr, Amin MB, et al. The 2005 international society of urological pathology (ISUP) consensus conference on Gleason grading of prostatic carcinoma. Am J Surg Pathol 2005; 29(9):1228–42.

20. Egevad L, Delahunt B, Evans AJ, et al. international society of urological pathology (ISUP) grading of prostate cancer. Am J Surg Pathol 2016;40(6): 858–61.

21. Gansler T, Fedewa SA, Lin CC, et al. Trends in diagnosis of Gleason score 2 through 4 prostate cancer in the national cancer database, 1990-2013. Arch Pathol Lab Med 2017;141(12):1686–96.

22. Fine SW, Epstein JI. A contemporary study correlating prostate needle biopsy and radical prostatectomy Gleason score. J Urol 2008;179(4):1335–8, [discussion: 1338–9].

23. Ghani KR, Grigor K, Tulloch DN, et al. Trends in reporting Gleason score 1991 to 2001: changes in the pathologist's practice. Eur Urol 2005;47(2): 196–201.

24. Amin MB, Lin DW, Gore JL, et al. The critical role of the pathologist in determining eligibility for active surveillance as a management option in patients with prostate cancer: consensus statement with recommendations supported by the College of American Pathologists, International Society of Urological Pathology, Association of Directors of Anatomic and Surgical Pathology, the New Zealand Society of Pathologists, and the Prostate Cancer Foundation. Arch Pathol Lab Med 2014;138(10): 1387–405.

25. Choy B, Pearce SM, Anderson BB, et al. Prognostic significance of percentage and architectural types of contemporary Gleason pattern 4 prostate cancer in radical prostatectomy. Am J Surg Pathol 2016; 40(10):1400–6.

26. Kweldam CF, Wildhagen MF, Steyerberg EW, et al. Cribriform growth is highly predictive for postoperative metastasis and disease-specific death in Gleason score 7 prostate cancer. Mod Pathol 2015; 28(3):457–64.

27. Kweldam CF, Kummerlin IP, Nieboer D, et al. Presence of invasive cribriform or intraductal growth at biopsy outperforms percentage grade 4 in predicting outcome of Gleason score 3+4=7 prostate cancer. Mod Pathol 2017;30(8):1126–32.

28. Siadat F, Sykes J, Zlotta AR, et al. Not all Gleason pattern 4 prostate cancers are created equal: a study of latent prostatic carcinomas in a cystoprostatectomy and autopsy series. Prostate 2015; 75(12):1277–84.

29. Kryvenko ON, Gupta NS, Virani N, et al. Gleason score 7 adenocarcinoma of the prostate with lymph node metastases: analysis of 184 radical prostatectomy specimens. Arch Pathol Lab Med 2013;137(5): 610–7.

30. Zhou M, Li J, Cheng L, et al. Diagnosis of "poorly formed glands" Gleason pattern 4 prostatic adenocarcinoma on needle biopsy: an interobserver reproducibility study among urologic pathologists with recommendations. Am J Surg Pathol 2015;39(10): 1331–9.

31. Meliti A, Sadimin E, Diolombi M, et al. accuracy of grading Gleason score 7 prostatic adenocarcinoma on needle biopsy: influence of percent pattern 4 and other histological factors. Prostate 2017;77(6): 681–5.

32. Lane BR, Magi-Galluzzi C, Reuther AM, et al. Mucinous adenocarcinoma of the prostate does not confer poor prognosis. Urology 2006;68(4): 825–30.

33. Ali TZ, Epstein JI. Basal cell carcinoma of the prostate: a clinicopathologic study of 29 cases. Am J Surg Pathol 2007;31(5):697–705.

34. Tavora F, Epstein JI. High-grade prostatic intraepithelial neoplasialike ductal adenocarcinoma of the prostate: a clinicopathologic study of 28 cases. Am J Surg Pathol 2008;32(7):1060–7.

35. Zhou M. High-grade prostatic intraepithelial neoplasia, PIN-like carcinoma, ductal carcinoma, and intraductal carcinoma of the prostate. Mod Pathol 2018;31(S1):S71–9.

36. Epstein JI, Amin MB, Beltran H, et al. Proposed morphologic classification of prostate cancer with neuroendocrine differentiation. Am J Surg Pathol 2014;38(6):756–67.

37. Fine SW. Neuroendocrine tumors of the prostate. Mod Pathol 2018;31(S1):S122–32.

38. So JS, Gordetsky J, Epstein JI. Variant of prostatic adenocarcinoma with Paneth cell-like neuroendocrine differentiation readily misdiagnosed as Gleason pattern 5. Hum Pathol 2014;45(12): 2388–93.

39. Nadal R, Schweizer M, Kryvenko ON, et al. Small cell carcinoma of the prostate. Nat Rev Urol 2014; 11(4):213–9.

40. Guo CC, Epstein JI. Intraductal carcinoma of the prostate on needle biopsy: histologic features and

clinical significance. Mod Pathol 2006;19(12): 1528–35.

41. Miyai K, Divatia MK, Shen SS, et al. Heterogeneous clinicopathological features of intraductal carcinoma of the prostate: a comparison between "precursor-like" and "regular type" lesions. Int J Clin Exp Pathol 2014;7(5):2518–26.

42. Robinson BD, Epstein JI. Intraductal carcinoma of the prostate without invasive carcinoma on needle biopsy: emphasis on radical prostatectomy findings. J Urol 2010;184(4):1328–33.

43. Crook JM, Malone S, Perry G, et al. Twenty-four-month postradiation prostate biopsies are strongly predictive of 7-year disease-free survival: results from a Canadian randomized trial. Cancer 2009; 115(3):673–9.

44. Biermann K, Montironi R, Lopez-Beltran A, et al. His-topathological findings after treatment of prostate cancer using high-intensity focused ultrasound (HIFU). Prostate 2010;70(11):1196–200.

45. Epstein JI, Kryvenko ON. In reply. Arch Pathol Lab Med 2017;141(2):183–4.

46. Humphrey PA, Moch H, Cubilla AL, et al. The 2016 who classification of tumours of the urinary system and male genital organs-part b: prostate and bladder tumours. Eur Urol 2016;70(1):106–19.

47. Delahunt B, Egevad L, Srigley JR, et al. Validation of International Society of Urological Pathology (ISUP) grading for prostatic adenocarcinoma in thin core biopsies using TROG 03.04 'RADAR' trial clinical data. Pathology 2015;47(6):520–5.

48. Kryvenko ON, Epstein JI. Changes in prostate cancer grading: including a new patient-centric grading system. Prostate 2016;76(5):427–33.

49. Dong F, Wang C, Farris AB, et al. Impact on the clinical outcome of prostate cancer by the 2005 international society of urological pathology modified Gleason grading system. Am J Surg Pathol 2012; 36(6):838–43.

50. van den Bergh RC, van der Kwast TH, de Jong J, et al. Validation of the novel International Society of Urological Pathology 2014 five-tier Gleason grade grouping: biochemical recurrence rates for 3+5 disease may be overestimated. BJU Int 2016;118(4): 502–5.

51. Mahal BA, Muralidhar V, Chen YW, et al. Gleason score 5 + 3 = 8 prostate cancer: much more like Gleason score 9? BJU Int 2016;118(1):95–101.

52. Harding-Jackson N, Kryvenko ON, Whittington EE, et al. Outcome of Gleason 3 + 5 = 8 prostate cancer diagnosed on needle biopsy: prognostic comparison with Gleason 4 + 4 = 8. J Urol 2016;196(4): 1076–81.

53. Gandaglia G, Karnes RJ, Sivaraman A, et al. Are all grade group 4 prostate cancers created equal? Implications for the applicability of the novel grade grouping. Urol Oncol 2017;35(7):461.e7–14.

54. Huynh MA, Chen MH, Wu J, et al. Gleason score 3 + 5 or 5 + 3 versus 4 + 4 prostate cancer: the risk of death. Eur Urol 2016;69(6):976–9.

55. Kryvenko ON, Diaz M, Meier FA, et al. Findings in 12-core transrectal ultrasound-guided prostate needle biopsy that predict more advanced cancer at prostatectomy: analysis of 388 biopsy-prostatectomy pairs. Am J Clin Pathol 2012;137(5): 739–46.

56. Sauter G, Steurer S, Clauditz TS, et al. clinical utility of quantitative Gleason grading in prostate biopsies and prostatectomy specimens. Eur Urol 2016;69(4): 592–8.

57. Arias-Stella JA 3rd, Varma KR, Montoya-Cerrillo D, et al. Does discontinuous involvement of a prostatic needle biopsy core by adenocarcinoma correlate with a large tumor focus at radical prostatectomy? Am J Surg Pathol 2015;39(2):281–6.

58. Lucca I, Shariat SF, Briganti A, et al. Validation of tertiary Gleason pattern 5 in Gleason score 7 prostate cancer as an independent predictor of biochemical recurrence and development of a prognostic model. Urol Oncol 2015;33(2):71.e21-6.

59. Sauter G, Clauditz T, Steurer S, et al. Integrating tertiary Gleason 5 patterns into quantitative Gleason grading in prostate biopsies and prostatectomy specimens. Eur Urol 2018;73(5):674–83.

60. Ross HM, Kryvenko ON, Cowan JE, et al. Do adeno-carcinomas of the prostate with Gleason score (GS) </=6 have the potential to metastasize to lymph nodes? Am J Surg Pathol 2012;36(9):1346–52.

61. Kryvenko ON, Epstein JI. Definition of insignificant tumor volume of Gleason score 3 + 3 = 6 (grade group 1) prostate cancer at radical prostatectomy-is it time to increase the threshold? J Urol 2016; 196(6):1664–9.

62. Kryvenko ON, Carter HB, Trock BJ, et al. Biopsy criteria for determining appropriateness for active surveillance in the modern era. Urology 2014; 83(4):869–74.

63. Kryvenko ON, Epstein JI. Improving the evaluation and diagnosis of clinically significant prostate cancer. Curr Opin Urol 2017;27(3):191–7.

64. Magi-Galluzzi C, Evans AJ, Delahunt B, et al. International society of urological pathology (ISUP) consensus conference on handling and staging of radical prostatectomy specimens. Working group 3: extraprostatic extension, lymphovascular invasion and locally advanced disease. Mod Pathol 2011; 24(1):26–38.

65. Paluru S, Epstein JI. Does the distance between tumor and margin in radical prostatectomy specimens correlate with prognosis: relation to tumor location. Hum Pathol 2016;56:11–5.

66. Arias-Stella JA 3rd, Shah AB, Montoya-Cerrillo D, et al. Prostate biopsy and radical prostatectomy Gleason score correlation in heterogenous

tumors: proposal for a composite Gleason score. Am J Surg Pathol 2015;39(9):1213–8.

67. Patologist CoA. Protocol for the Examination of Specimens From Patients With Carcinoma of the Prostate Gland. 2017. Available at: http://www.cap.org/ShowProperty?nodePath=/UCMCon/Contribution Folders/WebContent/pdf/cp-prostate-17protocol-4020.pdf. Accessed April 23, 2018.

68. Moschini M, Spahn M, Mattei A, et al. Incorporation of tissue-based genomic biomarkers into localized prostate cancer clinics. BMC Med 2016;14:67.

69. Klein EA, Cooperberg MR, Magi-Galluzzi C, et al. A 17-gene assay to predict prostate cancer aggressiveness in the context of Gleason grade heterogeneity, tumor multifocality, and biopsy undersampling. Eur Urol 2014;66(3):550–60.

70. Cooperberg MR, Simko JP, Cowan JE, et al. Validation of a cell-cycle progression gene panel to improve risk stratification in a contemporary prostatectomy cohort. J Clin Oncol 2013;31(11):1428–34.

71. Klein EA, Haddad Z, Yousefi K, et al. Decipher genomic classifier measured on prostate biopsy predicts metastasis risk. Urology 2016;90:148–52.

72. Dalela D, Santiago-Jimenez M, Yousefi K, et al. Genomic classifier augments the role of pathological features in identifying optimal candidates for adjuvant radiation therapy in patients with prostate cancer: development and internal validation of a multivariable prognostic model. J Clin Oncol 2017; 35(18):1982–90.

73. Wei L, Wang J, Lampert E, et al. Intratumoral and intertumoral genomic heterogeneity of multifocal localized prostate cancer impacts molecular classifications and genomic prognosticators. Eur Urol 2017;71(2):183–92.

74. Radtke JP, Takhar M, Bonekamp D, et al. Transcriptome wide analysis of magnetic resonance imaging-targeted biopsy and matching surgical specimens from high-risk prostate cancer patients treated with radical prostatectomy: the target must be hit. Eur Urol Focus 2017, [Epub ahead of print].

Contemporary Grading and Staging of Urothelial Neoplasms of the Urinary Bladder
New Concepts and Approaches to Challenging Scenarios

Alexander J. Gallan, MD[a], Bonnie Choy, MD[a], Gladell P. Paner, MD[a,b],*

KEYWORDS

• Urinary • Bladder • Urothelial • Grade • Stage • WHO • TNM • Transurethral

---

Key points

- New facets in grading of noninvasive urothelial neoplasms in the new 4th edition of the World Health Organization classification and International Consultation on Urological Diseases–European Association of Urology recommendations are described.

- New approaches and recommendations to staging of urothelial neoplasms in the urinary bladder according to the new 8th edition of the American Joint Committee *Cancer Staging Manual* on Cancer TNM staging are explained.

- Challenges and problematic situations in grading and staging of urothelial neoplasms in the urinary bladder are highlighted, and the practical approaches in handling and reporting of these issues are provided.

ABSTRACT

G rading and staging of urothelial neoplasm are the most crucial factors in risk stratification and management; both necessitate optimal accuracy and consistency. Several updates and recommendations have been provided though recent publications of the 4th edition of the World Health Organization classification, the 8th edition of the American Joint Committee on Cancer staging system, and the International Consultation on Urological Diseases–European Association of Urology updates on bladder cancer. Updates and recent studies have provided better insights into and approaches to the challenging scenarios in grading and staging of urothelial neoplasm; however, there remain aspects that need further investigation and refinement.

OVERVIEW

Urothelial carcinoma of the bladder is among the most common cancers in the United States and is

---

The authors have nothing to disclose regarding any commercial or financial conflicts of interest and any funding sources.

[a] Department of Pathology, University of Chicago, 5841 South Maryland Avenue, AMB S626-MC6101, Chicago, IL 60637, USA; [b] Department of Surgery, Section of Urology, University of Chicago, 5841 South Maryland Avenue, AMB S626-MC6101, Chicago, IL 60637, USA

* Corresponding author. Department of Pathology, University of Chicago, 5841 South Maryland Avenue, AMB S626-MC6101, Chicago, IL 60637.

E-mail address: gladell.paner@uchospitals.edu

1875-9181/18/© 2018 Elsevier Inc. All rights reserved.

routinely encountered by general surgical patholo-gists in transurethral resection (TUR) and radical cystectomy (RC) specimens. Proper categorization, grading, and staging of urothelial neoplasms are important drivers of optimal patient management, prognostication, and surveillance follow-up.[1–5] In 2016, the 4th edition of the World Health Organiza-tion (WHO) classification of urinary bladder tumors was released, which includes some refinements in grading of noninvasive urothelial neoplasms.[6] In 2012, under the auspices of the International Consultation on Urological Diseases (ICUD), expert genitourinary pathologists offered consensus rec-ommendations, including newer concepts, when grading challenging and problematic situations in urothelial neoplasms.[7,8] Furthermore, on January 1, 2018, use of the 8th edition of American Joint Committee on Cancer (AJCC) TNM *Cancer Staging Manual* (8E AJCC) for clinical practice and cancer registry reporting was implemented, providing evidence-based recommendations and clarifica-tions of stage categories.[9,10] In light of these up-dates, this article presents a review of the most recent grading and staging of urothelial neoplasms, with emphasis on problematic and clinically impact-ful issues encountered in routine practice.

GRADING OF UROTHELIAL NEOPLASIA

The primary purpose of grading in urothelial neo-plasms is to stratify tumor behavior, including pro-gression and recurrence, and is most applicable to noninvasive carcinomas.[1,2,11] Historically, grading was performed in accordance with the 1973 WHO classification, which is still occasionally used in some parts of the world, particularly in Europe.[12] The 1998 International Society of Urological Pa-thology (ISUP) grading criteria,[13] which was adop-ted in the 2004 WHO classification,[14] represented a significant step forward in the grading of these tumors, and the current 2016 WHO system ex-pands on these principles of tumor grading (**Ta-ble 1**).[6] The current system recognizes 3 basic tumor growth patterns: flat, papillary, and inverted. As set forth by the ICUD–European Association of Urology (EAU) 2012 update, each of these patterns has an analogous morphologic spectrum of uro-thelial lesions, with increasing risks of progression to invasive urothelial carcinoma (**Table 2**).[7,8] These different urothelial lesions occasionally may pre-sent with difficulties in categorization and distinc-tion from mimics related to their pattern and grade.

PAPILLARY LESIONS

Urothelial papilloma is lined by urothelium of normal layer (basal to umbrella cells) and

Table 1
Comparison of the 2004 and 2016 World Health Organization classifications of noninvasive urothelial neoplasms

2004 World Health Organization	2016 World Health Organization
Noninvasive PUC, HG	Noninvasive PUC, HG
Noninvasive PUC, LG	Noninvasive PUC, LG
Noninvasive PUNLMP	PUNLMP
Urothelial papilloma	Urothelial papilloma
Inverted urothelial papilloma	Inverted urothelial papilloma
Urothelial CIS	Urothelial CIS
	Urothelial dysplasia
	Urothelial proliferation of uncertain malignant potential

thickness (up to 7 cell layers) without cytologic atypia. Papillary urothelial neoplasm of low malig-nant potential (PUNLMP) is characterized by an increased number of cell layers with retained po-larity and minimal cytologic atypia. This category has been a source of significant controversy, but most studies show that it is associated with a small but real risk of tumor progression (1%) and a significant risk for recurrence (20%–28%).[15] Noninvasive low-grade (LG) papillary uro-thelial carcinoma (PUC) is characterized by some loss of polarity and mild cytologic atypia. Occa-sional mitoses may be seen but tend to occur in the lower half of the epithelium. Noninvasive high-grade (HG) PUC shows obvious loss of po-larity; moderate to severe cytologic atypia, including marked pleomorphism; prominent nucleoli; and mitoses at any level, including at the upper half of the epithelium. Although grading is principally based on the degree of cellular aty-pia and organization, there is also some correla-tion with the extent of papillary growth; the tumor usually becomes larger and the papillae

Table 2
Morphologic analogy of the different urothelial neoplasms and lesions

Flat	Papillary (Exophytic)	Inverted
Normal	Papilloma	Inverted papilloma
Hyperplasia	PUNLMP	Inverted PUNLMP
Dysplasia	PUC, LG	Inverted PUC, LG
CIS	PUC, HG	Inverted PUC, HG

more complex with further branching and fusion with increasing grade. Aggregate data show recurrence rates and progression rates for noninvasive LG PUC of 43% and 4%, respectively, compared with 58% and 19%, respectively, for HG PUC.[15]

One confounding issue in categorization is the presence of grade heterogeneity in papillary neoplasms, particularly with admixed HG features. A mixture of noninvasive HG and LG features in a PUC is encountered in approximately 25% of cases (**Fig. 1**A).[16,17] Although the 2016 WHO system does not offer official recommendations in grading, limited data suggest that predominantly LG PUCs with less than 5% or even less than 10% HG morphology may have rates of progression similar to pure LG PUCs.[18,19] Despite the lack of supporting evidence, the 1998 ISUP consensus recommended ignoring a miniscule amount of HG in mixed tumors and classifying those with significant amount as HG.[13]

> ### Key Features
> ### PUC WITH MIXED HG
> ### AND LG FEATURES
>
> - Due to limited data and uncertainty of the cutoff for HG in PUC with mixed grades, the authors' approach in practice is to (1) mention the presence of HG even when focal and (2) provide some estimation of the HG component (either by approximation [eg, focal, predominant] or by percentages) in the report.

This approach provides clarity to urologists, who also have to take into account other risk factors (eg, tumor size, multifocality, recurrence status, concomitant carcinoma in situ [CIS], and urethral involvement) with the TUR for management.[1,2,5] Mixed PUNLMP and LG tumors also may occur in approximately 8% of cases[16]; however, distinction from pure PUNLMP or LG is not as crucial for management as with admixed HG.

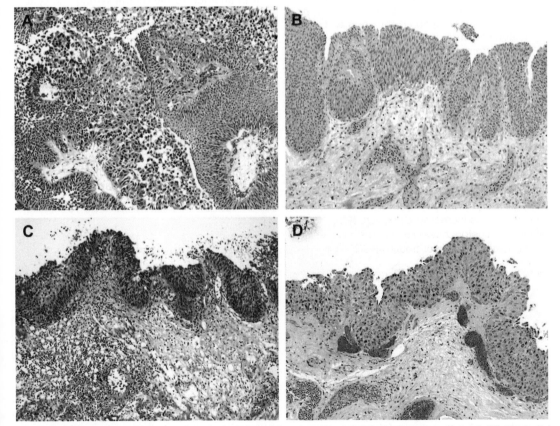

Fig. 1. (*A*) Mixed HG and LG PUC. (*B*) Urothelial proliferation of uncertain malignant potential. (*C*) Urothelial dysplasia with early papillary formation. (*D*) Urothelial CIS with early papillary formation (H&E, original magnification [*A–D*] ×200).

It is not uncommon during surveillance cystoscopy in patients with previous PUCs to encounter hyperplastic-appearing urothelial lesions lacking cytologic atypia and are usually undulating or show tenting but with no definitive fibrovascular core or true papillary formation (**Fig. 1B**). There is evidence revealing that these lesions are clonal or neoplastic and that it may represent the shoulder of a prior resected papillary neoplasm. These lesions are also previously referred to as papillary urothelial hyperplasia in the literature and have a significant risk (27%) for progression, mostly into LG papillary neoplasm.[20,21]

Key Features
UROTHELIAL PROLIFERATION OF
UNCERTAIN MALIGNANT POTENTIAL

- These hyperplastic-appearing urothelial lesions are now officially designated "urothelial proliferation of uncertain malignant potential" in the 2016 WHO classification, supplanting urothelial hyperplasia.

- Because of its novelty and the "uncertain malignant" designation, the authors recommend commenting on (1) the absence of HG features to make it clearer to (perhaps unfamiliar) urologists that this is within the spectrum of lower risk lesions and (2) the need to have a follow-up.

Occasionally during surveillance cystoscopy, problematic urothelial lesions are also encountered that may exhibit either (LG) dysplastic or noninvasive carcinoma features and with undulations or small fronds equivocal for the designation as a papillary tumor. The neoplastic urothelium typically shows increased cell layers (**Fig. 1C, D**). Other investigators have described similar lesions as "truncated papillae of treated PUC."[22]

Key Features
UROTHELIAL NEOPLASMS WITH
EARLY PAPILLARY FORMATION

- These forme fruste lesions are recommended by experts to be labeled, depending on the degree of atypia, as either *urothelial dysplasia with early papillary formation* or *urothelial CIS with early papillary formation*, with the belief that many of these may represent incipient papillary tumors.[8]

It is best that these lesions are given such a descriptive diagnosis because the clinical significance and validity of these entities remain to be seen, while in keeping with the current ISUP/WHO terminologies.

Other lesions in the bladder, such as polypoid cystitis (**Fig. 2A**) and nephrogenic adenoma (**Fig. 2B**), also may exhibit pure or predominant papillary growth, and distinction, particularly from LG papillary urothelial neoplasms, can be challenging.[23,24] Polypoid cystitis may develop as a response to mucosal irritation, such as catheterization, stone, and inflammation, and, thus, is most common along the trigonal area. Urologists may clinically suspect these lesions as inflammatory or non-neoplastic in nature because of their cystoscopy appearance of multiple and confluent edematous blebs and small projections.

Differential Diagnosis
PAPILLARY UROTHELIAL NEOPLASM

- In addition to the clinical setting and cystoscopic findings, polypoid cystitis can be identified histologically by larger broad-based papillae, edematous stroma, minimal architectural complexity or branching, associated chronic inflammation, and urothelium that lacks atypia.

The urothelial lining in polypoid cystitis also may be hyperplastic. The papillae with time may undergo fibrosis and thinning of the core (papillary cystitis), augmenting the difficulty in distinguishing from papillary urothelial neoplasm.

Differential Diagnosis
PAPILLARY UROTHELIAL
NEOPLASM

- In cases of papillary cystitis, presence of admixed more typical polypoid cystitis, lack of structural complexity, and absence of urothelial atypia are helpful in its diagnosis.

Nephrogenic adenoma with prominent or predominant exophytic papillary growth also may mimic papillary urothelial neoplasms, in particular papillary tumors with marked epithelial denudation.

> △△ **Differential Diagnosis**
> NEPHROGENIC ADENOMA
>
> - Unlike papillary urothelial neoplasms, nephrogenic adenoma is lined by a monolayer of cells, including with hobnailed appearance, lacks significant nuclear atypia, and has concomitant underlying tubuloglandular growth (biphasic pattern).

Nephrogenic adenoma is typically positive for PAX8 or PAX2 and negative for p63 in contrast to papillary urothelial neoplasms (**Fig. 2C**),[25–27] although often distinction can be made by morphology alone. Up to 40% of nephrogenic adenoma also may express the urothelial marker GATA3 and awareness of this pitfall is important to avoid a misdiagnosis.[25] In cases of denuded PUC, a search for preserved stratified atypical urothelium helps facilitate the diagnosis (**Fig. 2D**). Denudation in PUC occurs more often in HG

PUC, necessitating a search for residual detached HG cells if this feature is present.[28]

FLAT LESIONS

Flat urothelium of normal thickness and without cytologic atypia is simply normal urothelium. Urothelial dysplasia characteristically shows mild loss of cellular polarity and mild cellular atypia, akin to the cytologic changes in LG PUC. Urothelial CIS shows more pronounced architectural disorder with significant cellular atypia, including marked pleomorphism, similar to the cytologic changes in HG PUC. Diagnosis of dysplasia has been hampered by poor diagnostic reproducibility. The implications of dysplasia in risk stratification and management, however, are not as established as in CIS. The vast majority of dysplasia is encountered on follow-up after diagnosis of papillary neoplasm (or not de novo), which already dictates a follow-up surveillance protocol.

CIS may creep through a background of benign or lower-grade urothelium and only partially involve the cell layer to exhibit unique patterns, such as

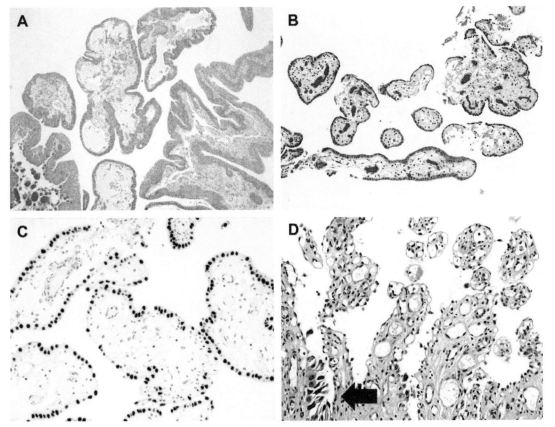

Fig. 2. (*A*) Polypoid/papillary cystitis (H&E, original magnification ×40). (*B*) Nephrogenic adenoma (H&E, original magnification ×100). (*C*) PAX8 positivity in nephrogenic adenoma (H&E, original magnification ×200). (*D*) Extensively denuded PUC, with focal residual attached stratified cells (*arrow*) (H&E, original magnification ×200).

pagetoid, undermining, or overriding patterns.[29] Diagnosis of pagetoid or single cells and small clusters spread can be challenging if present focally and without concomitant usual CIS in the TUR (**Fig. 3**A).

Key Features
ISOLATED PAGETOID CIS

- Recognition of isolated pagetoid CIS can be facilitated by seeing enlarged and atypical cells near or juxtaposed to the basement membrane (lower half of epithelium), in contrast to the benign umbrella cells that, although to certain extent may mimic the cytologic alterations, are confined only to the surface.

Identification of isolated CIS cells can be facilitated by immunopositivity for cytokeratin (CK) 20, which typically stains only the umbrella cells at the surface of a normal urothelium (**Fig. 3**B).[30]

CK20-positive cells in benign urothelium should not be situated immediately adjacent to the basement membrane. For the same reason, in markedly denuded CIS, CK20 positivity is helpful in highlighting the few clinging CIS cells attached to the basement membrane (**Fig. 3**C, D). The use of CK20 can be enhanced by the addition of CD44 (negative in CIS cells) and p53 (diffusely positive in CIS cell layer) as a panel.[30–33] CD44 and p53, however, may show greater variability in staining compared with CK20.[31]

Identification of CIS concurrent to HG PUC in TUR is important for risk stratification (high risk) and may have implications to the management.[1,2] A potential problematic situation is when seeing noninvasive HG PUC admixed with concurrent separate tissue fragment(s) containing flat carcinoma pattern. Distinction as concurrent CIS (**Fig. 4**) versus a detached shoulder of a fragmented HG PUC can be difficult if the flat carcinoma is limited or focal. In this situation, correlation with cystoscopy (eg, multiple lesions and gross appearance of lesions) and

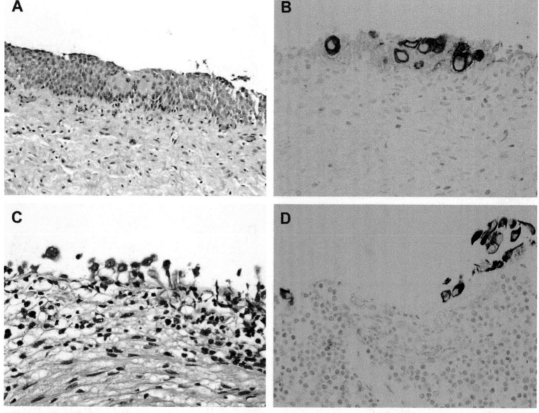

Fig. 3. (*A*) Focal pagetoid cell cluster of urothelial carcinoma, note an atypical cell next to the basement membrane (H&E, original magnification ×200). (*B*) CK20 highlights the pagetoid cells (H&E, original magnification ×400). (*C*) Clinging urothelial CIS (H&E, original magnification ×400). (*D*) CK20 highlights denuded urothelial CIS (H&E, original magnification ×400).

Fig. 4. HG PUC (*right inset*) with concurrent CIS (*left inset* and *rectangles*) present in the same container (H&E, original magnification ×20).

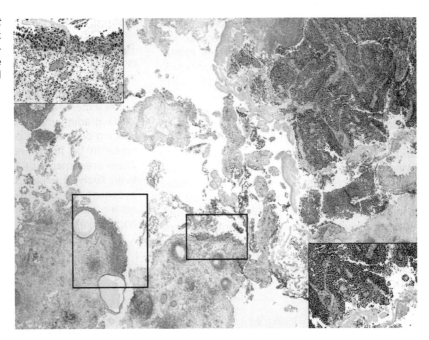

manner of specimen submission (same or separate containers) can be helpful.

> ### Key Features
> ### CONCURRENT CIS AND HG PUC LESIONS
>
> - In addition to review of cystoscopy and specimen submission, flat carcinoma pattern, when diffuse, presents in multiple tissue fragments, not thickened, or with pagetoid or other unique CIS patterns and is supportive for the diagnosis of concurrent CIS to the HG PUC in the container.

Advising urologists to place multiple separate TURs (with nonpapillary lesions) and mapping cold cup biopsies in different containers helps alleviate this problematic situation. It remains unclear, however, as to what extent a lateral flat continuation from an HG PUC would be enough to merit a concurrent CIS designation.

The most recognized and frequently discussed challenging scenario in TUR or biopsy is when distinguishing CIS from reactive atypia, including inflammatory and radiation atypia. The morphologic clues and immunohistochemical (eg, CK20, CD44, and p53) staining patterns helpful to make the distinction have been addressed extensively in textbooks and prior publications.[29–36]

INVERTED LESIONS

Inverted or endophytic lesions follow an analogous concept to the exophytic papillary and flat lesions.[7,8] Inverted growth into the lamina propria (LP) is characterized by having a regular boundary, sharp epithelial to stromal interface, and absence of stromal (desmoplastic) reaction. Inverted papilloma represents an endophytic growth with thin trabeculae or cords representing 2 apposed urothelium with minimal cytologic atypia. The apposed urothelium results in the characteristic peripheral palisading (basal/parabasal cells) and central streaming (surface umbrella cells) pattern (**Fig. 5**A). Inverted PUNLMP is an endophytic papillary lesion containing an increased number of cell layers but maintaining polarity with minimal cytologic atypia. Thickened trabeculae or cords essentially exclude a papilloma (**Fig. 5**B). Grading as PUNLMP, LG, or HG essentially follows the cytomorphology-based assessment similar for their exophytic counterparts (**Fig. 5**C, D).

> ### Pitfall
> ### INVERTED LESIONS
>
> ! Care should be exercised not to misdiagnose inverted PUC (pTa as carcinoma invading into the LP (pT1), because management can be different.

Unlike inverted PUC, invasive (conventional) urothelial carcinoma exhibits irregular or jagged pattern, single cell or small cell cluster infiltration, squamoid or more dense eosinophilic cytoplasm (paradoxic differentiation), and desmoplasia.

The unusual large nested variant of urothelial carcinoma can be difficult to distinguish from inverted PUC.[37,38] This tumor is characterized by invasive large nests of deceptively bland-appearing cells with a broad or somewhat pushing invasive front (**Fig. 6**). Most large nested variants have a surface papillary component and also may have concomitant conventional or variants urothelial carcinoma. A majority of these tumors are diagnosed as muscularis propria (MP)-invasive disease (pT2) at TUR and greater than 50% are locally aggressive tumors (>pT2) at RC.

> ### Key Features
> #### NESTED UROTHELIAL CARCINOMA
>
> - Because most large nested variants are MP invasive, adequate sampling of MP (deep bite) in TUR is vital to help establish the diagnosis (presence of MP involvement).

Communication with urologists regarding the predicament in diagnosis particularly in a superficial sample and the need for ample amount of MP should be made. In general, the guidelines for TUR require sampling of MP as a surrogate measure of adequacy of the resection, and for staging.[1,2]

> ### Pitfall
> #### INVERTED LESIONS
>
> ! Inverted urothelial neoplasm may also mimic florid von Brunn nests, which can extend deep into the LP.

Unlike von Brunn nests, inverted papillary neoplasms may also have an exophytic papillary component, have more trabecular or elongated inward growth, and can be more confluent and complex with branching and fusion of the endophytic extensions. von Brunn nests are usually more distinct rounded nests and may have concomitant cystitis cystica and cystitis glandularis, including goblet cells.

INVASIVE CARCINOMA

The vast majority of invasive urothelial carcinoma is graded as HG (>95%).[15] Rare invasive LG tumors have been reported in TUR, mostly (>85%) showing LP invasion only (pT1).[39,40] Some experts argue that this is where the 1973 WHO grading may outperform the ISUP/WHO grading because the latter allows invasive carcinoma to be further separated as G2 or G3.[15] There are variants of urothelial carcinoma, however, such as nested and microcytic, that have a deceptively bland or benign cellular appearance but paradoxically can behave aggressively.[41–44]

> ### Differential Diagnosis
> #### INVASIVE UROTHELIAL CARCINOMA
>
> - Invasive carcinoma must be distinguished from other mimics, such as CIS extending into von Brunn nests, cystitis cystica, or cystitis glandularis and also pseudocarcinomatous epithelial hyperplasia.

von Brunn nests with CIS show a regular circumscribed boundary and lack the features of invasion, such as desmoplasia, jagged irregular nests, and single or small cluster of cells with squamoid features (**Fig. 7**A). Presence of non-neoplastic von Brunn nest and cystitis cystica or glandularis in the background is also helpful. Pseudocarcinomatous epithelial hyperplasia is usually seen in the setting of prior irradiation and, thus, the bladder may also show changes of radiation cystitis.[45,46] The lesion is characterized by pseudoinfiltrative urothelial nests that characteristically wrap around vessels with fibrin (**Fig. 7**B). The cells usually exhibit mild to moderate atypia with no increase in mitosis, and with nests that do not reach the MP.

STAGING OF UROTHELIAL NEOPLASIA

PATHOLOGIC STAGE

As with other hollow organs, the staging schema for urothelial carcinoma of the bladder is based on the depth of invasion.[47] Treatment of urothelial carcinoma is highly dependent on pT staging. Nonmuscle invasive (pT1) urothelial carcinoma in TUR is considered high risk and is usually treated with intravesical instillation of chemotherapy or bacillus Calmette-Guérin.[1,2,5] Invasion of the tumor into MP (pT2) is the major indication for aggressive therapy, including RC with bilateral

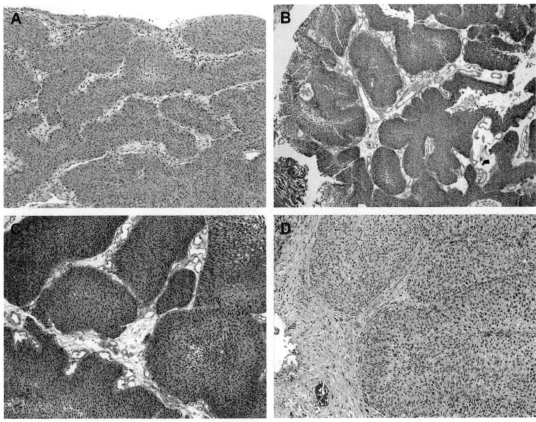

Fig. 5. (*A*) Inverted papilloma (H&E, original magnification ×200). (*B*) Thickened trabecular growth is incompatible with papilloma (H&E, original magnification ×100). (*C*) Inverted LG PUC (H&E, original magnification ×200). (*D*) Inverted HG PUC (H&E, original magnification ×200).

Fig. 6. Large nested urothelial carcinoma, invading into the MP (H&E, original magnification ×40).

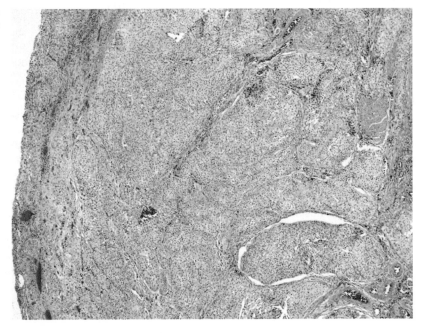

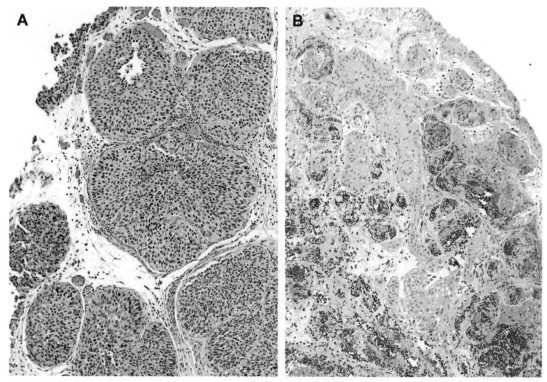

Fig. 7. (*A*) Urothelial CIS involving von Brunn nests. (*B*) Pseudocarcinomatous epithelial hyperplasia (H&E, original magnification [*A,B*] ×200).

pelvic lymphadenectomy and neoadjuvant chemotherapy,[3–5] although HG pT1 with concurrent CIS, multiple or large (>3 cm), as recurrence of a previous tumor, and with variant histologies (such as sarcomatoid, micropapillary, and plasmacytoid) also may be considered for RC.[1,2,5] Patients with non–organ-confined disease (>pT2) at RC without prior neoadjuvant chemotherapy are offered adjuvant chemotherapy.[4,5] Although the new TNM staging does not include any actual changes to the T categories, the 8E AJCC has made several clarifications and recommendations (**Table 3**).[9,10]

pT1 Tumors

Urothelial carcinoma invasive into the LP but not involving the MP layer is staged as pT1.

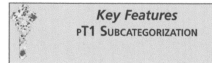

Key Features
PT1 SUBCATEGORIZATION

- The new AJCC notes the importance of pT1 subcategorization yet acknowledges that more research is needed to determine an optimal system for subcategorization.

Table 3
Updates and recommendations in the 8th edition of the American Joint Committee on Cancer TNM staging system

Stage Category	Details
pT1	Subcategorization of pT1 recommended, but no specific approach has been officially endorsed.
pT2	Staging of diverticular cancers skips pT2 (from pT1 to pT3).
pT4	Prostatic stromal invasion must be transmural extension from the bladder and intraurethral prostatic stromal invasion is staged as pT2 (by urethral cancer staging).
N1	Perivesical lymph node added into regional lymph nodes.
M1	Distant metastasis divided into nonregional lymph node only (M1a) and non–lymph node distant metastases (M1b).

Data from Amin MB, Edge SB, Greene FL, et al. AJCC cancer staging manual. 8th edition. New York: Springer Nature; 2017.

Approximately 50% of pT1 tumors are upstaged to pT2 or higher at the time of RC, and 33% are upstaged to non–organ-confined (>pT2) disease.[48,49] Subcategorization of pT1 tumors aims to better stratify this heterogeneous group of tumors in TUR and, therefore, is highly recommended. Although the approach is yet to be standardized, 2 major methods have been studied. The most studied is histoanatomic substaging, which uses the muscularis mucosae (MM) and/or vascular plexus as landmarks to divide the extent of LP invasion.[47,50–52] Both 3-tiered (above [pT1a], into [pT1b], and below [pT1c]) and 2-tiered (above [pT1a] and below [pT1b]) systems have been used, and most studies using the 2-tiered system demonstrate worse outcomes in pT1b tumors. The inherent problem with this approach is that the MM is often discontinuous or absent, with significant temporal variation (present in dome in 75% of cases vs 10% in trigone).[53] Although the vascular plexus may be used as a surrogate, its location is also variable. Overall, histoanatomic substaging was feasible in 43% to 100% of studies. The second method is micrometric substaging, which measures the extent of invasion. The most recognized approach uses a 0.5-mm (1 high-power field) cutoff (measured from the basement membrane) to divide pT1 into pT1m (microinvasive) and pT1e (extensive) (**Fig. 8**).[47,54,55] Unlike histoanatomic substaging, micrometric substaging using 0.5 mm was feasible in 100% of cases.[51,54–59] Multiple studies have shown micrometric substage to be an independent predictor of outcome in pT1 tumors.[51,54–59] Other studies have also used different micrometric cutoffs to divide pT1, such as 1-mm (×200 field), 1.5-mm, 3-mm depth, and 6-mm diameter of invasion.[51,57,60,61]

Recent studies also suggest that measuring the aggregate length of invasive carcinoma involving 1 or multiple TUR fragments is a superior method for pT1 subcategorization.[62,63] A cutoff of 2.3 mm has been suggested as the best predictor of progression. This proposal, however, needs further validation.[62]

pT2 Tumors

Urothelial carcinoma extending into the MP layer is staged as pT2. Diagnosis of pT2 tumor on TUR is the major criteria for RC and, therefore, proper diagnosis of MP invasion is critical.[3,4] A major diagnostic dilemma, however, is the distinction between MP and MM muscle bundle involvement by tumor.[47] The MM is not infrequently hyperplastic

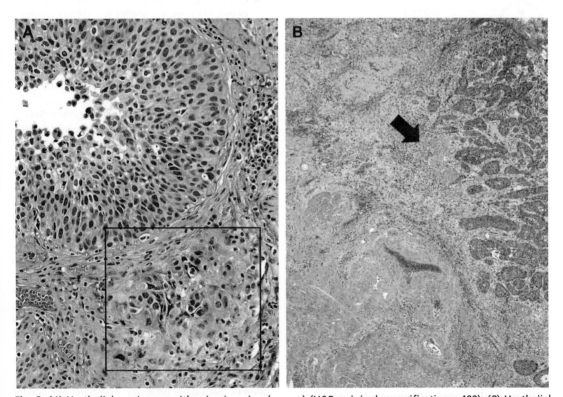

Fig. 8. (*A*) Urothelial carcinoma with microinvasion (*square*) (H&E, original magnification ×400). (*B*) Urothelial carcinoma with more extensive LP invasion, including MM involvement (*arrow*) (H&E, original magnification ×100).

and, therefore, can mimic MP in a poorly oriented TUR specimen. Additionally, in approximately 50% of cases, the hyperplastic MM has compact parallel muscle fibers and regular outlines, further mimicking MP appearance (MP-like).[53]

Key Features
MM

- Helpful morphologic clues for MM include its closeness to the surface epithelium, relationship to the vascular plexus, nonintermingling with adipose tissue (more common in deep LP), and typically occurring as isolated or few separate muscle bundles, even when hyperplastic.

MP in contrast is typically a tight aggregate of several larger muscle bundles of approximately similar size and shape displayed both vertically and horizontally. The presence of adjacent adipose tissue can be a helpful feature in identifying MP.[53,64]

Pitfall
MP INVASION

- Infiltrating carcinoma may also cause extensive fraying and fracturing of the MP, and the fragmented MP fibers can resemble MM bundles (Fig. 9A).

Care should be taken to appreciate the overall rounded outline of the frayed MP bundle on low-power view, better highlighted amid the infiltrating carcinoma and desmoplasia by use of smooth muscle markers, such as smoothelin or desmin.[31,47,65]

The immunohistochemical marker smoothelin has been suggested as a tool to distinguish hyperplastic MM from MP in difficult cases, because several studies have shown that it usually shows unequal staining of MP (usually strong) and MM (usually weak or absent).[31,65–70] The staining is highly dependent, however, on laboratory-dependent staining protocols and some overlap in staining does exist. Thus, care should be exercised in interpreting smoothelin when discriminating MP versus MM, particularly if the muscle of interest is not staining strongly and there is no internal MP control with strong staining. Correlation of the strong staining to the usual MP outline is also essential.

Key Features
IMMUNOSTAINING FOR FRAYED MP

- Because of its unequal MP and MM staining property, lack of staining in myofibroblasts or desmoplasia, and retention of staining in cauterized muscles, smoothelin, in the authors', experience is preferable (compared with desmin) in highlighting frayed MP muscle bundles (described previously).[31,65,67]

The MP layer in the bladder not only is composed of smooth muscle bundle but also contains fibroconnective tissue, adipose tissue, and vessels in-between the muscle bundles. Although carcinoma infiltrating into an MP muscle bundle is a definitive pT2 disease, tumor situated in-between MP muscle bundles within the MP layer should also be staged as pT2.

Key Features
STAGING pT2 WITHOUT MP
MUSCLE BUNDLE INFILTRATION

- Carcinoma that has infiltrated into spaces between MP muscle bundles and clearly crosses the LP–inner MP boundary in an orientable specimen, including TUR, should be staged as pT2, even in the absence of direct MP muscle bundle infiltration.

For example, in TURs where fragmentation is common, invasive carcinoma nests surrounded by MP muscle bundles should be categorized as pT2, even without MP muscle infiltration (Fig. 9B). Likewise, invasive carcinoma surrounding an MP muscle bundle in the absence of infiltration should be categorized as pT2 (Fig. 9C). The principle of defining the LP–inner MP boundary (for pT1 vs pT2) should also follow the common approach in demarcating the outer MP–perivesical tissue boundary (for pT2b vs pT3a)[47,71] (discussed later).

In RC, pT2 stage is subclassified as pT2a (involving inner half of MP) and pT2b (extending to outer half of MP), and involvement of perivesical soft tissue is staged as pT3 disease. Involvement of adipose tissue clearly within the MP layer remains as pT2 (Fig. 9D).[64] The outer boundary of MP bordering the perivesical soft tissue is another point of diagnostic difficulty. The outer MP border can be irregular, with MP muscle bundles positioned at varying levels separated by adipose or

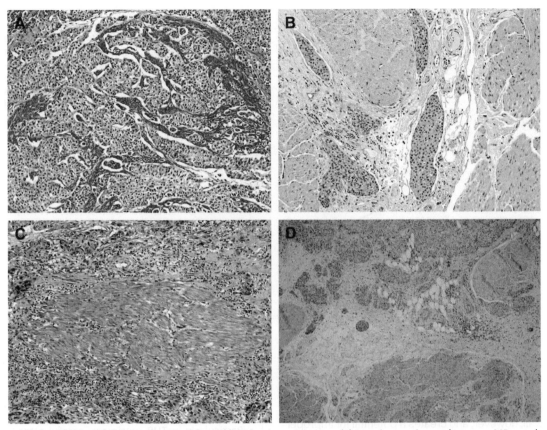

Fig. 9. (*A*) MP extensively involved and frayed by invasive carcinoma. (*B*) Invasive carcinoma between MP muscle bundles. (*C*) Invasive carcinoma surrounding a MP muscle bundle. (*D*) Involvement of adipose tissue by carcinoma within the MP layer (H&E, original magnification [*A-C*] ×200, [*D*] ×100).

fibrous tissues, creating difficulty when distinguishing pT2b from pT3a disease.[71] pT3 disease is usually treated with adjuvant chemotherapy and, therefore, represents a crucial distinction for patient management.[3,4]

> ### Key Features
> #### DEFINITION OF OUTER MP AND PERIVESICAL SOFT TISSUE BOUNDARY
>
> - In cases of irregular outer MP–perivesical soft tissue boundary, most experts advocate for interconnecting the outmost aspect of the MP muscle bundles with a straight line to define the boundary.[71]

Therefore, tumors that focally involve adipose tissue but without crossing this line are staged by more experts as pT2b (**Fig. 10**). Although this schema has not yet been validated with clinical data, the approach provides consistency and better accuracy when classifying patients with non–organ-confined disease, important for giving

adjuvant chemotherapy and for enrollment in clinical chemotherapeutic trials.

Diverticular Tumors

The 8E AJCC provided clarification regarding staging of urothelial carcinomas arising within bladder diverticula.[9] Because most bladder diverticula in adults are acquired and, therefore, lack an MP layer, the tumor invades directly from the LP into the perivesical soft tissue.[72–77]

>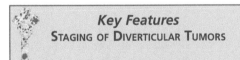
>
> ### Key Features
> #### STAGING OF DIVERTICULAR TUMORS
>
> - Therefore, the 8E AJCC specifically advises skipping the pT2 stage and staging as pT3 if the tumor has spread beyond the LP (**Fig. 11**).

The absence of an MP layer is believed to allow more aggressive tumor invasion, but limited studies suggest comparable outcomes to nondiverticular urothelial carcinoma.[74,77]

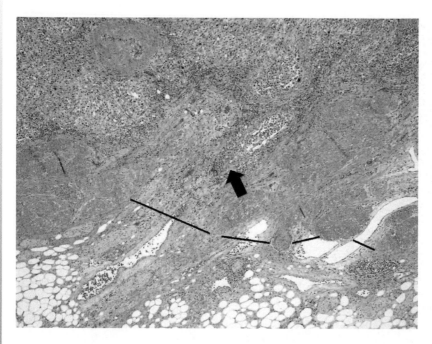

Fig. 10. Outer MP muscle bundles are interconnected to define the boundary; the furthest extent of the tumor (*arrow*) does not cross the line and is staged as pT2b (H&E, original magnification ×40).

pT3 Tumors

Urothelial carcinoma extending into the perivesical soft tissue constitutes pT3 disease. Adipose tissue can also be present in other layers of the bladder wall, however, and creates a potential for improper staging.[53,64] Adipose tissue is present in the LP of greater than 50% of cystectomies and in the MP in 100% of RCs.[64]

Key Features
STAGING OF CARCINOMA
INVOLVING ADIPOSE TISSUE

- Particularly in TUR specimens, careful attention should be paid to avoid overinterpreting adipose tissue involvement as pT3 disease.

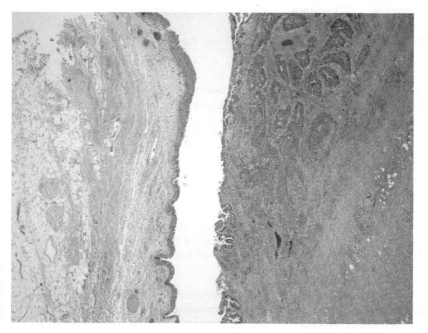

Fig. 11. Bladder diverticulum with urothelial carcinoma invasive into the peri-diverticular soft tissue (pT3). Note the CIS at the opposite wall (H&E, original magnification ×40).

Because the adipose tissue is usually present in the deep LP and between MP muscle bundles, this can also be used as a landmark on a TUR specimen to carefully search for nearby MP muscle fibers and associated invasion by tumor cells.[53]

Stage pT3 is subcategorized into pT3a and pT3b, which represents microscopic (pT3a) and macroscopically (pT3b) visible tumor. pT3b substaging has been shown in most studies to be an independent predictor of worse patient outcomes, including disease recurrence and cancer-specific death.[78–82]

KEY Features
MACROSCOPIC PERIVESICAL SOFT TISSUE INVASION

- Appropriate use of the pT3b subcategory relies predominantly on careful scrutinization of the gross bladder specimen.

In centers where RC specimens are grossly examined by house staff or pathology assistants, education as to the importance of identifying the gross extent and sampling of perivesical invasion is of paramount importance, and gross photography can also be helpful. Lack of documentation or sampling of macroscopic perivesical soft tissue invasion may lead to understaging.[83] In contrast, reactive changes, fibrosis, and inflammation around the tumor may result in gross overestimation as a macroscopic tumor. The recognition of bulky perivesical soft tissue involvement on the slides without documentation of macroscopic involvement should prompt re-examination of the gross specimen.

pT4 Tumors

Urothelial carcinoma invading through the bladder wall and into adjacent organs or structures is designated as pT4. Stage pT4 is subcategorized into pT4a (direct invasion of prostate, uterus, or vagina) and pT4b (pelvic or abdominal walls). Several studies in pT4a tumors have shown gender-related differences in outcome after RC with poorer prognosis in women than in men.[84–86] The reason for the gender disparity is unclear and is likely multifactorial, including due to anatomic factors.[47] Seminal vesicle invasion is categorized as pT4 without further distinction, although data suggest a behavior comparable to pT4b tumors.[87–89]

The new 8E AJCC clarifies staging of prostatic involvement by urothelial carcinoma, which occurs in 13% to 29% of bladder cancers.[47] There are 2 distinct mechanisms of prostatic stromal invasion: (1) direct transmural spread of urothelial carcinoma through the bladder wall the perivesicular soft tissue into the prostatic stroma and (2) intraurethral spread of urothelial carcinoma to the prostate with subsequent prostatic stromal invasion (**Fig. 12**).[90–96] As might be expected, direct transmural spread of deeply invasive urothelial carcinomas is associated with a higher rate of lymph node (LN) involvement and worse cancer-specific and overall survival compared with intraurethral spread.[90–96]

Key Features
STAGING BLADDER CANCER WITH PROSTATE INVASION

- Because of the differences in mechanism and patient outcomes, 2 different staging schemes (bladder and urethral cancer pT staging) should be used in bladder cancer with intraurethral spread to prostate.

Direct transmural spread of urothelial carcinoma into the prostatic stroma should be categorized as pT4a. The 8E AJCC clarified, however, that intraurethral spread of urothelial carcinoma with prostatic stromal invasion should be categorized as pT2 according to the urethral pT staging (not the bladder pT staging).[9] The bladder tumor should then be assigned a separate pT stage according to bladder pT staging, resulting in 2 separate pT stages for the specimen.

Key Features
STAGING UROTHELIAL CARCINOMA IN TUR OF PROSTATE

- In the scenario of prostatic stromal invasion of urothelial carcinoma discovered in a prostate TUR specimen, the authors recommend that a pT stage should not be rendered, and clinical correlation should be performed.

A comment stating that clinical correlation is required for appropriate staging should be provided and should note that in the absence of direct transmural spread, the prostatic stromal invasion should be staged as pT2 according to the urethral cancer staging.[47] Some transmural invasion into the prostate by bladder cancer may not be visible within the bladder by cystoscopy.[97]

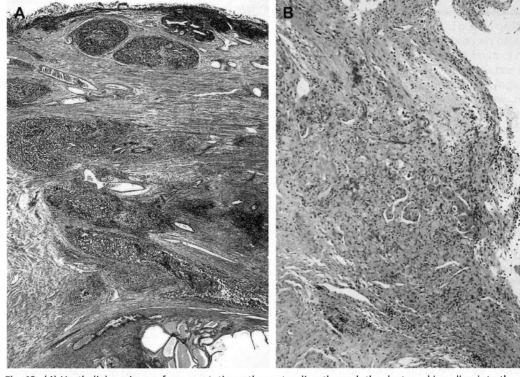

Fig. 12. (*A*) Urothelial carcinoma from prostatic urethra extending through the ducts and invading into the prostatic stroma (pT2 by urethral cancer staging) (H&E, original magnification ×40). (*B*) Bladder proper contains residual invasive urothelial carcinoma in the LP (pT1) (H&E, original magnification ×200).

REGIONAL LYMPH NODES

Nodal staging in urothelial carcinoma is determined by the location and number of positive LNs. pN1 describes a single regional LN metastasis in the true pelvis. In the previous AJCC edition, this included only hypogastric, obturator, external iliac, and presacral LNs. Perivesical LNs, however, are a major source of lymphatic draining from the bladder and may be identified in up to half of RC specimens. Although not typically excised separately by the surgeon, perivesical LNs are positive in up to 10% of RCs and have been shown an independent predictor of survival.[98,99]

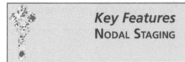

Key Features
NODAL STAGING

- Perivesical LNs are now considered regional nodes and involvement by tumor is staged as pN1.

Multiple positive regional LNs are staged as pN2. Metastases to the common iliac LNs are staged as pN3. Additionally, prognostic stage group III has been subdivided into IIIA and IIIB based on the pN subcategory (stage group III with pN1–IIIA, stage group III with pN2/3–IIIB).

METASTASES

In the previous AJCC, a stage of pM1 was designated for both nonregional LN metastases and distant non-LN metastases. The presence of distant non-nodal metastases, however, is now known to be independently predictive of worse outcomes in metastatic or unresectable disease, even when treated with chemotherapy.[100–104] Alternatively, better outcomes have been observed in patients with metastasis limited to nonregional LNs (5-year survival 20.9% vs 6.8% in those with visceral or bone metastases, respectively), and a subset of patients become long-term survivors after systemic chemotherapy.[100,101]

Key Features
METASTASIS STAGING

- 8E AJCC now distinguishes between LN positivity beyond the common iliac (pM1a) and all other non-LN metastases (pM1b).

Additionally, prognostic stage group IV has been subdivided into IVA and IVB based on the pM1 subcategory (stage group III with pM1a–pMIVA, stage group IV with pM1b–pMIVB).

REFERENCES

1. Babjuk M, Bohle A, Burger M, et al. EAU guidelines on non-muscle-invasive urothelial carcinoma of the bladder: update 2016. Eur Urol 2017;71(3):447–61.
2. Chang SS, Boorjian SA, Chou R, et al. Diagnosis and treatment of non-muscle invasive bladder cancer: AUA/SUO guideline. J Urol 2016;196(4):1021–9.
3. Chang SS, Bochner BH, Chou R, et al. Treatment of non-metastatic muscle-invasive bladder cancer: AUA/ASCO/ASTRO/SUO guideline. J Urol 2017;198(3):552–9.
4. Alfred Witjes J, Lebret T, Comperat EM, et al. Updated 2016 EAU guidelines on muscle-invasive and metastatic bladder cancer. Eur Urol 2017;71(3):462–75.
5. NCCN Clinical practical guidelines in oncology (NCCN Guidelines). 2018. Available at: https://www.nccn.org/professionals/physician_gls/pdf/bladder.pdf. Accessed May 16, 2018.
6. Moch H, Humphrey PA, Ulbright TM, et al. WHO classification of tumours of the urinary system and male genital organs. 4th edition. Geneva (Switzerland): WHO Press; 2016.
7. Amin MB, McKenney JK, Paner GP, et al. ICUD-EAU international consultation on bladder cancer 2012: pathology. Eur Urol 2013;63(1):16–35.
8. Amin MB, Smith SC, Reuter VE, et al. Update for the practicing pathologist: the international consultation on urologic disease-european association of urology consultation on bladder cancer. Mod Pathol 2015;28(5):612–30.
9. Amin MB, Edge SB, Greene FL, et al. AJCC cancer staging manual. 8th edition. Chicago: Springer; 2016.
10. Paner GP, Stadler WM, Hansel DE, et al. Updates in the eighth edition of the tumor-node-metastasis staging classification for urologic cancers. Eur Urol 2018;73(4):560–9.
11. Comperat EM, Burger M, Gontero P, et al. Grading of urothelial carcinoma and the new "World Health Organisation classification of tumours of the urinary system and male genital organs 2016. Eur Urol Focus 2018. https://doi.org/10.1016/j.euf.2018.01.003.
12. Mostofi FK, Sobin L, Torloni H. International histological classification of tumours. Histological typing of urinary bladder tumours. Geneva (Switzerland): World Health Organization; 1973.
13. Epstein JI, Amin MB, Reuter VR, et al. The World Health Organization/international society of urological pathology consensus classification of urothelial (transitional cell) neoplasms of the urinary bladder. bladder consensus conference committee. Am J Surg Pathol 1998;22(12):1435–48.
14. Eble JN, Sauter G, Epstein JI, et al. World Health Organization classification of tumours. pathology & genetics. tumours of the urinary system and male genital organs. Geneva (Switzerland): World Health Organization; 2004.
15. Soukup V, Capoun O, Cohen D, et al. Prognostic performance and reproducibility of the 1973 and 2004/2016 World Health Organization grading classification systems in non-muscle-invasive bladder cancer: a european association of urology non-muscle invasive bladder cancer guidelines panel systematic review. Eur Urol 2017;72(5):801–13.
16. Cheng L, Neumann RM, Nehra A, et al. Cancer heterogeneity and its biologic implications in the grading of urothelial carcinoma. Cancer 2000;88(7):1663–70.
17. Billis A, Carvalho RB, Mattos AC, et al. Tumor grade heterogeneity in urothelial bladder carcinoma–proposal of a system using combined numbers. Scand J Urol Nephrol 2001;35(4):275–9.
18. Reis LO, Taheri D, Chaux A, et al. Significance of a minor high-grade component in a low-grade noninvasive papillary urothelial carcinoma of bladder. Hum Pathol 2016;47(1):20–5.
19. Gofrit ON, Pizov G, Shapiro A, et al. Mixed high and low grade bladder tumors–are they clinically high or low grade? J Urol 2014;191(6):1693–6.
20. Taylor DC, Bhagavan BS, Larsen MP, et al. Papillary urothelial hyperplasia. A precursor to papillary neoplasms. Am J Surg Pathol 1996;20(12):1481–8.
21. Readal N, Epstein JI. Papillary urothelial hyperplasia: relationship to urothelial neoplasms. Pathology 2010;42(4):360–3.
22. Amin MB, McKenney JK. An approach to the diagnosis of flat intraepithelial lesions of the urinary bladder using the World Health Organization/international society of urological pathology consensus classification system. Adv Anat Pathol 2002;9(4):222–32.
23. Lane Z, Epstein JI. Polypoid/papillary cystitis: a series of 41 cases misdiagnosed as papillary urothelial neoplasia. Am J Surg Pathol 2008;32(5):758–64.
24. Oliva E, Young RH. Nephrogenic adenoma of the urinary tract: a review of the microscopic appearance of 80 cases with emphasis on unusual features. Mod Pathol 1995;8(7):722–30.
25. McDaniel AS, Chinnaiyan AM, Siddiqui J, et al. Immunohistochemical staining characteristics of nephrogenic adenoma using the PIN-4 cocktail (p63, AMACR, and CK903) and GATA-3. Am J Surg Pathol 2014;38(12):1664–71.

26. Tong GX, Weeden EM, Hamele-Bena D, et al. Expression of PAX8 in nephrogenic adenoma and clear cell adenocarcinoma of the lower urinary tract: evidence of related histogenesis? Am J Surg Pathol 2008;32(9):1380–7.

27. Tong GX, Melamed J, Mansukhani M, et al. PAX2: a reliable marker for nephrogenic adenoma. Mod Pathol 2006;19(3):356–63.

28. Owens CL, Epstein JI. Significance of denuded urothelium in papillary urothelial lesions. Am J Surg Pathol 2007;31(2):298–303.

29. McKenney JK, Gomez JA, Desai S, et al. Morphologic expressions of urothelial carcinoma in situ: a detailed evaluation of its histologic patterns with emphasis on carcinoma in situ with microinvasion. Am J Surg Pathol 2001;25(3):356–62.

30. McKenney JK, Desai S, Cohen C, et al. Discriminatory immunohistochemical staining of urothelial carcinoma in situ and non-neoplastic urothelium: an analysis of cytokeratin 20, p53, and CD44 antigens. Am J Surg Pathol 2001;25(8):1074–8.

31. Amin MB, Trpkov K, Lopez-Beltran A, et al. Members of the IIiDUPG. Best practices recommendations in the application of immunohistochemistry in the bladder lesions: report from the International Society of Urologic Pathology consensus conference. Am J Surg Pathol 2014;38(8):e20–34.

32. Lawless ME, Tretiakova MS, True LD, et al. Flat urothelial lesions with atypia: interobserver concordance and added value of immunohistochemical profiling. Appl Immunohistochem Mol Morphol 2018;26(3):180–5.

33. Aron M, Luthringer DJ, McKenney JK, et al. Utility of a triple antibody cocktail intraurothelial neoplasm-3 (IUN-3-CK20/CD44s/p53) and alpha-methylacyl-CoA racemase (AMACR) in the distinction of urothelial carcinoma in situ (CIS) and reactive urothelial atypia. Am J Surg Pathol 2013; 37(12):1815–23.

34. Oliva E, Pinheiro NF, Heney NM, et al. Immunohistochemistry as an adjunct in the differential diagnosis of radiation-induced atypia versus urothelial carcinoma in situ of the bladder: a study of 45 cases. Hum Pathol 2013;44(5):860–6.

35. Amin MBT, Tickoo SK, McKenney JK, et al. Diagnostic pathology. Genitourinary. 2nd edition. Salt Lake City (UT): Elsevier, Inc; 2016.

36. Epstein JIA, Reuter VE, Amin MB. Biopsy interpretation of the bladder. 3rd edition. Philadelphia: Wolters Kluwer; 2017.

37. Cox R, Epstein JI. Large nested variant of urothelial carcinoma: 23 cases mimicking von Brunn nests and inverted growth pattern of noninvasive papillary urothelial carcinoma. Am J Surg Pathol 2011; 35(9):1337–42.

38. Comperat E, McKenney JK, Hartmann A, et al. Large nested variant of urothelial carcinoma: a clinicopathological study of 36 cases. Histopathology 2017;71(5):703–10.

39. Tian W, Epstein JI. Invasive low-grade papillary urothelial carcinoma: an immunohistochemical study of 26 cases. Hum Pathol 2015;46(12):1836–41.

40. Watts KE, Montironi R, Mazzucchelli R, et al. Clinicopathologic characteristics of 23 cases of invasive low-grade papillary urothelial carcinoma. Urology 2012;80(2):361–6.

41. Linder BJ, Frank I, Cheville JC, et al. Outcomes following radical cystectomy for nested variant of urothelial carcinoma: a matched cohort analysis. J Urol 2013;189(5):1670–5.

42. Wasco MJ, Daignault S, Bradley D, et al. Nested variant of urothelial carcinoma: a clinicopathologic and immunohistochemical study of 30 pure and mixed cases. Hum Pathol 2010;41(2):163–71.

43. Lin O, Cardillo M, Dalbagni G, et al. Nested variant of urothelial carcinoma: a clinicopathologic and immunohistochemical study of 12 cases. Mod Pathol 2003;16(12):1289–98.

44. Lopez Beltran A, Montironi R, Cheng L. Microcystic urothelial carcinoma: morphology, immunohistochemistry and clinical behaviour. Histopathology 2014;64(6):872–9.

45. Kryvenko ON, Epstein JI. Pseudocarcinomatous urothelial hyperplasia of the bladder: clinical findings and followup of 70 patients. J Urol 2013;189(6): 2083–6.

46. Chan TY, Epstein JI. Radiation or chemotherapy cystitis with "pseudocarcinomatous" features. Am J Surg Pathol 2004;28(7):909–13.

47. Paner GP, Montironi R, Amin MB. Challenges in pathologic staging of bladder cancer: proposals for fresh approaches of assessing pathologic stage in light of recent studies and observations pertaining to bladder histoanatomic variances. Adv Anat Pathol 2017;24(3):113–27.

48. Fritsche HM, Burger M, Svatek RS, et al. Characteristics and outcomes of patients with clinical T1 grade 3 urothelial carcinoma treated with radical cystectomy: results from an international cohort. Eur Urol 2010;57(2):300–9.

49. Shariat SF, Palapattu GS, Karakiewicz PI, et al. Discrepancy between clinical and pathologic stage: impact on prognosis after radical cystectomy. Eur Urol 2007;51(1):137–49, [discussion: 149–51].

50. Roupret M, Seisen T, Comperat E, et al. Prognostic interest in discriminating muscularis mucosa invasion (T1a vs T1b) in nonmuscle invasive bladder carcinoma: French national multicenter study with central pathology review. J Urol 2013;189(6): 2069–76.

51. Patriarca C, Hurle R, Moschini M, et al. Usefulness of pT1 substaging in papillary urothelial bladder carcinoma. Diagn Pathol 2016;11:6.

52. Orsola A, Werner L, de Torres I, et al. Reexamining treatment of high-grade T1 bladder cancer according to depth of lamina propria invasion: a prospective trial of 200 patients. Br J Cancer 2015;112(3): 468–74.

53. Paner GP, Ro JY, Wojcik EM, et al. Further characterization of the muscle layers and lamina propria of the urinary bladder by systematic histologic mapping: implications for pathologic staging of invasive urothelial carcinoma. Am J Surg Pathol 2007;31(9): 1420–9.

54. van Rhijn BW, van der Kwast TH, Alkhateeb SS, et al. A new and highly prognostic system to discern T1 bladder cancer substage. Eur Urol 2012;61(2):378–84.

55. van der Aa MN, van Leenders GJ, Steyerberg EW, et al. A new system for substaging pT1 papillary bladder cancer: a prognostic evaluation. Hum Pathol 2005;36(9):981–6.

56. Bertz S, Denzinger S, Otto W, et al. Substaging by estimating the size of invasive tumour can improve risk stratification in pT1 urothelial bladder cancer-evaluation of a large hospital-based single-centre series. Histopathology 2011;59(4):722–32.

57. Chang WC, Chang YH, Pan CC. Prognostic significance in substaging ofT1 urinary bladder urothelial carcinoma on transurethral resection. Am J Surg Pathol 2012;36(3):454–61.

58. Nishiyama N, Kitamura H, Maeda T, et al. Clinico-pathological analysis of patients with non-muscle-invasive bladder cancer: prognostic value and clinical reliability of the 2004 WHO classification system. Jpn J Clin Oncol 2013;43(11):1124–31.

59. DE Marco V, Cerruto MA, D'Elia C, et al. Prognostic role of substaging in T1G3 transitional cell carcinoma of the urinary bladder. Mol Clin Oncol 2014; 2(4):575–80.

60. Cheng L, Neumann RM, Weaver AL, et al. Predicting cancer progression in patients with stage T1 bladder carcinoma. J Clin Oncol 1999;17(10): 3182–7.

61. Brimo F, Wu C, Zeizafoun N, et al. Prognostic factors in T1 bladder urothelial carcinoma: the value of recording millimetric depth of invasion, diameter of invasive carcinoma, and muscularis mucosa invasion. Hum Pathol 2013;44(1):95–102.

62. Leivo MZ, Sahoo D, Hamilton Z, et al. Analysis of T1 bladder cancer on biopsy and transurethral resection specimens: comparison and ranking of T1 quantification approaches to predict progression to muscularis propria invasion. Am J Surg Pathol 2018;42(1):e1–10.

63. Hu Z, Mudaliar K, Quek ML, et al. Measuring the dimension of invasive component in pT1 urothelial carcinoma in transurethral resection specimens can predict time to recurrence. Ann Diagn Pathol 2014;18(2):49–52.

64. Philip AT, Amin MB, Tamboli P, et al. Intravesical adipose tissue: a quantitative study of its presence and location with implications for therapy and prognosis. Am J Surg Pathol 2000;24(9):1286–90.

65. Paner GP, Brown JG, Lapetino S, et al. Diagnostic use of antibody to smoothelin in the recognition of muscularis propria in transurethral resection of urinary bladder tumor (TURBT) specimens. Am J Surg Pathol 2010;34(6):792–9.

66. Council L, Hameed O. Differential expression of immunohistochemical markers in bladder smooth muscle and myofibroblasts, and the potential utility of desmin, smoothelin, and vimentin in staging of bladder carcinoma. Mod Pathol 2009;22(5): 639–50.

67. Paner GP, Shen SS, Lapetino S, et al. Diagnostic utility of antibody to smoothelin in the distinction of muscularis propria from muscularis mucosae of the urinary bladder: a potential ancillary tool in the pathologic staging of invasive urothelial carcinoma. Am J Surg Pathol 2009;33(1):91–8.

68. Bovio IM, Al-Quran SZ, Rosser CJ, et al. Smoothelin immunohistochemistry is a useful adjunct for assessing muscularis propria invasion in bladder carcinoma. Histopathology 2010;56(7):951–6.

69. Miyamoto H, Sharma RB, Illei PB, et al. Pitfalls in the use of smoothelin to identify muscularis propria invasion by urothelial carcinoma. Am J Surg Pathol 2010;34(3):418–22.

70. Chakravarthy R, Ahmed K, Abbasi S, et al. In response–a modified staining protocol for Smoothelin immunostaining. Virchows Arch 2011;459(1): 119–20.

71. Ananthanarayanan V, Pan Y, Tretiakova M, et al. Influence of histologic criteria and confounding factors in staging equivocal cases for microscopic perivesical tissue invasion (pT3a): an interobserver study among genitourinary pathologists. Am J Surg Pathol 2014;38(2):167–75.

72. Walker NF, Gan C, Olsburgh J, et al. Diagnosis and management of intradiverticular bladder tumours. Nat Rev Urol 2014;11(7):383–90.

73. Hansel DE, Paner GP, Nese N, et al. Limited smoothelin expression within the muscularis mucosae: validation in bladder diverticula. Hum Pathol 2011;42(11):1770–6.

74. Golijanin D, Yossepowitch O, Beck SD, et al. Carcinoma in a bladder diverticulum: presentation and treatment outcome. J Urol 2003;170(5):1761–4.

75. Idrees MT, Alexander RE, Kum JB, et al. The spectrum of histopathologic findings in vesical diverticulum: implications for pathogenesis and staging. Hum Pathol 2013;44(7):1223–32.

76. Tamas EF, Stephenson AJ, Campbell SC, et al. Histopathologic features and clinical outcomes in 71 cases of bladder diverticula. Arch Pathol Lab Med 2009;133(5):791–6.

77. Hu B, Satkunasivam R, Schuckman A, et al. Urothelial carcinoma in bladder diverticula: outcomes after radical cystectomy. World J Urol 2015;33(10): 1397–402.

78. Scosyrev E, Yao J, Messing E. Microscopic invasion of perivesical fat by urothelial carcinoma: implications for prognosis and pathology practice. Urology 2010;76(4):908–13, [discussion: 914].

79. Neuzillet Y, Lebret T, Molinie V, et al. Perivesical fat invasion in bladder cancer: implications for prognosis comparing pT2b, pT3a and pT3b stages and consequences for adjuvant chemotherapy indications. BJU Int 2012;110(11): 1736–41.

80. Bastian PJ, Hutterer GC, Shariat SF, et al. Macroscopic, but not microscopic, perivesical fat invasion at radical cystectomy is an adverse predictor of recurrence and survival. BJU Int 2008;101(4): 450–4.

81. Sonpavde G, Khan MM, Svatek RS, et al. Prognostic risk stratification of pathological stage T3N0 bladder cancer after radical cystectomy. J Urol 2011;185(4):1216–21.

82. Tilki D, Svatek RS, Karakiewicz PI, et al. pT3 Substaging is a prognostic indicator for lymph node negative urothelial carcinoma of the bladder. J Urol 2010;184(2):470–4.

83. Tretter EM, Ebel JJ, Pohar KS, et al. Does the gross prosector impact pT3 subclassification or lymph node counts in bladder cancer? Hum Pathol 2017;61:190–8.

84. Aziz A, Shariat SF, Roghmann F, et al. Prediction of cancer-specific survival after radical cystectomy in pT4a urothelial carcinoma of the bladder: development of a tool for clinical decision-making. BJU Int 2016;117(2):272–9.

85. May M, Bastian PJ, Brookman-May S, et al. Gender-specific differences in cancer-specific survival after radical cystectomy for patients with urothelial carcinoma of the urinary bladder in pathologic tumor stage T4a. Urol Oncol 2013; 31(7):1141–7.

86. Tilki D, Reich O, Svatek RS, et al. Characteristics and outcomes of patients with clinical carcinoma in situ only treated with radical cystectomy: an international study of 243 patients. J Urol 2010; 183(5):1757–63.

87. You D, Kim SC, Jeong IG, et al. Urothelial carcinoma of the bladder with seminal vesicle invasion: prognostic significance. BJU Int 2010;106(11): 1657–61.

88. May M, Brookman-May S, Burger M, et al. Concomitant seminal vesicle invasion in pT4a urothelial carcinoma of the bladder with contiguous prostatic infiltration is an adverse prognosticator for cancer-specific survival after radical cystectomy. Ann Surg Oncol 2014;21(12):4034–40.

89. Daneshmand S, Stein JP, Lesser T, et al. Prognosis of seminal vesicle involvement by transitional cell carcinoma of the bladder. J Urol 2004; 172(1):81–4.

90. Knoedler JJ, Boorjian SA, Tollefson MK, et al. Urothelial carcinoma involving the prostate: the association of revised tumour stage and coexistent bladder cancer with survival after radical cystectomy. BJU Int 2014;114(6):832–6.

91. Njinou Ngninkeu B, Lorge F, Moulin P, et al. Transitional cell carcinoma involving the prostate: a clinicopathological retrospective study of 76 cases. J Urol 2003;169(1):149–52.

92. Esrig D, Freeman JA, Elmajian DA, et al. Transitional cell carcinoma involving the prostate with a proposed staging classification for stromal invasion. J Urol 1996;156(3):1071–6.

93. Ayyathurai R, Gomez P, Luongo T, et al. Prostatic involvement by urothelial carcinoma of the bladder: clinicopathological features and outcome after radical cystectomy. BJU Int 2007; 100(5):1021–5.

94. Pagano F, Bassi P, Ferrante GL, et al. Is stage pT4a (D1) reliable in assessing transitional cell carcinoma involvement of the prostate in patients with a concurrent bladder cancer? A necessary distinction for contiguous or noncontiguous involvement. J Urol 1996;155(1):244–7.

95. Vallo S, Gilfrich C, Burger M, et al. Comparative analysis of the effect of prostatic invasion patterns on cancer-specific mortality after radical cystectomy in pT4a urothelial carcinoma of the bladder. Urol Oncol 2016;34(10):432.e1-8.

96. Patel AR, Cohn JA, Abd El Latif A, et al. Validation of new AJCC exclusion criteria for subepithelial prostatic stromal invasion from pT4a bladder urothelial carcinoma. J Urol 2013; 189(1):53–8.

97. Donat SM, Genega EM, Herr HW, et al. Mechanisms of prostatic stromal invasion in patients with bladder cancer: clinical significance. J Urol 2001; 165(4):1117–20.

98. Bella AJ, Stitt LW, Chin JL, et al. The prognostic significance of metastatic perivesical lymph nodes identified in radical cystectomy specimens for transitional cell carcinoma of the bladder. J Urol 2003; 170(6 Pt 1):2253–7.

99. Hu B, Satkunasivam R, Schuckman A, et al. Significance of perivesical lymph nodes in radical cystectomy for bladder cancer. Urol Oncol 2014; 32(8):1158–65.

100. von der Maase H, Sengelov L, Roberts JT, et al. Long-term survival results of a randomized trial comparing gemcitabine plus cisplatin, with methotrexate, vinblastine, doxorubicin, plus cisplatin in patients with bladder cancer. J Clin Oncol 2005; 23(21):4602–8.

101. Galsky MD, Moshier E, Krege S, et al. Nomogram for predicting survival in patients with unresectable and/or metastatic urothelial cancer who are treated with cisplatin-based chemotherapy. Cancer 2013; 119(16):3012–9.

102. Stadler WM, Hayden A, von der Maase H, et al. Long-term survival in phase II trials of gemcitabine plus cisplatin for advanced transitional cell cancer. Urol Oncol 2002;7(4):153–7.

103. Bajorin DF, Dodd PM, Mazumdar M, et al. Long-term survival in metastatic transitional-cell carcinoma and prognostic factors predicting outcome of therapy. J Clin Oncol 1999;17(10):3173–81.

104. Apolo AB, Ostrovnaya I, Halabi S, et al. Prognostic model for predicting survival of patients with metastatic urothelial cancer treated with cisplatin-based chemotherapy. J Natl Cancer Inst 2013;105(7): 499–503.

Updates in Pathologic Staging and Histologic Grading of Renal Cell Carcinoma

Kanika Taneja, MD[a], Sean R. Williamson, MD[a,b],*

KEYWORDS

- Renal tumors • TNM staging • Staging neoplasms • Prognostic parameters • Renal cell carcinoma

---

Key points

- Renal cell carcinoma differs from other cancers, in that invasion of structures, in particular veins, can manifest as subtle tongue-like outpouchings.
- The likelihood of renal sinus invasion increases dramatically with increased tumor size.
- Larger tumors (>4–5 cm) should be carefully assessed for the possibility of renal sinus invasion.
- The current American Joint Commission on Cancer staging system removes the requirements that renal vein invasion be identified grossly and that vein walls must contain muscle to qualify for pT3a.
- Satellite nodules adjacent to, or away from, a large renal mass often represent retrograde spread of tumor within vein branches and should be regarded as multifocal tumors only after this has been excluded.

ABSTRACT

The most important prognostic parameter in renal cell carcinoma is tumor stage. Although pathologic primary tumor (pT) categories are influenced by tumor size (pT1–pT2), critical elements (≥pT3) are dictated by invasion of structures, including renal sinus, perinephric fat, and the renal vein or segmental branches. Because this invasion can be subtle, awareness of the unique characteristics of renal cell carcinoma is critical for the pathologist to aid in clinical decision making. This review addresses challenges in pathologic stage and grade reporting and updates to the World Health Organization and American Joint Commission on Cancer classification schemes.

OVERVIEW

Renal cell carcinoma (RCC) is the ninth and the fourteenth most common cancer in American men and women, respectively, and is the most lethal of the genitourinary tumors.[1] It is, however, not a single entity but rather a collection of diverse tumors believed to recapitulate the phenotypes of several parts of the nephron, each with distinct histologic and genetic features. Renal tumors, in contrast to many other invasive cancers with irregular or infiltrative configuration, are often spherical with subtle tongue-like extensions into renal veins,[2] renal sinus, or perinephric tissue, often without desmoplastic or destructive infiltrative response. As such, this potentially can

---

Disclosure Statement: The authors have no disclosures relevant to this work.
[a] Department of Pathology and Laboratory Medicine, Henry Ford Health System, Henry Ford Hospital, K6, W615, 2799 West Grand Boulevard, Detroit, MI 48202, USA; [b] Department of Pathology and Laboratory Medicine, Wayne State University School of Medicine, 2799 West Grand Boulevard, Detroit, MI 48202, USA
* Corresponding author.
E-mail address: swilli25@hfhs.org

surgpath.theclinics.com

be subtle compared with cancers of other organs. Thorough understanding of renal anatomy, adequate sampling of tissue, and anticipation of and careful search for the these findings important during gross examination and microscopic analysis.[3]

With the advancement in imaging techniques, a majority of renal masses now present incidentally.[4,5] Clinical and pathologic staging of RCC has often been revised to reflect this changing presentation[6,7] as well as better understanding of prognostic features.[4,8] This article reviews the prognostic factors in RCC in the context of American Joint Committee on Cancer (AJCC), 8th edition,[9] TNM staging system. The methodology of gross and microscopic examination relevant to staging and grading of RCC also are reviewed.

IMPORTANCE OF PATHOLOGIC STAGING OF RENAL CANCER

Cancer staging in general uses the available tumor characteristics to stratify patients into clinically meaningful and prognostically relevant categories. Other outcome prediction models[10,11] that include stage as a variable have been developed to improve on prognostic information provided by stage alone. These tools can predict survival, metastases, and pattern of disease recurrence. At the same time, staging provides an easy to reference and nearly uniformly adopted prognostic tool. This also translates into a common language for treatment, prognostication, and publication purposes. Clinical staging is important to weigh treatment options, like nephron-sparing surgery versus radical nephrectomy,[12] especially in scenarios like solitary kidney[13] and decreased renal function. Pathologic staging, on the other hand, is a valuable tool that can guide clinical follow-up schedules, patient counseling, and enrollment in clinical trials.[14] The AJCC TNM system is the most recent and commonly used staging system. The 8th edition of AJCC staging system[9] (summarized in **Table 1**) defines TNM as local extension of the primary tumor (T), involvement of regional lymph nodes (N), and presence of distant metastasis (M). T stage is determined by tumor size and its extension into neighboring structures. Based on these pTNM categories, the system categorizes renal masses into stages I to IV. Surveillance, Epidemiology, and End Results statistics show that there has been a stage migration in presentation of RCC over the years. Currently, most RCC presents in the localized stage (65%), with 16% having regional lymph node spread and 16%

having distant metastases. The 5-year overall survival for localized disease is 92.6%, falling precipitously with regional spread (66.7%) and metastases (11.7%).[15]

TUMOR SIZE (T1/T2)

Most oncological staging systems are based on the size and anatomic extent of disease. Staging in RCC is similar to staging of other cancers in terms of tumor size; however, features, including renal sinus invasion,[16] vein invasion,[17] perinephric fat invasion,[18] and tumor thrombus,[19] can potentially upstage cases, which, based on size alone, would have been classified as lower-stage tumors. Tumor size has been shown to be associated with survival in multiple studies.[20–24] It is known that the survival is decreased by a factor of 3.5 when the tumor size is doubled.[24] Because 7 cm seems predictive of poor outcomes,[25] the 8th edition of the AJCC staging manual continues to classify tumors greater than 7 cm as pathologic primary tumor (pT) 2. It is prudent to note, however, that more than 90% of clear cell RCCs greater than or equal to 7 cm are found to invade the renal sinus, which increases the tumor to pT3a.[26] As such, it has been argued that at this size, it is rare for RCC to be confined to the kidney.[27] In the 8th edition of AJCC, tumor size greater than 10 cm is classified as pT2b; however, again, this is quite rare, at least for clear cell RCC, because almost all of these tumors would be found to have renal sinus, vein, or perinephric invasion with careful sampling.[27,28] Some tumors of this size may represent the phenomenon of retrograde venous invasion, discussed later, in which confluent intravenous growth may lead to confusion as to where the primary tumor ends and venous spread begins.[28,29]

As a convention, tumor size is generally measured in the fresh gross pathologic specimen.[3] There may be some variability, however, between radiologic and pathologic tumor measurements. For example, Tran and colleagues[30] assessed tumor size in fresh RCC specimens and compared it with postfixation specimens and the size reported by imaging. It was found that the maximum tumor diameter by imaging was 12.1% greater than the measurement in fresh specimens, which, in turn, was 4.6% larger than formalin-fixed specimens. Tumor size may be recorded after bisecting the specimen along the long axis, preferably in a plane through either the venous or collecting system, and measuring the greatest dimension of the tumor with a ruler (**Fig. 1**). The distance of tumor reaching beyond the kidney into perinephric tissue and the renal sinus is by convention included in this

Table 1
Changes in American Joint Committee on Cancer proposed TNM classification

	4th Edition	5th Edition	6th Edition	7th Edition	8th Edition
Publication year	1992	1997	2002	2009	2016
Effective year	1993	1998	2003	2010	2018
T1	Organ confined ≤2.5 cm	Organ confined ≤7 cm	Organ confined ≤7 cm	Organ confined ≤7 cm	Organ confined ≤7 cm
pT1a	Not defined	Not defined	Organ confined ≤4 cm	Organ confined ≤4 cm	Organ confined ≤4 cm
pT1b	Not defined	Not defined	Organ confined 4 cm–7 cm	Organ confined 4 cm–7 cm	Organ confined 4–7 cm
pT2	Organ confined >2.5 cm	Organ confined >7 cm	Organ confined >7 cm	Organ confined >7 cm	Organ confined >7 cm
pT2a	Not defined	Not defined	Not defined	Organ confined 7 cm–10 cm	Organ confined 7 cm–10 cm
pT2b	Not defined	Not defined	Not defined	Organ confined >10 cm	Organ confined >10 cm
pT3a	Perinephric tissue or contiguous into adrenal gland but not beyond Gerota fascia	Perinephric tissue or contiguous into adrenal gland but not beyond Gerota fascia	Perinephric tissue, renal sinus, or contiguous into adrenal gland but not beyond Gerota fascia	Perinephric tissue, renal sinus, or renal vein (including segmental, muscle-containing branches) but not beyond Gerota fascia	Perinephric tissue, renal sinus, renal vein/ segmental veins, or pelvicalyceal system but not beyond Gerota fascia
pT3b	Renal vein	Renal vein or vena cava below diaphragm	Renal vein or vena cava below diaphragm	Vena cava below diaphragm (without wall invasion)	Vena cava below diaphragm (without wall invasion)
pT3c	Vena cava below diaphragm	Vena cava above diaphragm	Vena cava above diaphragm	Vena cava above diaphragm or wall of vena cava at any level	Vena cava above diaphragm or wall of vena cava at any level

(continued on next page)

Table 1
(continued)

	4th Edition	5th Edition	6th Edition	7th Edition	8th Edition
pT4	Beyond Gerota fascia or vena cava above diaphragm	Beyond Gerota fascia	Beyond Gerota fascia	Beyond Gerota fascia or directly into adrenal gland	Beyond Gerota fascia or directly into adrenal gland
N0	No regional lymph node metastasis	No regional lymph node metastasis	No regional lymph node metastasis	No regional lymph node metastasis	No regional lymph node metastasis
N1	Metastasis in 1 lymph node ≤2 cm in greatest dimension	Metastasis in a single regional lymph node	Metastasis in a single regional lymph node	Metastasis in 1 or more lymph nodes	Metastasis in 1 or more lymph nodes
N2	Metastasis in 1 lymph node >2 but ≤5 cm in greatest dimension, or multiple lymph nodes, none >5 cm	Metastasis in more than 1 regional lymph node	Metastasis in more than 1 regional lymph node	NA	NA
N3	Metastasis in 1 lymph node >5 cm in greatest dimension	NA	NA	NA	NA
M1	Distant metastasis	Distant metastasis	Distant metastasis	Distant metastasis	Distant metastasis

Fig. 1. Tumor size is an important factor in pT1–pT2 RCC. This clear cell RCC tumor is greater than 4 cm and bulges beyond the kidney; however, no definite outpouchings to indicate extrarenal extension are evident grossly.

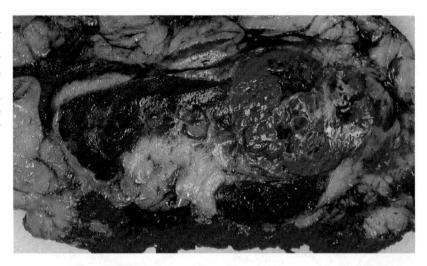

measurement; however, renal vein or vena cava tumor extension is excluded from the measurement.[3] When multiple tumors are present, the International Society of Urological Pathology (ISUP) guidelines recommend sampling and measuring at least the 5 largest tumors.[3]

RENAL SINUS INVASION

Renal sinus fat is the central fat compartment that is located between the pelvicalyceal system and the renal parenchyma, which contains the main lymphovascular supply of the kidney.[31,32] The most critical step of RCC pathologic staging is determining whether a tumor is limited to the kidney or invades the perinephric fat, renal veins, or the renal sinus.[3] This is based on decreased cancer-specific survival in patients with renal sinus invasion,[16] although it is debated whether or not renal sinus invasion is an independent prognostic factor.[33] The 8th edition of AJCC TNM staging system classifies the presence of renal sinus invasion as pT3a.[9] This has been added to the pT category since the 2002 revision of the TNM classification, with several works by Bonsib and colleagues[2,26,34] contributing greatly to the understanding of renal sinus invasion as one of the important routes for extrarenal extension of clear cell RCC.

Renal sinus invasion potentially is subtle and may have significant interobserver variability.[14] Its identification, however, is likely critically important (**Fig. 2**). In an interesting study, Thompson and colleagues[35] retrieved 49 patients with RCC tumors originally reported as pT1 yet who died of renal cancer. Of these patients, 33 had their preserved specimens analyzed retrospectively and compared with a control group of 33 patients who did not die from RCC. In total, 22 (67%) patients who died from RCC had unrecognized renal

sinus fat or small vein invasion compared with 7 (21%) of the controls (*P*<.001). This highlights that sinus fat or vascular invasion may go undiagnosed by histopathology if aggressive search is not undertaken and that this may have significant prognostic implications.

In the AJCC 8th edition staging manual, renal sinus and perinephric fat infiltration continue to be considered under same category (pT3a); however, there is some evidence that there may be a difference in prognosis between the two.[36,37] The authors' experience is that in clear cell RCC, perinephric fat invasion alone is uncommon in the absence of vein branch or renal sinus invasion.[28] The authors' practice is to submit at least 2 to 3 histologic sections of the renal sinus interface for tumors with no grossly definite invasion. In larger tumors, however, or those with equivocal vascular invasion on gross examination, extensive sampling or the entire renal sinus interface should be strongly considered, particularly for tumors larger than 5 cm.[28,32]

 Pitfalls

! The likelihood of renal sinus invasion increases with increasing tumor size, especially over 5 cm.

! The authors' practice is to sample at least 2 to 3 sections of renal sinus interface for smaller tumors with no gross suspicion for renal sinus invasion.

! Submitting the entire renal sinus interface may be considered for larger tumors, especially clear cell RCC.

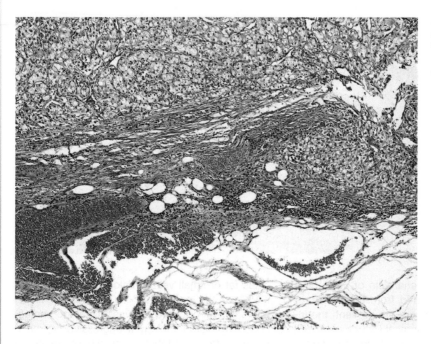

Fig. 2. Renal sinus invasion can include direct invasion or LVI within the renal sinus. This clear cell RCC directly invades renal sinus fat (original magnification ×100).

SEGMENTAL RENAL VEIN BRANCH AND MAIN RENAL VEIN INVASION

RCC, especially clear cell RCC,[17] has a predilection for intravenous growth in the form of so-called tumor thrombus (finger-like outpouching or extension into veins or vein branches),[38] which may be present in 4% to 10% of newly diagnosed patients.[38] The 8th edition of AJCC classifies segmental or main renal vein invasion as pT3a. This was changed from pT3b in AJCC 6th edition, because the prognostic impact of isolated renal vein involvement is comparable to other prognostic features in stage pT3a, with which it was grouped.[39,40]

Ball and colleagues[19] evaluated the extent of vein invasion and found that the 3-year recurrence-free survival rates for segmental vein invasion alone and main renal vein invasion were 93.9% and 67.9%, respectively, and the cancer-specific survival rates were 93.5% and 80.8%, respectively. Furthermore, when followed for a period of 37 months, segmental renal vein invasion (**Fig. 3**) without main renal vein invasion behaved similarly to pT2 disease, whereas main renal vein invasion (**Fig. 4**) behaved similarly to pT3b disease in their study group. As such, it was suggested that the current pT3a may be further substratified in the future, based on whether segmental veins or the main renal vein is involved. Overall, there is likely some prognostic difference between early vein invasion and more obvious vein invasion.

In previous editions of AJCC TNM staging, the demonstration of muscle in segmental veins was required, as was identification of vein invasion by gross examination. The AJCC 8th edition has removed the phrase, "muscle-containing," because the diameter of sinus veins or the presence or absence of muscle in sinus veins is considered a poor indicator of the involved vein segment or its relationship to main renal vein. The word, "grossly," has also been removed, because it is believed that whenever renal vein invasion is present, it is always visible grossly. In the event that it was not appreciated by the individual performing the gross dissection, the intravenous nature can often be appreciated by microscopic examination.[9]

Key Features

- Venous invasion by RCC often manifests as finger-like outpouching with an intact endothelial layer.

- The requirement that vein invasion be identified grossly has been removed from the AJCC 8th edition staging.

- The requirement that veins contain muscle to warrant pT3a has been removed, because small veins may have inconspicuous or attenuated muscle.

Fig. 3. Early vein branch invasion can be difficult to detect in RCC. This tumor has a mushroom-shaped outpouching that bulges beyond the fibromuscular pseudo-capsule of the tumor. Traction on this area (area illustrated with forceps) reveals a cleft-like space with smooth lining, supporting interpretation as early vein branch invasion.

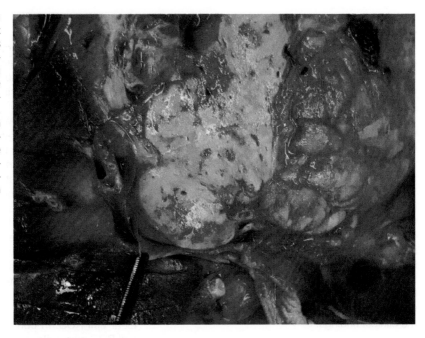

There has also been some interest in the prognostic significance of the consistency of tumor thrombus. It is believed that friable tumor thrombus is an independent predictor of cancer-specific survival.[41]

INFERIOR VENA CAVA TUMOR INVOLVEMENT

Tumor can extend to inferior vena cava (IVC) superiorly up to the right atrium of the heart. When this tumor does not invade the venous wall, however, it can sometimes be retracted back from this location and resected with the specimen. As such, the prognostic importance of the cranial extent of IVC thrombus is debated. Kim and colleagues,[42] in a study of 654 patients undergoing nephrectomy, out of whom 117 patients had renal vein

involvement without IVC extension and 109 patients had IVC tumor extension, found that the risk of recurrence of RCC is increased if there is tumor thrombus versus no tumor thrombus. Additionally, the cancer-specific survival of localized RCC was similar to patients with subdiaphragmatic extension of tumor thrombus. Supradiaphragmatic extension, however, was associated with a significantly worse survival even after controlling for grade and performance status. The 8th edition of AJCC classifies subdiaphragmatic extension of IVC tumor as pT3b, whereas extension above the level of diaphragm is classified as pT3c.[9] On the other hand, Moinzadeh and Libertino[39] found that the level of IVC tumor thrombus did not have an impact on survival in patients with N_0M_0 disease. Patients with isolated renal

Fig. 4. This large, finger-like extension of a clear cell RCC tumor shows extension in a polypoid fashion into the venous system (original magnification ×200).

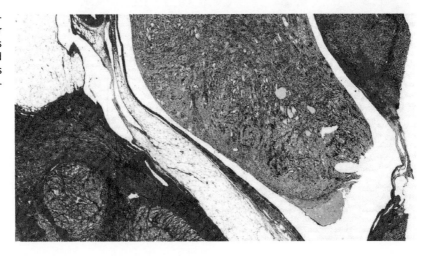

vein involvement, however, had better survival compared with tumor in the IVC.

Because tumor invading the wall of the IVC is categorized together with supradiaphragmatic involvement as pT3c, it is important to also evaluate for wall invasion. As such, if IVC specimen is sent for histopathologic examination, the authors' approach is to search for vein wall tissue within or adherent to the tumor and to correlate these histologic findings with the clinical impression of adherence to vein wall before arriving at an overall interpretation of pT3c stage category. Likewise, taking clinical and radiographic findings into account may be necessary for specimens that have main renal vein involvement with a surgical or radiographic impression of early extension into the IVC. If it is not clear whether IVC tissue is included part of the pathologic specimen, but if the surgical impression is of extension into the lumen, the authors report the specimen as pT3b with comment that IVC involvement is based on the clinical findings.

Key Features

- IVC and renal vein involvement often can be diagnosed by imaging, but segmental vein involvement often may be a subtle gross or microscopic finding.

- For separately received vena cava tumor specimen, select several histologic sections to assess for possible involvement of vein wall.

RETROGRADE VENOUS INVASION

In addition to antegrade spread of tumor thrombus into major veins, tumor may grow in a retrograde fashion into the proximal tributaries of the renal vein, especially when the main renal vein is occluded by the tumor thrombus.[29] This, in turn, may lead to growth of cortical nodules in noncontiguous areas, separate from the original tumor (Fig. 5). When present, this has been termed *retrograde vein invasion*. Bonsib and Bhalodia[29] were the first to describe the pathology of retrograde venous invasion in detail, which can be a cause of misinterpretation of tumor as multifocal or of larger size, if the intravenous spread is not recognized as such. The authors of this review have recently studied retrograde venous invasion in a series of 300 consecutive renal tumor specimens.[28] Retrograde venous invasion was found in 15 of 300 (5%) cases, of which almost all (13/15) were clear cell RCC. In contrast, true multifocal clear cell RCC was quite rare, with only a single equivocal case. Other histologies, however, such as papillary RCC or clear cell papillary RCC, have a proclivity to be multifocal.[28] Therefore, any case of clear cell RCC with satellite lesions should be approached with caution, considering the possibility that these may represent a hereditary syndrome (such as von Hippel–Lindau disease), intravenous spread, or a variant mimicking clear cell RCC, especially clear cell papillary RCC. Although retrograde venous invasion is not considered differently from vein invasion in the AJCC 8th edition staging of RCC,

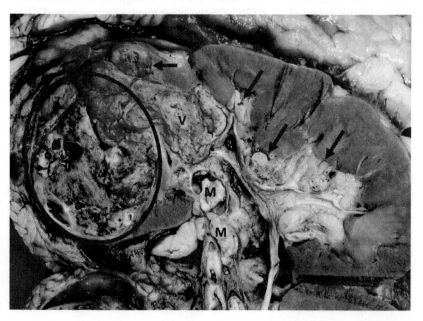

Fig. 5. Retrograde venous invasion in RCC can exhibit a complex constellation of features. In this case, the presumed site of the primary tumor is marked with the circle. An area of confluent venous invasion (V) leads into invasion of the main renal vein (M). Multiple nodules of retrograde invasion are highlighted by arrows in sites both adjacent to, and distant from, the primary tumor.

knowledge of this phenomenon is important to prevent misdiagnosis of multifocal or lower-stage (but larger) RCC. Retrograde venous invasion is principally diagnosed at gross examination. That is, if satellite tumor nodules adjacent to a main mass are present in locations that conform to the normal venous outflow of the kidney (between renal pyramids or at the cortico-medullary junction), the findings are supportive of retrograde venous invasion. Microscopic confirmation of this phenomenon requires a combination of location, relationship to veins, and ideally evidence of preexisting vein.

Pitfalls

! Multiple satellite nodules associated with a large mass are unlikely to be secondary tumors and are most likely retrograde venous spread.

! Multifocal clear cell RCC in the sporadic setting is uncommon—the possibilities of venous invasion or variant histology (such as clear cell papillary RCC) should be considered.

! Microscopic diagnosis of retrograde venous invasion is based on a combination of location, relationship to veins, and evidence of preexisting veins.

RENAL VEIN OR INFERIOR VENA CAVA MARGIN

Because RCC tumors are often present within blood vessels as finger-like extensions, they can sometimes be retracted back by a surgeon to a level at which the vessel can be transected and the tumor removed, without transecting the tumor. Combining this with artifacts of specimen fixation and vascular clipping or stapling by the surgeon, it is not unusual to encounter RCC specimens for which tumor is extending beyond the renal vein margin, or where a so-called tumor thrombus extends close to the vein margin (**Fig. 6**). The authors' approach in this situation is to either dissect the distal-most vein rim (if freely mobile from the tumor) and examine it microscopically to verify that no tumor is adherent to it or, alternatively, to amputate the distal-most section of vein wall containing tumor, to verify in the histologic section that the tumor is not microscopically adherent to the vein wall. In either of these approaches, if the tumor is not adherent to, or invading, the vein wall, the authors interpret the vein margin as negative.[14]

LYMPHOVASCULAR INVASION

Along with macrovascular invasion into the renal veins, RCC can have microvascular invasion, which refers to the presence of tumor within the microscopic blood vessels or lymphatics (**Fig. 7**). Belsante and colleagues,[43] in a single-institution

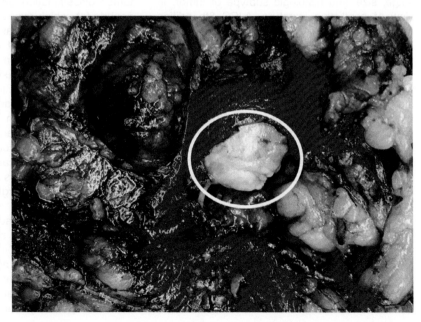

Fig. 6. On removing the staples or clips that ligate the renal vein, tumors with main renal vein invasion may exhibit a finger-like extension that approximates the vein margin (*circle*). The authors' approach is to either dissect off the rim of vein wall (if freely mobile) and submit it for histologic examination to ensure absence of adherent tumor or alternatively to amputate the tip of the protruding tumor (while also capturing the entire vein wall) and evaluate it for adherence or invasion.

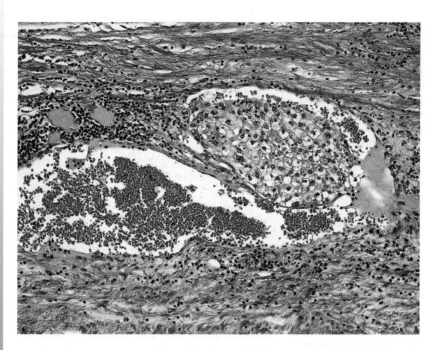

Fig. 7. LVI does not necessarily alter the pathologic tumor stage category, unless it is present in the renal sinus, which is considered renal sinus invasion in the ISUP recommendations. The authors recommend that this be reported, when present (original magnification ×200).

study of 419 patients, found lymphovascular invasion (LVI) in 14.3% of patients. The presence of LVI was found a significant predictor of poorer disease-free survival and cancer-specific survival. The patients with organ-confined RCC with LVI had a similar disease-free survival compared with patients with locally advanced tumors (pT3–pT4, any N, M0). On the other hand, Katz and colleagues[44] found that LVI was not significantly associated with metastasis-free, disease-free, or overall survival after controlling for Fuhrman grade, stage, size, and histologic subtype of tumor. In view of conflicting literature, AJCC 8th edition mentions the significance of LVI, both in predicting cancer-specific survival and disease-specific survival, but this is not specifically included in the staging system. It is recommended to report LVI whenever present.[3] The incidence of LVI in recent studies also may differ from older literature, with more recent literature on this subject using markers like podoplanin (D2-40) to define LVI.[9,45] ISUP recommendations also note that any LVI within the renal sinus should be classified as renal sinus invasion (pT3a).[3]

PERINEPHRIC FAT INVASION

In addition to the findings discussed previously, the AJCC 8th edition again includes perinephric fat invasion in the pT3a stage category. In the authors' experience, perinephric fat invasion is uncommon in the absence of venous or renal sinus invasion in clear cell RCC.[28] The authors' criteria

for this, however, includes tumor cells in contact with fat or irregular tongues or nodules into the perinephric tissue (**Fig. 8**), with or without desmoplasia.[3]

In theory, the renal capsule may represent more of a barrier to extrarenal spread than the renal sinus, which is composed of loose fibrovascular and adipose tissue directly in contact with the kidney. Because the renal sinus also contains abundant veins and lymphatics, this may also provide increased opportunity for tumor dissemination compared with the perinephric fat, which raises the possibility of differences in significance as well as differences in incidence of invasion at these 2 sites.[45] Thompson and colleagues,[36] in a study of 162 patients with perinephric fat invasion and 43 patients with renal sinus fat invasion, found that 95 (59%) and 31 (72%), respectively, died of RCC. The patients with renal sinus invasion were 63% more likely to die of RCC compared with perinephric fat invasion. Jeon and colleagues[46] investigated the prognostic significance of perinephric fat involvement in small size tumors. The study group included 946 surgical specimens of pT1–pT3b N_0M_0 RCC, out of which patients with only pT3a stage with isolated perinephric invasion were subselected and further divided into 2 categories using a 7-cm cutoff. Tumors with size greater than 7 cm and perinephric fat invasion had 5-year disease-free survival and cancer-specific survival rates of 49.5% and 58.5%, respectively. Tumors with size less than

Fig. 8. Perinephric fat invasion in clear cell RCC is less common in the absence of renal sinus or renal vein invasion. The authors regard an irregular outpouching or herniation beyond the contour of the kidney into the plane of fat as perinephric invasion (original magnification ×200).

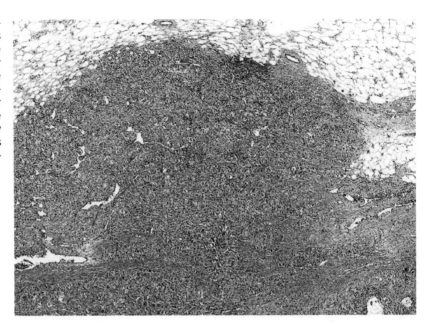

7 cm and perinephric fat invasion had 77.2% disease-free survival and 95.6% cancer-specific survival. Multivariate analysis also showed that perinephric fat invasion when present in tumor less than 7 cm was not a significant predictor of disease-free or cancer-specific survival. Zhang and colleagues,[45] in a metanalysis, calculated the odds ratio and hazard ratio [HR] to differentiate prognostic significance of renal sinus and perinephric fat invasion. Six studies, including 1031 patients, qualified for the analysis. Sinus fat invasion in pT3a NX/NM subgroup had a significantly poorer survival than perinephric fat invasion (HR 1.47; 95% CI, 1.19–1.83; *P*<.001) and worse prognosis (HR 1.94; 95% CI, 1.21–3.12; *P* 0.006). The main limitation of this analysis, however, was small number of studies included due to the limited literature available. At present, the AJCC 8th edition continues to classify both of these under the pT3a category.[9]

Another peculiar feature of RCC is that tumors can bulge well beyond the normal contour of the kidney and that sometimes this bulge remains encapsulated by a layer of normal or atrophic kidney tissue, arguing against invasion. In an online survey conducted among genitourinary pathologists assessing challenges in pathologic staging, there was a strong agreement (90%) that a spherical mass bulging well into the perinephric tissue did not necessarily constitute perinephric fat invasion, especially if a layer of compressed normal structures could be appreciated microscopically surrounding the tumor.[14]

Pitfalls

! Isolated perinephric fat invasion is uncommon in clear cell RCC and is best assessed using multiple perpendicular sections.

! Perinephric fat invasion usually coexists with renal sinus or vein invasion in clear cell RCC.

RENAL CAPSULE INVASION

The renal capsule is the tough fibrous membrane surrounding the renal parenchyma and located below the adipose tissue or perirenal fat. RCC tumors are also often surrounded by a pseudocapsule at the interface with the renal parenchyma, which may be complete or incomplete. This has been a subject of interest in recent years with implications for partial nephrectomy techniques.[47] Renal capsule invasion is defined as the presence of tumor cells within the fibrous renal capsule yet without perirenal fat tissue infiltration. The significance of renal capsule invasion has been debated, with some studies showing impact on recurrence and others not. Ha and colleagues[48] evaluated the independent prognostic significance of renal capsule invasion in a large multi-institutional cohort of 6849 patients of RCC using statistical models that combine proportional hazard regression and propensity score matching. Renal capsule invasion was seen in 603 patients. Recurrence was observed in 75 (12.4%) patients with renal capsule invasion and 134 (6.3%) patients without renal capsule invasion. Renal capsule invasion was significantly associated with an increased risk of recurrence. In the absence of perinephric fat invasion, the AJCC 8th edition does not include any specific categories for renal capsule invasion.[9]

RENAL PELVIS INVASION

Renal pelvis invasion by RCC is uncommon and had not been specifically addressed in prior AJCC systems,[3] until the 8th edition, in which it has been added to the pT3a category.[9] Prognosis for pelvis invasion is still considered debatable. A renal cell tumor that invades the renal pelvis would have likely extended through other structures, such as renal sinus in most cases; however, theoretically, extension to the tip of the medullary papilla could be a mechanism that leads to renal pelvis extension without involving the renal sinus. Terrone and colleagues,[49] in a 2-institution–based study on 671 patients, found invasion of the renal pelvis in 8.8%. Univariate analysis showed decreased survival rates for tumors with renal pelvis invasion compared to those without (42.8% vs 60.8% overall 5-year survival and 45.5% vs 64.7% cause-specific survival). At multivariate analysis, however, renal pelvis invasion was not found an independent prognostic factor. In contrast, Klatte and colleagues,[50] in a study of 519 patients with intracapsular RCC, found invasion of renal capsule in 21.6% and invasion of collecting system in 7.5% of patients. Both capsular invasion and pelvis/pelvicalyceal system invasion were found to have significant impact on recurrence-free survival ($P = .007$ and $P<.001$, respectively) and were independent predictors of recurrence-free survival on multivariate analysis with reported risk ratios of 1.84 and 3.78, respectively.

ADRENAL GLAND INVOLVEMENT

In modern surgical practice and in contrast to historical approaches, the adrenal gland is typically resected only if imaging or intraoperative findings suspect involvement.[9] Adrenal gland involvement by renal cancer can be direct (invasion) or indirect (metastasis). Every attempt should be made on gross examination to distinguish these, because they are reported in different categories. As in previous editions, the AJCC 8th edition staging system continues to classify direct adrenal gland invasion as pT4, in contrast to indirect invasion (a metastatic nodule) as pM1.[9] Direct adrenal gland invasion is rare, with an incidence of only 2.5%, as shown by Han and colleagues.[51] Median survival for patients with pT3a disease was 36 months with 36% cancer-specific survival, which dropped to 12.6 months, and 0% cancer-specific survival with involvement of adrenal gland.[16]

LYMPH NODES

Lymph node dissections have demonstrated that 7% to 17% of RCC tumors have hilar or locoregional lymph node metastases, including caval and aortic lymph nodes.[3] In current practice, however, dissection is generally considered unnecessary in patients with clinically negative lymph nodes, because it offers extremely limited staging information and no benefit in terms of survival or disease recurrence.[52] Lymph node dissection is more frequently performed in younger patients, locally advanced disease, and cases of open surgery.[53] Previously, the N category has been divided on the basis on size of involved lymph nodes, but in further revisions this has been reduced to 2 categories only (positive and negative).[9] In routine resection specimens (without specifically resected lymph node regions), palpation and dissection emphasizing the hilar area specifically is generally sufficient; however, occasionally, lymph nodes can be found in other areas.[54] Random histologic sections of fat that does not contain grossly appreciable lymph nodes are generally not necessary due to the low likelihood of identifying positive lymph nodes in incidental microscopic lymph nodes.[54]

HISTOLOGIC GRADING

The Fuhrman grading system has been replaced with the modified ISUP grading system, which now places most of the emphasis in tumor grade on the nucleolar prominence, particularly whether the nucleoli are prominent at ×100 magnification (×10 microscope objective) or only at higher magnification or not at all, to distinguish grades 1 to 3. This leaves grade 4, including tumors with extreme nuclear pleomorphism, multinucleated giant cells, or sarcomatoid or rhabdoid features (**Fig. 9**).[55,56]

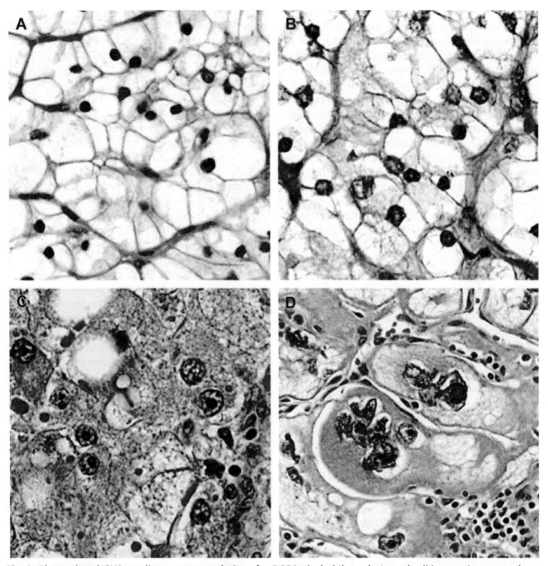

Fig. 9. The updated ISUP grading recommendations for RCC include (*A*) grade 1: nucleoli inconspicuous or absent at ×400 (objective magnification ×40); (*B*) grade 2: nucleoli prominent at ×400 magnification but not ×100; (*C*) grade 3: nucleoli prominent at ×100 magnification; and (*D*) grade 4: extreme nuclear pleomorphism, multinucleated giant cells, sarcomatoid or rhabdoid change (original magnification ×400).

Key Features
RENAL CELL
CARCINOMA GRADING

Grade 1: nucleoli inconspicuous or absent at ×400 (objective magnification ×40)

Grade 2: nucleoli prominent at ×400 magnification but not ×100 (objective magnification ×10)

Grade 3: nucleoli prominent at ×100 magnification

Grade 4: extreme nuclear pleomorphism, multinucleated giant cells, sarcomatoid or rhabdoid change

TUMOR NECROSIS

Tumor necrosis has also emerged as a potentially important prognostic parameter.[57–59] One study proposed a combined grading scheme that includes both the tumor histologic grade and presence or absence of necrosis into a single system. Proposed grades in this scheme were defined as grade 1: ISUP grade 1 and ISUP grade 2 without necrosis; grade 2: ISUP grade 2 with necrosis and ISUP grade 3 without necrosis; grade 3: ISUP grade 3 with necrosis and ISUP grade 4 without necrosis; and grade 4: ISUP grade 4 with necrosis or sarcomatoid/rhabdoid tumors. There was a significant difference in survival rates between each of the grades for clear cell RCC, and the concordance index was superior to that of ISUP grading. The proposed grading system also outperformed the ISUP grading system when cases were stratified according to the TNM stage. Similar results were not obtained for papillary RCC or chromophobe RCC.[60] Overall, however, this system has not gained widespread use at present. Nonetheless, current recommendations are to grade based on nucleolar prominence, report the presence or absence of necrosis, and use the ISUP system for clear cell, papillary, and other RCCs, whereas not to use it for chromophobe RCC (which has inherent cytologic atypia but often nonaggressive behavior).[56]

REFERENCES

1. Moch H, Cubilla AL, Humphrey PA, et al. The 2016 WHO classification of tumours of the urinary system and male genital organs—part A: renal, penile, and testicular tumours. Eur Urol 2016;70: 93–105.

2. Bonsib SM, Gibson D, Mhoon M, et al. Renal sinus involvement in renal cell carcinomas. Am J Surg Pathol 2000;24:451–8.

3. Trpkov K, Grignon DJ, Bonsib SM, et al. Handling and staging of renal cell carcinoma: the International Society of Urological Pathology Consensus (ISUP) conference recommendations. Am J Surg Pathol 2013;37:1505–17.

4. Pichler M, Hutterer GC, Chromecki TF, et al. Comparison of the 2002 and 2010 TNM classification systems regarding outcome prediction in clear cell and papillary renal cell carcinoma. Histopathology 2013;62:237–46.

5. Hollingsworth JM, Miller DC, Daignault S, et al. Rising incidence of small renal masses: a need to reassess treatment effect. J Natl Cancer Inst 2006;98: 1331–4.

6. Moch H, Artibani W, Delahunt B, et al. Reassessing the current UICC/AJCC TNM staging for renal cell carcinoma. Eur Urol 2009;56:636–43.

7. Gospodarowicz MK, Miller D, Groome PA, et al. The process for continuous improvement of the TNM classification. Cancer 2004;100:1–5.

8. Lee C, You D, Park J, et al. Validation of the 2009 TNM classification for renal cell carcinoma: comparison with the 2002 TNM classification by concordance index. Korean J Urol 2011;52:524–30.

9. Rini BI, McKiernan JM, Chang SS, et al. Kidney. In: Amin MB, Edge SB, Greene FL, et al, editors. AJCC cancer staging manual. 8th edition. Switzerland: Springer; 2017. p. 739–48.

10. Leibovich BC, Lohse CM, Cheville JC, et al. Predicting oncologic outcomes in renal cell carcinoma after surgery. Eur Urol 2018;73:772–80.

11. Karakiewicz PI, Briganti A, Chun FK-H, et al. Multi-institutional validation of a new renal cancer–specific survival nomogram. J Clin Oncol 2007;25: 1316–22.

12. Abdollah F, Arora S, von Landenberg N, et al. Testing the external validity of the EORTC randomized trial 30904 comparing overall survival after radical nephrectomy vs nephron-sparing surgery in contemporary North American patients with renal cell cancer. BJU Int 2018;121:345–7.

13. Arora S, Abaza R, Adshead JM, et al. 'Trifecta' outcomes of robot-assisted partial nephrectomy in solitary kidney: a Vattikuti Collective Quality Initiative (VCQI) database analysis. BJU Int 2018;121: 119–23.

14. Williamson SR, Rao P, Hes O, et al. Challenges in pathologic staging of renal cell carcinoma. Am J Surg Pathol 2018, [Epub ahead of print].

15. SEER cancer stat facts: kidney and renal pelvis cancer. Bethesda (MD): National Cancer Institute. Available at: http://seer.cancer.gov/statfacts/html/kidrp. html. Accessed April 4, 2018.

16. Thompson RH, Cheville JC, Lohse CM, et al. Reclassification of patients with pT3 and pT4 renal cell carcinoma improves prognostic accuracy. Cancer 2005;104:53–60.

17. Bonsib SM. Renal veins and venous extension in clear cell renal cell carcinoma. Mod Pathol 2007; 20:44–53.

18. Süer E, Baltaci S, Burgu B, et al. Significance of tumor size in renal cell cancer with perinephric fat infiltration: Is TNM staging system adequate for predicting prognosis? Urol J 2013;10:774–9.

19. Ball MW, Gorin MA, Harris KT, et al. Extent of renal vein invasion influences prognosis in patients with renal cell carcinoma. BJU Int 2016;118:112–7.

20. Hafez KS, Fergany AF, Novick AC. Nephron sparing surgery for localized renal cell carcinoma: Impact of tumor size on patient survival, tumor recurrence and TNM staging. J Urol 1999;162:1930–3.

21. Kinouchi T, Saiki S, Meguro N, et al. Impact of tumor size on the clinical outcomes of patients with Robson Stage I renal cell carcinoma. Cancer 1999;85: 689–95.

22. Gettman MT, Blute ML, Spotts B, et al. Pathologic staging of renal cell carcinoma: Significance of tumor classification with the 1997 TNM staging system. Cancer 2001;91:354–61.

23. Zisman A, Pantuck AJ, Chao D, et al. Reevaluation of the 1997 TNM classification for renal cell carcinoma: T1 and T2 cutoff point at 4.5 rather than 7 cm. Better correlates with clinical outcome. J Urol 2001;166:54–8.

24. Delahunt B, Kittelson JM, McCredie MRE, et al. Prognostic importance of tumor size for localized conventional (clear cell) renal cell carcinoma: assessment of TNM T1 and T2 tumor categories

and comparison with other prognostic parameters. Cancer 2002;94:658–64.

25. Bedke J, Pritsch M, Buse S, et al. Prognostic stratification of localized renal cell carcinoma by tumor size. J Urol 2008;180:62–7.

26. Bonsib SM. The renal sinus is the principal invasive pathway: a prospective study of 100 renal cell carcinomas. Am J Surg Pathol 2004;28:1594–600.

27. Bonsib SM. T2 clear cell renal cell carcinoma is a rare entity: a study of 120 clear cell renal cell carcinomas. J Urol 2005;174(4 Pt 1):1199–202.

28. Taneja K, Arora S, Rogers CG, et al. Pathologic staging of renal cell carcinoma: a review of 300 consecutive cases with emphasis on retrograde venous invasion. Histopathology 2018, [Epub ahead of print].

29. Bonsib SM, Bhalodia A. Retrograde venous invasion in renal cell carcinoma: a complication of sinus vein and main renal vein invasion. Mod Pathol 2011;24:1578–85.

30. Tran T, Sundaram CP, Bahler CD, et al. Correcting the shrinkage effects of formalin fixation and tissue processing for renal tumors: Toward standardization of pathological reporting of tumor size. J Cancer 2015;6:759–66.

31. Siegel R, Miller K, Jemal A. Cancer statistics, 2015. CA Cancer J Clin 2015;65:29.

32. Bonsib SM. Macroscopic assessment, dissection protocols and histologic sampling strategy for renal cell carcinoma. Diagn Histopathol 2008;14:151–6.

33. Poon SA, Gonzalez JR, Benson MC, et al. Invasion of renal sinus fat is not an independent predictor of survival in pT3a renal cell carcinoma. BJU Int 2009;103:1622–5.

34. Grignon D, Paner GP. Renal cell carcinoma and the renal sinus. Adv Anat Pathol 2007;14:63–8.

35. Thompson RH, Blute ML, Krambeck AE, et al. Patients with pT1 renal cell carcinoma who die from disease after nephrectomy may have unrecognized renal sinus fat invasion. Am J Surg Pathol 2007;31:1089–93.

36. Thompson RH, Leibovich BC, Cheville JC, et al. Is renal sinus fat invasion the same as perinephric fat invasion for pT3a renal cell carcinoma? J Urol 2005;174:1218–21.

37. Bedke J, Buse S, Pritsch M, et al. Perinephric and renal sinus fat infiltration in pT3a renal cell carcinoma: possible prognostic differences. BJU Int 2009;103:1349–54.

38. Hatcher PA, Anderson EE, Paulson DF, et al. Surgical management and prognosis of renal cell carcinoma invading the vena cava. J Urol 1991;145:20–3, [discussion: 23–4].

39. Moinzadeh A, Libertino JA. Prognostic significance of tumor thrombus level in patients with renal cell carcinoma and venous tumor thrombus extension. Is all T3b the same? J Urol 2004;171:598–601.

40. Leibovich BC, Cheville JC, Lohse CM, et al. Cancer specific survival for patients with pT3 renal cell carcinoma-can the 2002 primary tumor classification be improved? J Urol 2005;173:716–9.

41. Bertini R, Roscigno M, Freschi M, et al. Impact of venous tumour thrombus consistency (solid vs friable) on cancer-specific survival in patients with renal cell carcinoma. Eur Urol 2011;60:358–65.

42. Kim HL, Zisman A, Han KR, et al. Prognostic significance of venous thrombus in renal cell carcinoma. Are renal vein and inferior vena cava involvement different? J Urol 2004;171:588–91.

43. Belsante M, Darwish O, Youssef R, et al. Lymphovascular invasion in clear cell renal cell carcinoma–association with disease-free and cancer-specific survival. Urol Oncol 2014;32(1):30.e23-8.

44. Katz MD, Serrano MF, Humphrey PA, et al. The role of lymphovascular space invasion in renal cell carcinoma as a prognostic marker of survival after curative resection. Urol Oncol 2011;29:738–44.

45. Zhang Z, Yu C, Velet L, et al. The difference in prognosis between renal sinus fat and perinephric fat invasion for pT3a renal cell carcinoma: a meta-analysis. PLoS One 2016;11(2):e0149420.

46. Jeon HG, Jeong IG, Kwak C, et al. Reevaluation of renal cell carcinoma and perirenal fat invasion only. J Urol 2009;182:2137–43.

47. Jacob JM, Williamson SR, Gondim DD, et al. Characteristics of the peritumoral pseudocapsule vary predictably with histologic subtype of T1 renal neoplasms. Urology 2015;86:956–61.

48. Ha US, Lee KW, Jung JH, et al. Renal capsular invasion is a prognostic biomarker in localized clear cell renal cell carcinoma. Sci Rep 2018;8(1):202.

49. Terrone C, Cracco C, Guercio S, et al. Prognostic value of the involvement of the urinary collecting system in renal cell carcinoma. Eur Urol 2004;46:472–6.

50. Klatte T, Chung J, Leppert JT, et al. Prognostic relevance of capsular involvement and collecting system invasion in stage I and II renal cell carcinoma. BJU Int 2007;99:821–4.

51. Han KR, Bui MHT, Pantuck AJ, et al. TNM T3A renal cell carcinoma: adrenal gland involvement is not the same as renal fat invasion. J Urol 2003;169:899–903.

52. Blom JHM, van Poppel H, Maréchal JM, et al. Radical nephrectomy with and without lymph-node dissection: final results of European Organization for Research and Treatment of Cancer (EORTC) randomized phase 3 trial 30881. Eur Urol 2009;55:28–34.

53. Capitanio U, Stewart GD, Larcher A, et al. European temporal trends in the use of lymph node dissection in patients with renal cancer. Eur J Surg Oncol 2017;43(11):2184–92.

54. Mehta V, Mudaliar K, Ghai R, et al. Renal lymph nodes for tumor staging: appraisal of 871

nephrectomies with examination of hilar fat. Arch Pathol Lab Med 2013;137:1584–90.

55. Moch H. An overview of renal cell cancer: pathology and genetics. Semin Cancer Biol 2013;23:3–9.

56. Delahunt B, Cheville JC, Martignoni G, et al. The International Society of Urological Pathology (ISUP) grading system for renal cell carcinoma and other prognostic parameters. Am J Surg Pathol 2013;37:1490–504.

57. Khor LY, Dhakal HP, Jia X, et al. Tumor necrosis adds prognostically significant information to grade in clear cell renal cell carcinoma: a study of 842 consecutive cases from a single institution. Am J Surg Pathol 2016;40:1224–31.

58. Lohse CM, Gupta S, Cheville JC. Outcome prediction for patients with renal cell carcinoma. Semin Diagn Pathol 2015;32:172–83.

59. Sengupta S, Lohse CM, Leibovich BC, et al. Histologic coagulative tumor necrosis as a prognostic indicator of renal cell carcinoma aggressiveness. Cancer 2005;104:511–20.

60. Delahunt B, McKenney JK, Lohse CM, et al. A novel grading system for clear cell renal cell carcinoma incorporating tumor necrosis. Am J Surg Pathol 2013;37:311–22.

Updates in Staging and Reporting of Testicular Cancer

Martin J. Magers, MD, Muhammad T. Idrees, MD, MBBS*

KEYWORDS

- TNM classification • Testis • Paratestis • Scrotum • Tunica vaginalis

---

Key points

- Testis germ cell tumors should be staged according to the American Joint Committee for Cancer (AJCC) eighth edition staging manual.

- The AJCC eighth edition incorporated several critical changes compared with the seventh edition.

- Although some important changes and clarifications were made in the AJCC eighth edition, several challenges remain.

- Unfortunately, the Union for International Cancer Control eighth edition did not incorporate the same changes as the AJCC eighth edition, and these discrepancies need resolution to avoid confusion.

ABSTRACT

The American Joint Committee for Cancer eighth edition staging manual incorporated several critical changes regarding staging of testis germ cell tumors, and these changes are summarized and discussed in this article. Further challenges, however, remain, and these are also highlighted.

OVERVIEW

The TNM classification (tumor, node, and metastasis) of malignant tumors is a standardized and widely accepted staging system that has evolved as a fundamental concept and makes possible evidence-based cancer management. Current guidelines for tumor treatment are therefore based on the TNM system, thereby permitting consistent and uniform treatment strategies among various institutions worldwide.

Professor Pierre Denoix[1] at The Institute Gustave-Roussy in France developed fundamentals of the TNM classification of cancer between 1943 and 1952. Dr Denoix, in collaboration with Union for International Cancer Control (UICC), chaired a special committee on clinical stage classification to further refine and develop the TNM classification. This committee and a subsidiary committee, "The UICC TNM Prognostic Factors Project," refined the definition for TNM classification over several years. Because of these efforts, the UICC published a pocket book, "Livre de Poche," in 1968, which is now in its eighth edition. Around the same time, the American Joint Committee for Cancer (AJCC) began developing separate definitions of the TNM categories. The first TNM AJCC Cancer Staging Manual was published in 1977. In 1987, the UICC and the AJCC TNM classifications were aligned and the classification systems were unified. Currently, UICC, AJCC, and the International Federation of Gynecology

---

Disclosure Statement: Nothing to disclose.
Pathology and Laboratory Medicine, Indiana University School of Medicine, 350 West 11th Street, Room 4010, Indianapolis, IN 46202, USA
* Corresponding author.
E-mail address: midrees@iupui.edu

Surgical Pathology 11 (2018) 813–824
https://doi.org/10.1016/j.path.2018.07.005
1875-9181/18/© 2018 Elsevier Inc. All rights reserved.

and Obstetrics (FIGO) oversee, collaborate, and agree on the staging classifications for all organ systems, including genitourinary malignancies. The AJCC eighth edition is a product of extensive collaborative efforts of UICC and AJCC to standardize and harmonize the staging system. However, the recent UICC staging manual published after the AJCC manual (eighth edition) did not incorporate many of the changes that are suggested by AJCC.[2,3] This caused tremendous confusion and frustration among pathologists and created a perception that these organizations are taking diverging pathways. Because many of these changes concern testicular staging, it is certain that serious challenges and issues will be faced by physicians as well as the pathologists if 2 differing classification systems are followed. There is an immense need for uniformity as soon as possible to resolve and remediate the major differences based on clinical and statistical evidence.

In the first testicular TNM AJCC staging, T stage was based on the progression of the tumor and the extent of involvement with adjacent structures. No evidence of primary tumor in the testis was T0, the primary tumor limited to the testis was T1, the primary tumor extending beyond the tunica albuginea was T2, the primary tumor involving the rete testis or epididymis was T3, invasion of the spermatic cord was T4a, and invasion of the scrotum was T4b. N and M staging had similar patterns. No involvement of regional lymph nodes was N0; involvement of a single ipsilateral regional lymph node, which is mobile if inguinal, was N1; involvement of a contralateral, bilateral, or multiple lymph nodes, which is/are mobile if inguinal, was N2; the presence of a palpable abdominal mass or fixed inguinal lymph nodes was N3; and involvement of juxtaregional lymph nodes was N4. Distant metastasis was stage M0 if no known distant metastases and M1 if a distant metastasis was present. All of the TNM classifiers also had an X stage, which was applied if that component could not be assessed.[4] As more data became available, later classifications incorporated several histologic parameters related to prognosis. This 1st edition (1977) served as the basis for later modifications and amendments that shaped the current AJCC staging system.[4]

As reflected in the current AJCC Staging Manual (eighth edition), the TNM classification of testicular tumors has undergone several significant changes (**Box 1**). Currently, only tumors related to germ cell neoplasia in situ (GCNIS) or malignant sex cord stromal tumors are staged according to the AJCC classification.[5] Broadly, the GCNIS-related germ cell tumors are divided into seminomatous and nonseminomatous categories. This division

Box 1
Details of change
In pure seminoma, T1 is subclassified to T1a and T1b according to tumor size using a 3-cm cutoff
Epididymal invasion is considered T2 rather than T1
Hilar soft tissue invasion is considered T2
Discontinuous involvement of the spermatic cord by vascular-lymphatic invasion represents M1 disease

is important, as pathologic prognostic factors differ in these 2 groups. It should be noted that seminoma can be a component of mixed germ cell tumors, which are broadly categorized as nonseminomatous germ cell tumors. The World Health Organization (WHO) 2016 classification has replaced the name of spermatocytic seminoma to spermatocytic tumor; hence, assignment of a stage is not required because of its indolent course. The sarcomatous transformation of spermatocytic tumor is not addressed in the eighth edition of AJCC. Fortunately, this occurrence is extremely rare and will not pose a great challenge for the vast majority of pathologists. Similarly, GCNIS has replaced the term "intratubular germ cell neoplasia in situ" (ITGCNU) in the WHO 2016 classification.[6] Only germ cell tumors associated with GCNIS are staged, whereas non–GCNIS-associated germ cell tumors are not. Prepubertal yolk sac tumor or mixed prepubertal tumors are not associated with GCNIS but their potential to metastasize and progress warrant staging, and, considering these facts, we recommend that the AJCC TNM staging system or alternatively "Pediatric Oncology Group" staging should be used. No AJCC staging is developed for paratesticular neoplasms. Occasionally, hematolymphoid malignancies arise as primary testicular neoplasms, and these should be staged according to the current AJCC staging system described for hematolymphoid malignancies.

In the eighth edition of the AJCC Staging Manual, major changes and clarifications are provided in the T-stage category. These changes are primarily based on recently reported pathologic data relevant to the prognosis. Three main modifications were made compared with the seventh edition, including documentation of tumor size, hilar soft tissue invasion, and the reorganization of pT1 and pT2 categories. Level of evidence (I–III) for new changes has been provided, which will serve as a baseline for future refinements.

Serum tumor markers are important in diagnosis and serve as indicators of disease spread. It is fundamental to use serum markers to guide management and predict prognosis of germ cell cancers. In contrast to cancers from other organs, the TNM staging system for male testicular gem cell tumors incorporated serum tumor marker elevation as a separate category (S) of staging information. Interestingly, the clinical and pathologic stage IV is eliminated in testicular staging because of its high cure rate regardless of locoregional or systemic spread of disease. The highest stage is thus Stage IIIC in the testis.

ANATOMY OF THE TESTIS AND PARATESTIS

The testes are paired organs suspended in the scrotum by the spermatic cord. The entire testis is surrounded by a thin membrane, the tunica vaginalis, which is composed of an external (parietal) layer, which apposes the internal spermatic fascia of the scrotum, and an internal (visceral) layer, which intimately covers the tunica albuginea. Between the 2 membrane layers of the tunica vaginalis is a potential space. The tunica albuginea is densely fibrotic and contains collagen, fibroblasts, and myocytes. Underlying the tunica albuginea is the tunica vasculosa, through which blood vessels and lymphatics course. In combination, the tunica layers function to protect the testis, maintain intratesticular pressure, and supply the testicular parenchyma with blood flow and lymphatic drainage. Emanating from the tunica albuginea are thin fibrous septae that divide the testis into approximately 250 lobules that are composed of seminiferous tubules containing germ cells and supporting sex cord cells (Sertoli cells). The seminiferous tubules are embedded in a collagenous stroma containing androgen-producing Leydig cells. The seminiferous tubules converge at the hilum of the testis, which is not covered by the tunica layers, to become the rete testis and subsequently the efferent ductules. The efferent ductules then merge into a single duct, the epididymis. The epididymis coils outside the testis and eventually drains into the vas deferens, which travels through the spermatic cord and eventually merges with the excretory duct of the seminal vesicle to drain into the ejaculatory duct in the prostate.

The tunica vasculosa is rich with blood vessels and lymphatic channels, and it is often the site of lymphovascular invasion. Invasion through the tunica albuginea and tunica vaginalis perforation is rare. Rather, the hilar region, which is not cloaked by the tunica albuginea, is the major route for tumor spread from the testis into hilar soft tissue. The hilar soft tissue is also rich with blood vessels and lymphatic channels. After coursing through the hilar soft tissue, the tumor can spread into the epididymis and superiorly into the spermatic cord. Because most tumors spread through the hilum, invasion through the tunica vaginalis without concomitant hilar invasion is quite rare (<5% of cases).[7] Gross and microscopic assessment of the extent of tumor invasion relative to these testicular and paratesticular structures is paramount for accurate staging and assessment of prognostic parameters.

GROSS ASSESSMENT OF TESTICULAR TUMORS

The gross assessment of testicular tumors is an essential first step in diagnosis and staging. For example, whether a tumor nodule within the spermatic cord represents direct extension of the tumor (ie, pT3) or a discontinuous metastatic deposit (ie, M1), requires a careful gross assessment. Additionally, germ cell tumors, which comprise the vast majority of testicular tumors, are notorious for artifactual spread of tumor cells, particularly in the case of seminoma. Indeed, nearly every pathologist who has reported a seminoma has witnessed artifactual transport of tumor cells beyond their true location into lymphovascular channels and paratesticular soft tissue (**Fig.** 1A, B). For these reasons, scrupulous macroscopic examination and microscopic evaluation is required for accurate stage assignment.

The first sections taken from an orchiectomy specimen should not be of the tumor. Rather, it is recommended that the spermatic cord margin section (ie, en face section of the most proximal portion of the spermatic cord) and a section of the distal spermatic cord (ie, across the cord where it emerges superior to the epididymal head) be the first sections taken to avoid artifactual transport of tumor cells into these sections. Additional sections should be taken if there is suggestion of spermatic cord involvement by tumor.

Once the spermatic cord sections have been taken, the sac enclosing the testis can be opened anteriorly by incising the parietal tunica vaginalis. At this point, the parietal tunica vaginalis should be closely inspected for any area of potential disruption by tumor. The testis can then be bisected parallel to the long axis through the anterior testis toward the hilum. It is advisable to then allow the bisected testis with exposed tumor to adequately fix in formalin to prevent artifactual tumor spread. Once fixed, the testis can be further sectioned.

Once the testis has been sectioned and carefully examined, tumor size, multifocality, location,

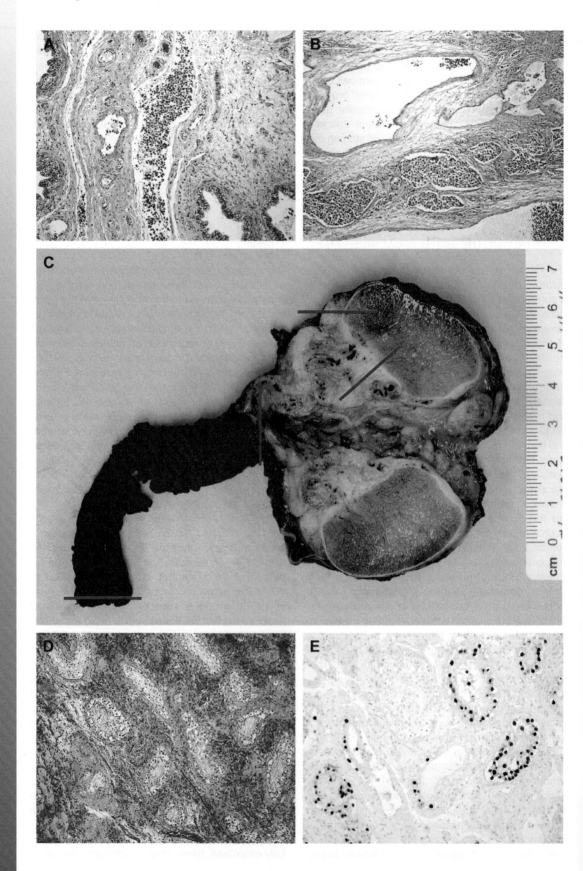

and presence or absence of invasion into adjacent structures (ie, hilum, tunica albuginea, tunica vaginalis, epididymis, and spermatic cord) should be documented. Adequate sampling of the tumor is necessary for histologic confirmation (**Fig.** 1C). The general rule is one section per centimeter of tumor, although tumors that are ≤2 cm should be entirely submitted, and, because germ cell tumors are often heterogeneous, it is important to generously sample different areas of the tumor. Included in these sections should also be the edge of tumor and nonneoplastic testicular parenchyma as well as the tumor's relationship to adjacent structures. Additionally, a section of testicular parenchyma uninvolved by the tumor should be submitted.

Specific staging issues will be discussed in further detail in the following sections, but it is no exaggeration to say that accurate diagnosis and staging begin with and are entirely reliant on a careful gross assessment.

Pitfalls
(GROSS ASSESSMENT OF
TESTICULAR TUMORS
SECTION)

! Placing the orchiectomy specimen in formalin without bivalving could cause autolysis and hamper proper evaluation.

! Failure to take spermatic cord margin section before incising the testis tumor can cause artifactual spread of neoplastic cells into the spermatic cord margin section.

! Failure to take sections demonstrating the tumor's relation to adjacent structures may result in inability to accurately stage the tumor.

! Inadequate sampling, particularly of heterogeneous areas, may result in failure to identify a component of a mixed germ cell tumor.

! Hemorrhage does not mean necrosis; it is a good idea to take sections from hemorrhagic areas to potentially sample choriocarcinoma, if clinically relevant based on serum HCG.

PRIMARY TUMOR: pT

The pathologic T stage is dependent on tumor size and extent into adjacent structures. In pathologic T staging, the pTx category is used only when the tissue is either not available or is insufficient to render a diagnosis. It is recommended to avoid this category, if possible. The pT0 category should be used only when no tumor is identified; this may occur with tumor regression (ie, scar in the testis). It is often difficult to relate a scar in the testicular parenchyma to tumor regression; however, several morphologic findings may help in making this distinction.[8] GCNIS in the absence of an invasive tumor should be assigned a pTis stage. In cases in which GCNIS is difficult to interpret or is present in rare tubules, immunohistochemical staining with OCT3/4 may be helpful (**Fig.** 1D, E).[9] Additional sections may need to be submitted when sufficient tubules are not available for evaluation.

Invasive tumors limited to the testis in the absence of lymphovascular invasion are classified as pT1. Pure seminomas are further divided into pT1a and pT1b based on a size cutoff of 3 cm (ie, <3 cm = pT1a, ≥3 cm = pT1b). The size of seminoma is important when considering adjuvant radiation or carboplatin-based chemotherapy, as several recent studies have emphasized that seminoma size is an independent factor for disease progression.[10–12] It is therefore justifiable to incorporate the size of a seminoma in the pT classification, and this determination of tumor size should typically be based on a careful gross assessment of the tumor size. Some ambiguity remains regarding the 3-cm size cutoff for seminoma, as many of the previous and recent publications recommend a larger size cutoff at least 4 cm; however, the 3-cm cutoff was conservatively adopted by the AJCC.[5,10–13] For nonseminomatous germ cell tumors, including mixed germ cell tumors that possess a component of seminoma, size is not a factor in the pT stage, and pT1 is not subdivided.

It has been pointed out in the past that rete testis invasion may be associated with a higher clinical stage; however, AJCC has taken the stance that currently there is not enough evidence to justify

Fig. 1. Artifactual smearing of neoplastic cells, particularly seminoma, into lymphovascular spaces (*A*) must be carefully distinguished from true lymphovascular invasion (LVI). [H&E, original magnification ×10] (*B*). It is helpful to assess for in peritumoral locations. Accurate assessment of pathologic stage begins with a careful gross assessment (*C*), and sampling of several important structures/locations (indicated by a red bar) is imperative. These include the cord margin (which should be the first section taken before incising the testis), the interface between the cord and hilum, the rete testis and hilar soft tissue, and the epididymis. GCNIS in the absence of an invasive tumor should be assigned a pTis stage (*D*). GCNIS may sometimes be difficult to identify, and immunohistochemical staining with OCT3/4 may be helpful (*E*).

upstaging based on rete testis invasion.[7,10,12,14,15] Additionally, uniformity regarding the definition and reporting of rete testis invasion is lacking. Although most pathologists report rete testis involvement, a significant minority (up to 21%) do not distinguish pagetoid spread from stromal invasion (**Fig. 2**A, B).[16] This may be an important distinction, as evidence is emerging that stromal

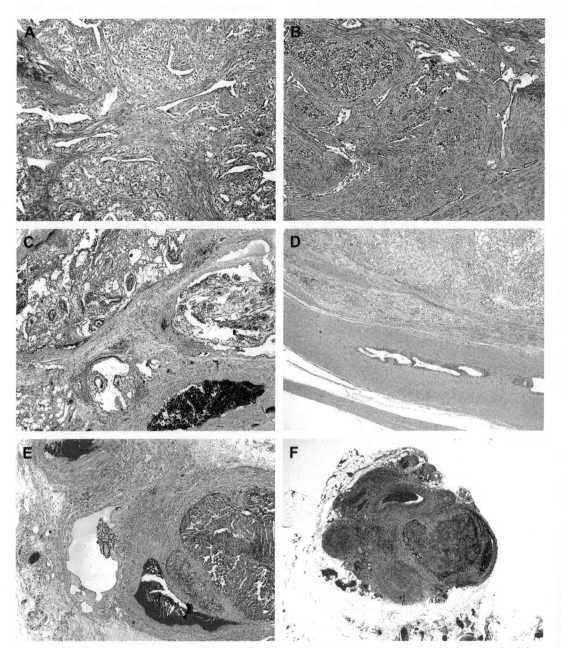

Fig. 2. Most pathologists distinguish pagetoid spread into rete testis (H&E, original magnification ×10) (*A*) from rete testis stromal invasion (H&E, original magnification ×10) (*B*). Although rete testis invasion is not currently a staging parameter, evidence suggests that stromal invasion of the rete testis is associated with advanced clinical stage. The hilum of the testis includes rete testis and hilar soft tissue, and invasion of hilar soft tissue is now considered pT2 (H&E, original magnification ×4) (*C*). When tumor has invaded through the hilar soft tissue and directly into the spermatic cord, stage pT3 is assigned (H&E, original magnification ×4) (*D*). When tumor is present in the spermatic cord only within lymphovascular spaces, however, the appropriate stage assignment is pT2 (H&E, original magnification ×4) (*E*). Finally, if there is tumor present within the spermatic cord that is not confined to lymphovascular spaces and is not in direct continuity with the main testis mass, the spermatic cord tumor is considered a metastasis (H&E, original magnification ×2) (pM1; *F*).

invasion of the rete testis is associated with advanced clinical stage. Because of this, further refinement and subdivision of pT1 may occur in the future.[7] Currently, though, rete testis invasion is not a staging parameter.

The presence of lymphovascular invasion was staged as pT2 in the AJCC seventh edition, and this is unchanged in the AJCC eighth edition. Lymphatic channels and blood vessels course through the testicular parenchyma between seminiferous tubules as well as within the tunica vasculosa at the periphery of the testis. Because of this, lymphovascular invasion often occurs in the absence of hilar, tunica vaginalis, or epididymal invasion, and in this scenario, the correct stage assignment is pT2. Specification of lymphatic versus vascular invasion is not necessary; both are considered pT2.[17–19] When assigning a stage of pT2 based on lymphovascular invasion alone, one should be completely certain that the lymphovascular invasion is real and not artifactually present. Displacement of tumor, particularly seminoma, into lymphovascular vessels and tumoral retraction are frequent artifacts that may mimic lymphovascular invasion.[20] For these reasons, it is helpful to assess for lymphovascular invasion in peritumoral locations, although unequivocal intratumoral lymphovascular invasion may occasionally be present. The importance of lymphovascular invasion in seminoma is much less significant as compared with nonseminomatous germ cell tumors.[10,12,14] The type of tumor involving lymphovascular space is not mandatory, as there is no existing evidence that reflects the significance of this determination.

Extratesticular extension of tumor most commonly occurs via invasion through the hilum of the testis, which consists of rete testis and hilar soft tissue (**Fig. 2**C). The rete testis drains into the efferent ductules, and hilar soft tissue is contiguous with the base of the spermatic cord adjacent to the head of epididymis. Staging of hilar soft tissue invasion is problematic, as no consensus exists among expert genitourinary pathologists. In the AJCC seventh edition, it was staged as pT1, but some evidence supports that it should be staged higher.[7] Due to the paucity of evidence and to avoid understaging or overstaging, a middle ground approach was taken to stage it as pT2 in the AJCC eighth edition until further data become available. Invasion of the hilar soft tissue is defined as invasion of the adipose and loose fibrous connective tissue present in this region. Differentiation of hilar soft tissue from the soft tissue of the spermatic cord, which is morphologically indistinguishable, is critical, and this will be addressed in the discussion of pT3 staging.

Epididymal invasion previously was placed in the pT1 category in the AJCC seventh edition; however, considering that epididymal invasion in most instances occurs after tumor invasion of the hilar soft tissue, it should be staged higher. Although there are limited data, it logically is appropriate to stage epididymal invasion as pT2, and this practice is recommended in the AJCC eighth edition.[21] Rarely, tumors may invade the epididymis via the tunica albuginea, bypassing the hilum altogether. The placement of epididymal invasion into the pT2 category ameliorates this potential staging problem.

Perforation of the visceral layer of the tunica vaginalis, which covers the external surface of tunica albuginea, also should be considered pT2. The AJCC eighth edition does not comment regarding the parietal layer of the tunica albuginea. In any case, this type of tumor spread is extremely rare, and, ironically, there is not sufficient evidence to support assignment of a higher stage based on invasion of the parietal layer.

Pathologic stage pT3 is defined in the AJCC eighth edition as invasion of the spermatic cord. As discussed previously, this typically occurs following invasion of the hilar soft tissue (pT2). Thus, assessment of whether the soft tissue involved by tumor is hilar or spermatic cord is critical for accurate staging in these cases. Correlation with the gross assessment and the location from which the tissue section was taken is often helpful. At our institution, soft tissue is considered spermatic cord if the section contains vas deferens. It is important to note that pT3 is assigned only when the tumor contiguously involves the spermatic cord (**Fig. 2**D). When there is discontinuous involvement of the spermatic cord, the portion of the tumor within the spermatic cord is considered a metastatic deposit, and the primary tumor is not assigned a pT3 stage (**Fig. 2**E, F); this is further discussed in the section regarding metastasis. There is some recent evidence that spermatic cord lymphovascular invasion may be related to higher clinical stage and recurrence; however, further studies are required to consolidate this observation.[22–24]

Invasion of the scrotum is rare in developed countries, and, when present, it is assigned a stage of pT4. The AJCC eighth edition does not discuss scrotal invasion in any detail; however, it should be noted that invasion of the parietal layer of the tunica vaginalis is not considered scrotal invasion. Rather, to assign a stage of pT4, the tumor must invade beyond the tunica vaginalis and spermatic fascia into soft tissue or skin of the scrotum.

Pitfalls
(THE PRIMARY TUMOR SECTION)

! Pure seminoma that lacks lymphovascular invasion and is confined to the testis is now substaged as pT1a (<3 cm) or pT1b (≥3 cm).

! Although not formally part of the AJCC staging system, invasion of the rete testis is usually reported, and pagetoid spread within the rete testis epithelium should be distinguished from rete testis stromal invasion.

! Germ cell tumor may be artifactually displaced into lymphovascular spaces, and care should be taken to avoid calling this lymphovascular invasion.

! Hilar soft tissue and epididymal invasion are now staged as pT2.

! Contiguous tumor within the spermatic cord is considered pT3, but discontiguous tumor within the spermatic cord does not affect the T stage and is rather either considered lymphovascular invasion (ie, pT2) or a metastatic deposit (ie, M1).

REGIONAL LYMPH NODES: pN

The lymphatic channels of the testis drain into retroperitoneal lymph nodes, and, with few exceptions, tumors first involve retroperitoneal lymph nodes before spreading to other regions. For the purposes of staging, interaortocaval, paraaortic (or periaortic), paracaval, preaortic, precaval, retroaortic, retrocaval, and lymph nodes along the spermatic vein are considered regional lymph nodes, and a pN stage is assigned to metastatic disease involving these lymph nodes. Additionally, intrapelvic, external iliac, and inguinal lymph nodes should be considered regional lymph nodes if the patient underwent scrotal or inguinal surgery before presentation of the testis tumor. All other lymph nodes are distant or nonregional nodes, such as those above the diaphragm, and an M stage is applied to these lymph node metastases.

A stage of pNx should be assigned to cases in which the regional lymph nodes cannot be assessed, such as in cases in which a retroperitoneal lymph node dissection is not performed. Radical orchiectomy is often performed as a separate procedure before a retroperitoneal lymph node dissection, with the decision of whether to perform a retroperitoneal lymph node dissection hinging on the pathologic findings within the testis, and pNx should be used in these cases. When regional lymph nodes are sampled, and no metastatic disease is identified, a stage of pN0 is assigned. Often, retroperitoneal lymph node dissection is performed following radiation or chemotherapy. In these cases, there may be no viable tumor remaining, but there may be treatment effect, such as necrosis, fibrosis, hemorrhage, and/or scarring. In these cases, pN0 remains the appropriate stage assignment, but the presence of treatment effect should be mentioned and quantified in the final report.

The pN stage is divided based on the number of lymph nodes involved by metastatic tumor, the size of the largest lymph node involved by tumor, the presence or absence of extranodal extension by the tumor. The size cutoffs are unchanged in the AJCC eighth edition from the AJCC seventh edition, but the pN stage dependence on both quantity of involved lymph nodes and extranodal extension are new in the AJCC eighth edition. Stage pN1 is defined as ≤5 lymph nodes positive with no single lymph node measuring larger than 2 cm in greatest dimension and without extranodal extension. Stage pN2 should be assigned when there are more than 5 lymph nodes positive, there is a positive lymph node larger than 2 cm but ≤5 cm in greatest dimension, and/or there is tumoral extranodal extension. Finally, pN3 is assigned when there is a lymph node measuring larger than 5 cm in greatest dimension.

It should be noted that the AJCC eighth edition emphasizes the size cutoffs refer to the size of the involved lymph node and not on the size of the metastatic deposit. For example, a lymph node that is radiologically or grossly measured 3 cm in greatest dimension, but that demonstrates only a 2-cm metastatic deposit based on microscopic examination should be staged as pN2.

Pitfalls
(THE REGIONAL LYMPH NODES SECTION)

! The N stage is dependent on the number of involved lymph nodes, size of involved lymph node, and the presence or absence of extranodal extension.

! Lymph nodes that demonstrate only treatment effect and lack residual viable tumor should be reported as such and assigned pN0.

DISTANT METASTASIS: M

Testis tumors typically metastasize first to retroperitoneal lymph nodes followed by spread to distant lymph nodes, lung, liver, bone, and other visceral sites. Radiology plays a significant role in providing accurate information regarding the extent of disease in retroperitoneum or elsewhere.[25,26] Distant metastases are assigned a stage of M1, whereas M0 is assigned to tumors without distant metastases. In practicality, when most orchiectomy specimens are examined, it is unknown to the pathologist whether distant metastases are present, as these are often not resected for histologic examination contemporaneously with the orchiectomy; in these cases, it is appropriate to designate "M stage–not applicable" or simply not comment on the M stage in the final report.

M1 is further subdivided into M1a (ie, nonretroperitoneal nodal or pulmonary metastases) and M1b (ie, nonpulmonary visceral metastases). The new M1a subcategory definition is slightly more defined than in the AJCC seventh edition, which defined nodal M1a disease as "nonregional" lymph nodes, but the lymph node groups considered regional or retroperitoneal remains unchanged in the AJCC eighth edition. This clarification of the M1a subcategory is, however, accompanied by a slightly more problematic new definition of M1b. The AJCC eighth edition defines M1b as nonpulmonary visceral metastases, compared with the AJCC seventh edition, which essentially defined any metastasis ineligible for the M1a subcategory as M1b. This new definition of M1b in the AJCC eighth edition raises the possibility of metastases that do not clearly fit into the new M1a or M1b subcategories (eg, discontinuous involvement of the spermatic cord), and this is discussed in greater detail in the section dealing with further challenges.

Pitfalls
(THE DISTANT METASTASIS SECTION)

! M1 is subdivided into M1a and M1b.

! Discontiguous tumor within the spermatic cord that is not confined to a lymphovascular space should be assigned M1, as it does not clearly fit into either M1a or M1b.

SERUM TUMOR MARKERS: S

Testis cancer is one of the few malignancies for which reliable serum markers are available, and they serve a critical role in diagnosis, prognosis, and disease management.[27,28] Because of their exceptional utility in testicular germ cell tumors,

the TNM staging system incorporates an additional category for serum tumor markers (S). Serum tumor markers should be obtained before orchiectomy, following orchiectomy, during treatment to assess response, and during surveillance to monitor for recurrence.

The 3 serum tumor markers included in the S category of TNM staging in the AJCC eighth edition are alpha fetoprotein (AFP), human chorionic gonadotropin (hCG), and lactate dehydrogenase (LDH). AFP is synthesized in the yolk sac, liver, and intestine of fetuses, with its major function being a serum-binding protein. Peak levels occur at approximately week 12 to 14 of gestation and subsequently decrease, such that 1 year after birth, serum AFP should be <15 ng/mL. In germ cell neoplasia, AFP is primarily produced by yolk sac tumor, but it also may be produced by embryonal carcinoma and teratoma, albeit to a lesser extent; pure choriocarcinoma and seminoma, however, do not produce AFP.[29] In fact, a patient with an elevated AFP should be regarded as having a nonseminomatous germ cell tumor, even if only seminoma is histologically identified. Serum levels of AFP should normalize 20 to 28 days after therapy.

Placental syncytiotrophoblasts normally produce hCG, and, in the setting of germ cell neoplasia, increased levels are associated with trophoblastic tumors, such as choriocarcinoma. Elevated serum hCG also may occur in embryonal carcinoma and seminoma, although compared with choriocarcinoma, embryonal carcinoma and seminoma produce less of an elevation.[29,30] Following surgery, serum levels of hCG should normalize within 4 to 6 days.

LDH is produced by many types of tissue throughout the body, including muscle, liver, kidney, and brain. Because of this, although LDH is often elevated in approximately half of men with testicular germ cell tumors, it is relatively nonspecific compared with AFP and hCG.[31] Nonetheless, elevations greater than 2000 U/L are consistent with bulky seminomatous disease, LDH level is related to tumor burden in nonseminomatous disease, and LDH may be the sole biochemical abnormality in approximately 10% of patients with persistent/recurrent nonseminomatous germ cell tumors.[32]

The S category is based on the pre-orchiectomy measurement of serum tumor markers. When serum tumor markers have not been performed or are not available, the category SX is assigned. The category of S0 is assigned when all serum tumor markers are within normal limits. If serum tumor markers are known to be elevated above the limits of normal, one of the categories of S1, S2, or S3 is applicable. S1 is assigned when at least 1 serum tumor marker is elevated above normal and all the following criteria are met: LDH less than 1.5 times the upper limit of normal, hCG (mIU/mL) <5000, and AFP (ng/mL) <1000. S2 is assigned when 1 of the following criteria is present: LDH 1.5 to 10 times the upper limit of normal, hCG is between 5000 and 50,000, or AFP is between 1000 and 10,000. S3 is then assigned when LDH, hCG, or AFP are greater than its respective limit for the S2 category.

ADDITIONAL REPORTING PARAMETERS AND FURTHER CHALLENGES

Several challenges remain in staging testicular germ cell tumors, and these issues merit brief discussion.

SUBCATEGORIZATION OF pT1 IN PURE SEMINOMA

New in the AJCC eighth edition is subcategorization of the pT1 stage of pure seminoma. It should be emphasized that this does not apply to nonseminomatous germ cell tumors, including mixed germ cell tumors with a seminomatous component. Pure seminomas that are confined to the testis and lack lymphovascular invasion are subcategorized based on a 3-cm cutoff, such that tumors smaller than 3 cm are stage pT1a and tumors that are ≥3 cm are stage pT1b. This is a welcome addition to the staging system, as several large studies have identified size of pure seminoma as an independent predictor of disease recurrence.[10–12,16] There is, however, some controversy regarding the 3-cm size cutoff for seminoma, as many of the previous and recent publications recommended a larger size cutoff of ≥4 cm.[12,13,33,34] The AJCC has conservatively accepted the 3-cm cutoff, which leaves room for criticism as well as providing an incentive for future studies to refine this data point.

STAGING OF METASTATIC DEPOSITS IN THE SPERMATIC CORD

Tumor adjacent to or surrounding the vas deferens constitutes spermatic cord invasion (stage pT3), but a discontinuous tumor deposit outside of a lymphovascular space in the mid or upper spermatic cord is considered a metastasis, warranting assignment as stage M1 in accordance with the AJCC staging eighth edition. There are no comprehensive data about this finding, but it is reported that it is strongly associated with vascular invasion. Although the AJCC eighth edition is clear that this situation warrants assignment of stage M1, it is unclear which, if either, M1 substage is applicable. As discussed previously, M1a is

defined as nonretroperitoneal nodal or pulmonary metastases, whereas M1b is defined as nonpulmonary visceral metastases. Given these definitions, neither M1a nor M1b seems strictly to apply to metastatic deposits in the spermatic cord. Clearly, it would intuitively make sense to assign M1a given the close proximity of the spermatic cord to the primary tumor relative to other potential metastatic sites. This ambiguity requires further clarification to either not sub stage, assign M1a, or perhaps create a third subcategory for spermatic cord metastases.

RISK CATEGORY STRATIFICATION AND RISK ASSESSMENT MODELS

AJCC also endorsed patient stratification into 3 risk categories (good, intermediate, poor) considering serum markers and visceral metastasis including mediastinal location, for which guidelines have been provided by International Germ Cell Consensus Classification Grouping. Similarly, AJCC established guidelines to evaluate published statistical prediction models and to endorse them for clinical purposes.[35,36]

ROLE OF UNION FOR INTERNATIONAL CANCER CONTROL IN STANDARDIZATION AND HARMONIZATION OF TNM STAGING CLASSIFICATION

More than a year after publication of the AJCC eighth edition and the UICC eighth edition, there is no clarity regarding what to expect in the future, as it has been widely criticized that UICC has not incorporated many of the changes that are now part of the AJCC staging classification despite having sound clinical data to support these additions/modifications.[2] UICC TNM staging is widely accepted and used globally, and there is a genuine fear that it will have ramifications for patient management approaches and an even more concerning dilemma is that questions will be raised as to the credibility of these organizations if no resolution is urgently provided.

SUMMARY

In the eighth edition of the AJCC Staging Manual, substantial changes and clarifications are provided for the TNM and S stage categories. These changes are primarily based on recently reported pathologic data relevant to prognosis. Although these changes improve on the prior staging system, several further challenges remain.

REFERENCES

1. Denoix PF. Bull Inst nag Hyg (Paris) 1944;1:69. 1944;2:82. 1950;5:81. 1952;7:743.

2. Delahunt B, Egevad L, Samaratunga H, et al. UICC drops the ball in the 8th edition TNM staging of urological cancers. Histopathology 2017;71(1):5–11.

3. Brierley JD, Gospodarowicz MK, Wittekind C. UICC TNM classification of malignant tumours. 8th edition. New York: Wiley Black-well; 2016.

4. Beahrs OH, Carr DT, Rubin P. Manual for staging of cancer 1977. 1st edition. Chicago: American Joint Committee; 1977.

5. Amin MB, Edge S, Geen F, et al. AJCC cancer staging manual. 8th edition. New York: Springer Verlag; 2016.

6. Moch H, Humphrey PA, Ulbright TM, et al. WHO classification of tumours of the urinary system and male genital organs. 4th edition. Lyon (France): IARC; 2016.

7. Yilmaz A, Cheng T, Zhang J, et al. Testicular hilum and vascular invasion predict advanced clinical stage in nonseminomatous germ cell tumors. Mod Pathol 2013;26(4):579–86.

8. Balzer BL, Ulbright TM. Spontaneous regression of testicular germ cell tumors: an analysis of 42 cases. Am J Surg Pathol 2006;30(7):858–65.

9. Emerson RE, Ulbright TM. Intratubular germ cell neoplasia of the testis and its associated cancers: the use of novel biomarkers. Pathology 2010;42(4): 344–55.

10. Chung P, Daugaard G, Tyldesley S, et al. Evaluation of a prognostic model for risk of relapse in stage I seminoma surveillance. Cancer Med 2015;4(1):155–60.

11. Aparicio J, Maroto P, Garcia del Muro X, et al. Prognostic factors for relapse in stage I seminoma: a new nomogram derived from three consecutive, risk-adapted studies from the Spanish Germ Cell Cancer Group (SGCCG). Ann Oncol 2014;25(11):2173–8.

12. Warde P, Specht L, Horwich A, et al. Prognostic factors for relapse in stage I seminoma managed by surveillance: a pooled analysis. J Clin Oncol 2002; 20(22):4448–52.

13. Mortensen MS, Lauritsen J, Gundgaard MG, et al. A nationwide cohort study of stage I seminoma patients followed on a surveillance program. Eur Urol 2014;66(6):1172–8.

14. Kamba T, Kamoto T, Okubo K, et al. Outcome of different post-orchiectomy management for stage I seminoma: Japanese multi-institutional study including 425 patients. Int J Urol 2010;17(12):980–7.

15. Vogt AP, Chen Z, Osunkoya AO. Rete testis invasion by malignant germ cell tumor and/or intratubular germ cell neoplasia: what is the significance of this finding? Hum Pathol 2010;41(9):1339–44.

16. Berney DM, Algaba F, Amin M, et al. Handling and reporting of orchidectomy specimens with testicular cancer: areas of consensus and variation among 25 experts and 225 European pathologists. Histopathology 2015;67(3):313–24.

17. Alexandre J, Fizazi K, Mahe C, et al. Stage I nonseminomatous germ-cell tumours of the testis: identification of a subgroup of patients with a very low risk of relapse. Eur J Cancer 2001;37(5):576–82.

18. Lu K. Surveillance for stage I nonseminoma testicular cancer: outcomes and long-term follow-up in a population-based cohort. J Clin Oncol 2015;33(20): 2322.

19. Daugaard G, Gundgaard MG, Mortensen MS, et al. Surveillance for stage I nonseminoma testicular cancer: outcomes and long-term follow-up in a population-based cohort. J Clin Oncol 2014;32(34):3817–23.

20. Nazeer T, Ro JY, Kee KH, et al. Spermatic cord contamination in testicular cancer. Mod Pathol 1996;9(7):762–6.

21. Verrill C, Yilmaz A, Srigley JR, et al. Reporting and staging of testicular germ cell tumors: The International Society of Urological Pathology (ISUP) testicular cancer consultation conference recommendations. Am J Surg Pathol 2017;41(6):e22–32.

22. McCleskey BC, Epstein JI, Albany C, et al. The significance of lymphovascular invasion of the spermatic cord in the absence of cord soft tissue invasion. Arch Pathol Lab Med 2017;141(6):824–9.

23. Gordetsky J, Sanfrancesco J, Epstein JI, et al. Do nonseminomatous germ cell tumors of the testis with lymphovascular invasion of the spermatic cord merit staging as pT3? Am J Surg Pathol 2017; 41(10):1397–402.

24. Sanfrancesco JM, Trevino KE, Xu H, et al. The significance of spermatic cord involvement by testicular germ cell tumors: should we be staging discontinuous invasion from involved lymphovascular spaces differently from direct extension? Am J Surg Pathol 2018;42(3):306–11.

25. Coursey Moreno C, Small WC, Camacho JC, et al. Testicular tumors: what radiologists need to know–differential diagnosis, staging, and management. Radiographics 2015;35(2):400–15.

26. Hedgire SS, Pargaonkar VK, Elmi A, et al. Pelvic nodal imaging. Radiol Clin North Am 2012;50(6):1111–25.

27. Ehrlich Y, Beck SD, Foster RS, et al. Serum tumor markers in testicular cancer. Urol Oncol 2013; 31(1):17–23.

28. Masterson TA, Rice KR, Beck SD. Current and future biologic markers for disease progression and relapse in testicular germ cell tumors: a review. Urol Oncol 2014;32(3):261–71.

29. Bosl GJ, Motzer RJ. Testicular germ-cell cancer. N Engl J Med 1997;337(4):242–53.

30. Gilbert SM, Daignault S, Weizer AZ, et al. The use of tumor markers in testis cancer in the United States: a potential quality issue. Urol Oncol 2008;26(2):153–7.

31. Gilligan TD, Seidenfeld J, Basch EM, et al. American Society of Clinical Oncology Clinical Practice Guideline on uses of serum tumor markers in adult males with germ cell tumors. J Clin Oncol 2010;28(20): 3388–404.

32. Skinner DG, Scardino PT. Relevance of biochemical tumor markers and lymphadenectomy in management of non-seminomatous testis tumors: current perspective. J Urol 1980;123(3):378–82.

33. Albers P, Albrecht W, Algaba F, et al. EAU guidelines on testicular cancer: 2011 update. European Association of Urology. Actas Urol Esp 2012;36(3): 127–45, [in Spanish].

34. Albers P, Albrecht W, Algaba F, et al. EAU guidelines on testicular cancer: 2011 update. Eur Urol 2011; 60(2):304–19.

35. International Germ Cell Consensus Classification. A prognostic factor-based staging system for metastatic germ cell cancers. International Germ Cell Cancer Collaborative Group. J Clin Oncol 1997; 15(2):594–603.

36. Kattan MW, Hess KR, Amin MB, et al. American Joint Committee on Cancer acceptance criteria for inclusion of risk models for individualized prognosis in the practice of precision medicine. CA Cancer J Clin 2016;66(5):370–4.

"Man in Istanbul" Lesions of the Urinary Tract (Known Entities in an Unusual Context)

Melanoma, Carcinoid Tumors, Epithelioid Angiosarcoma

Sameh Samaan, MD[a], M. Ruhul Quddus, MD[b],
Andres Matoso, MD[a,c,d],*

KEYWORDS

- Melanoma • Carcinoid tumor • Epithelioid angiosarcoma • Urethra • Bladder • Kidney

---

Key points

- Distal urethra is the most common site for melanoma, which may present as polypoid mass with surface ulceration.

- The most common patterns of growth of primary melanoma include diffuse followed by nested. Other patterns also seen are spindle-shaped cells growing in a storiform and fascicular pattern and large pleomorphic cells.

- Carcinoid tumors of the bladder and prostatic urethra are usually small submucosal nodules, and the overlying urothelium usually shows cystitis cystica glandularis and papillary hyperplasia. The most common architectural pattern is pseudoglandular.

- In contrast to carcinoid tumors of the bladder, renal carcinoid tumors develop metastasis in approximately 50% of patients, and the most common architectural pattern is tightly packed cords.

- Epithelioid angiosarcoma can present following radiation therapy or de novo. Tumor cells show highly atypical nuclei with scant to moderate amount of eosinophilic or amphophilic cytoplasm, immersed in a hemorrhagic background with fragments of erythrocytes between tumor cells.

ABSTRACT

Certain tumors are more difficult to recognize when they present in an unusual location. Within the urinary tract, primary melanomas, carcinoid tumors, or epithelioid angiosarcoma could present diagnostic challenges due to their infrequent occurrence. This article emphasizes the clinical and histopathologic features of these entities and their differential diagnoses including the immunophenotype and their prognoses.

Conflict of Interest: The authors declare no conflict of interest.

Source of Funding: This study was supported by the Department of Pathology of Johns Hopkins University.

[a] Department of Pathology, The Johns Hopkins Medical Institutions, Johns Hopkins Hospital, Weinberg 2242, 401 North Broadway, Baltimore, MD 21231-2410, USA; [b] Department of Pathology, Women and Infants Hospital of Rhode Island, 101 Dudley Street, Providence, RI 02903, USA; [c] Department of Urology, The Johns Hopkins Medical Institutions, Johns Hopkins Hospital, Weinberg 2242, 401 North Broadway, Baltimore, MD 21231-2410, USA; [d] Department of Oncology, The Johns Hopkins Medical Institutions, Johns Hopkins Hospital, Weinberg 2242, 401 North Broadway, Baltimore, MD 21231-2410, USA

* Corresponding author. Johns Hopkins Hospital, Weinberg 2242, 401 North Broadway, Baltimore, MD 21231-2410.

E-mail address: amatoso1@jhmi.edu

surgpath.theclinics.com

OVERVIEW

It is well known by all pathologists that recognition of a specific entity is facilitated when it is located in its expected surroundings. Some lesions that are not commonly seen within the urinary system may be misdiagnosed due to their "wrong location" despite otherwise classic histologic features. Dr Lauren V. Ackerman used to refer to this situation as the "Man from Istanbul." The story, as told by Dr Juan Rosai, is that of a man who lives in New York City and each morning he opened the door of his apartment to go to work and found himself facing the man living in the apartment in front of his, who went to work at exactly the same time. For decades, he would say "Good morning, Fred," hear the reply "Good morning, John," and go to his business. Until, 1 day, John was given an assignment in Istanbul. The first morning in Istanbul, he opened the door of his hotel room and found himself facing Fred, who has just opened the door of the room across from his. John's conscience told him it was unthinkable to that this person was his neighbor Fred, because he was in Istanbul; however, Fred had also been given an assignment in Istanbul.[1] It is unclear whether this story is true, but it is well known by any experienced pathologist that a lesion that would have been an easy "pattern recognition" diagnosis, when present in an unexpected location, it might be hard to recognize. In this review, we summarize several such lesions occasionally seen in the genitourinary tract and provide clues to arrive at the correct diagnosis.

PRIMARY MELANOMA

Primary melanoma of the genitourinary tract is very rare but well documented. The most common site of origin is the urethra and represents fewer than 1% of all melanomas.[2–4] It is more frequent in women than men with a female:male ratio of 3:1.[5,6] Melanoma most commonly affects the distal urethra and urethral meatus.[7] In men, more than half of the cases occur in the fossa navicularis, and the remaining are distributed in all different segments of the urethra, including in the prostatic urethra.[8] Rarely, they can present in the urinary bladder or renal pelvis and ureter.[9–11] They are thought to develop from ectopic melanocytes that have been arrested in the urothelium during embryonic neural crest migration.[3] The average age at presentation in the largest series published was 72 years (range 56–96) in women and 62 years (range 44–69) in men. The clinical presentation includes perineal mass and pain, dysuria, incontinence, hematuria, or local bleeding. Occasionally, if the mass is occluding the lumen of the urethra, the presenting symptoms could be voiding dysfunction.[3,5] One case had the diagnosis of lentigo of the meatus for several years.[6] The clinical presentation might include inguinal lymphadenopathy, due to reactive lymphoid hyperplasia due to infection of the primary lesion or lymph node enlargement due to metastasis.[12]

GROSS FEATURES

The gross findings of primary urethral melanoma range from pigmented nodular tumor, pedunculated tumor, or a pigmented hemorrhagic lesion in the posterior wall of the urethral meatus.[2,5] Cases resembling a caruncle or polyps have also been reported.[6,13] Multifocality is rare but reported.[6] In men, glans penis may also be affected by extension of melanoma from the urethra.[12] In women, the primary lesion could be located in the vagina or vulva and invade the urethra.[14]

MICROSCOPIC FEATURES

Histopathological examination most commonly reveals a polypoid tumor with overlying mucosal ulceration, partially covered with squamous mucosa. Tumor cells may be epithelioid or spindled and can be arranged in nests, or grow in a storiform and fascicular pattern and with large pleomorphic cells. The most common pattern of growth is diffuse, followed by nested. Prominent rhabdoid features have been observed in many cases. Pseudopapillary growth was also reported.[6] Due to surface ulceration, there could be an inflammatory infiltrate. Melanin deposition is not always present.[15] Mitoses and necrosis can be seen (**Fig. 1**).

DIFFERENTIAL DIAGNOSIS

Epithelioid melanomas should be differentiated from carcinomas. In the urethra, the most frequent carcinomas include squamous and urothelial carcinomas. Spindle-cell melanomas could be

> *Pathologic Key Features*
> OF PRIMARY MELANOMA
> OF THE URINARY TRACT
>
> 1. Most common location is the distal urethra and urethral meatus.
>
> 2. Can present as polypoid mass resembling a caruncle.
>
> 3. May show surface ulceration or be partially covered with squamous mucosa.
>
> 4. Some are pigmented but a proportion of them are not (amelanotic).

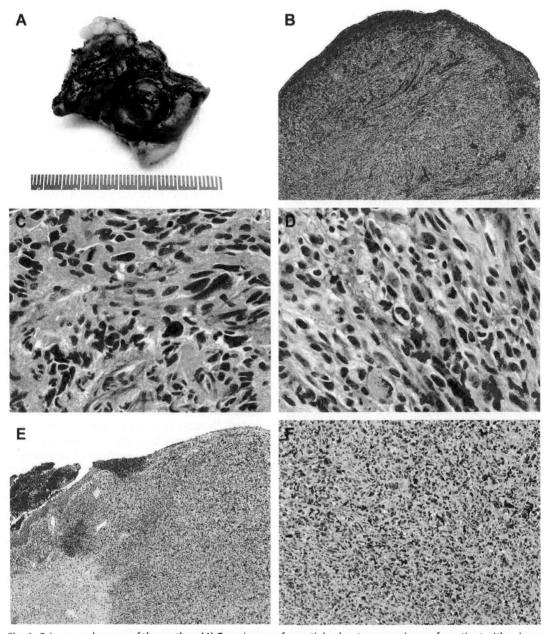

Fig. 1. Primary melanoma of the urethra. (*A*) Gross image of a partial vulvectomy specimen of a patient with primary melanoma of the urethra. The tumor is pigmented and bulges the mucosal surface. (*B*) Low-power view (H&E, original magnification ×40) of a urethral melanoma showing surface ulceration and underlying population of malignant cells with spindle morphology forming intersecting fascicles. (*C*) High power (H&E, original magnification ×400) of (*B*) showing focal pigment deposition where it is difficult to differentiate between melanin and hemosiderin. (*D*) High-power view (H&E, original magnification ×400) of (*B*) showing high-grade nuclear features, spindle-cell morphology, and mitotic figures. (*E*) Another urethral melanoma also characterized by mucosal ulceration and underlying population of highly atypical neoplastic cells. (H&E, original magnification ×40) (*F*) High-power view (H&E, original magnification ×400) of (*E*) shows highly pleomorphic population of cells. Note the absence of pigmentation.

misdiagnosed as sarcomatoid carcinoma. Neoplastic cells can show reactivity for one or more of melanoma markers including Melan-A, HMB45, SOX10, MITF, MART-1, and S100 protein.[2,16] Markers of urothelial or squamous differentiation including high molecular weight cytokeratin, p63, or GATA-3 are usually negative.[17] Metastatic melanoma to the urethra is rarely a clinically significant finding but it should be considered within the differential diagnosis. Of the patients included in the largest case series published, 2 (13%) of 15 had history of a

Pitfalls
IN THE DIAGNOSIS OF
PRIMARY URETHRAL MELANOMA

! Given its epithelioid/spindle morphology, melanomas are potential pitfalls for invasive carcinoma or sarcomatoid carcinoma, especially amelanotic ones.

! Some lesions are ulcerated and inflamed and if the biopsy is superficial it might obscure the visualization of tumor cells. Performing a cytokeratin immunostain could be misleading, as tumor cells will be negative in a case of melanoma that is occult within a brisk inflammatory infiltrate. Performing immunomarkers for melanocytes, including S100, Melan-A, HMB45, or SOX10, would be helpful in the identification of the tumor cells.

melanoma in another location but were thought to have a new primary in the urethra.[6]

DIAGNOSIS

Almost invariably, the diagnosis of primary melanoma of the urinary tract involves the use of immunohistochemistry stains to prove the melanocytic origin of malignant cells. These markers include HMB45, Melan-A, MART1, MITF1, S100, and SOX10. Due to its rarity, there are no well-established guidelines of histopathologic parameters that are expected to be included in the pathology report. Some basic information that should be mentioned in the report include size, depth of invasion (pathologic stage), vascular or perineural invasion, mitotic activity, and distance to margins.[18]

PROGNOSIS

Overall, primary melanoma of the urethra has a poor prognosis with high recurrence rates and systemic metastases.[6] The management options include radical urethrectomy followed by radiotherapy and/or systemic chemotherapy.[12,19,20] A study that investigated mutations in genitourinary melanomas in women identified 1 of 5 urethral melanomas with an *NRAS* mutation and none with a *KIT* or *BRAF* mutation.[21] There is an ongoing clinical trial with anti-CTLA-4 and anti-PD-1/PD-L1 for mucosal melanoma with promising results.[22]

PRIMARY CARCINOID TUMOR OF THE URINARY BLADDER AND PROSTATIC URETHRA

Primary carcinoid tumors of the bladder and prostatic urethra are extremely rare and the literature consists mostly of single case reports and 1 series of 6 cases.[23–29] The age at presentation varied from 30 to 73 years and there was a slight male predominance. Most cases presented with gross hematuria. They have a predilection for the trigone and bladder neck area and are usually very small.

GROSS FINDINGS

On cystoscopic evaluation, all reported cases were small, round, or polypoid nodules raging in size from 0.1 to 0.6 cm. There is 1 case in the literature with a size of 3.0 cm with muscularis propria invasion.

MICROSCOPIC FEATURES

Most of the cases are subepithelial lesions confined to the submucosa.[23] Rarely, the tumor may involve the muscularis propria (detrusor muscle).[30] Tumor cells are usually cuboidal or columnar and have a stippled chromatin with inconspicuous nucleoli. Paneth cell-like features are common. The most common architectural pattern is pseudoglandular structures including cribriform areas.[23,24] The case that presented with detrusor invasion showed a trabecular pattern in addition to pseudoglandular.[30] Mitotic activity is absent or only rare. Necrosis has not been reported. Occasional nuclear hyperchromasia or irregularities were noted. The overlying urothelium often shows papillary hyperplasia or cystitis cystica glandularis.[23] Neuroendocrine markers, such as chromogranin A and synaptophysin, are positive in most cases[23,24] (**Fig. 2**). There are 2 reported cases of positive immunostaining for prostatic-specific acid phosphatase (PSAP),[23,30] and 1 case that was positive for calcitonin.[27] The neuroendocrine markers also highlight the neuroendocrine cells within the cystitis cystica glandularis that overlies the carcinoid tumor. This close association has led to speculate that these neuroendocrine cells within cystitis cystica glandularis are the origin of the tumors.[23]

Pathologic Key Features
OF PRIMARY CARCINOID TUMOR
OF THE BLADDER AND URETHRA

1. Most of the cases are subepithelial lesions confined to the submucosa.

2. The most common architectural pattern is pseudoglandular structures including cribriform areas.

3. Neuroendocrine, chromogranin A, and synaptophysin are positive in most cases.

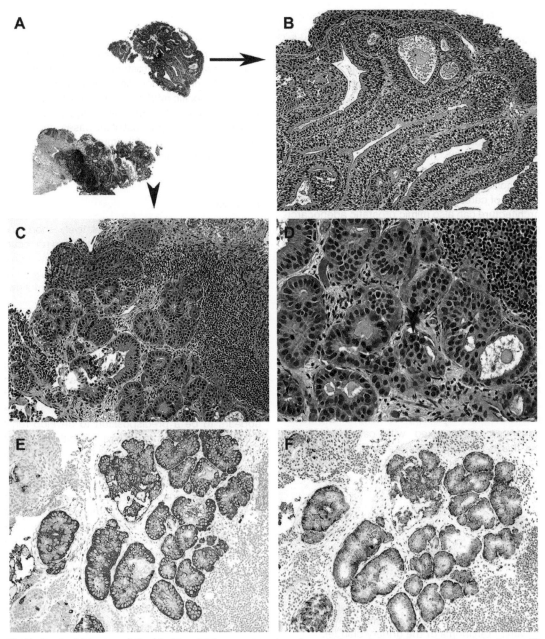

Fig. 2. Carcinoid tumor of the bladder. (*A*) Low-power view shows 2 fragments of tissue (H&E, original magnification ×20). The one on the top right corner is the overlying urothelium showing cystitis cystica (*arrow* points to magnification of upper right tissue fragment; *arrowhead* points to magnification of lower left tissue fragment). (*B*) Higher magnification (H&E, original magnification ×100) of top right corner of (*A*). This corresponds to the urothelium overlying the area of the carcinoid tumor. The benign urothelium is forming cystic spaces underlying the surface, characteristic of cystitis cystica, which is frequently associated with carcinoid tumors of the bladder. (*C*) Higher magnification (H&E, original magnification ×100) of lower left corner of (*A*). The tumor involves the lamina propria and is composed of glandularlike structures characteristic of the "pseudoglandular" pattern of carcinoid tumor. Note the surrounding associated chronic inflammation. (*D*) Higher magnification of (*C*) (H&E, original magnification ×400). Tumor cells show round to oval nuclei with smooth nuclear borders and inconspicuous nucleoli and eosinophilic cytoplasm. Mitotic activity can be seen (*arrowhead*) but is rare. (*E*) Immunohistochemistry for chromogranin shows diffuse staining of tumor cells. (*F*) Immunohistochemistry for synaptophysin is also diffusely positive in tumor cells.

DIFFERENTIAL DIAGNOSIS

Carcinoid tumors could mimic inverted urothelial papillomas cystoscopically given its polypoid appearance. Peripheral palisading of nuclei, which is characteristic of inverted urothelial papillomas, is not seen in carcinoid tumors. Additionally, cribriform glands, eosinophilic granules, and stippled chromatin are not features of inverted papilloma. Another important differential diagnosis is with nested variant of urothelial carcinoma, which can often show a tubular morphology, similar to the pseudoglandular pattern of carcinoid tumors. The pseudoglandular architecture can also mimic prostatic adenocarcinoma involving the bladder. The presence of positive immunostaining for PSAP in 2 of the reported cases could lead to the diagnostic pitfall if carcinoid tumor is not considered.[23,30] The opposite is also a potential pitfall, as prostate adenocarcinoma is often positive for neuroendocrine markers.[31] Last, the pseudoglandular differentiation could lead to the misdiagnosis of invasive urothelial carcinoma with glandular differentiation or primary adenocarcinoma of the bladder and urethra. Adenocarcinomas show more nuclear atypia, nuclear overlap, mitoses, and apoptosis and are usually negative for neuroendocrine markers. There is a reported case of a bladder adenocarcinoma mixed with carcinoid tumor, but this is not the typical presentation of neither adenocarcinoma nor carcinoid tumor.[32] Key diagnostic pitfalls are presented in.

Pitfalls
IN THE DIAGNOSIS OF
CARCINOID TUMORS OF THE BLADDER
AND URETHRA

! The pseudoglandular architecture of carcinoid tumors is a potential diagnostic pitfall for prostate adenocarcinoma or primary adenocarcinoma of the urinary bladder.

! Rare cases of carcinoid tumors have been reported to be prostate-specific acid phosphatase (PSAP) positive by immunohistochemistry; addition of other prostate-specific markers, including PSA, NKX3.1, or prostein, should prevent this misinterpretation.

! The pseudoglandular architecture could mimic the tubular type of invasive urothelial carcinoma, nested variant. The presence of cribriform areas and subnuclear eosinophilic granules characteristic of carcinoid tumor are not features of nested urothelial carcinoma.

DIAGNOSIS

By immunohistochemistry, carcinoid tumors are positive for neuroendocrine markers synaptophysin and chromogranin. Prostate cancer can also be positive for neuroendocrine markers, and therefore prostate-specific markers, including NKX3.1, prostein, and/or prostate-specific antigen should be considered. Although most of the cases are submucosal without invasion of the muscularis propria, the presence or absence of detrusor invasion should be reported.

PROGNOSIS

Although the follow-up was relatively short, the cases of the largest series published had no recurrence or evidence of disease progression.[23] One case that presented with invasion of the detrusor showed a millimetric tumor recurrence in follow-up cystoscopy.[30]

CARCINOID TUMOR OF THE KIDNEY

Primary carcinoid tumors of the kidney are very uncommon but there are many cases reported in the literature, including a series of 21 cases.[33,34] There is an equal gender distribution.[33,35] There appears to be a predisposition to develop renal carcinoids in patients with a clinical history of horseshoe kidney, although the mechanisms involved in that association are unclear.[21,35–40] Other associations include polycystic kidney disease and teratomas.[41–43] Some cases have been associated with intestinal metaplasia within the renal pelvis.[35,44] The clinical presentation is variable and common to any renal tumor, including hematuria, palpable mass, and pain or discomfort. Some patients have reported to experience Cushing syndrome and flushing.[35]

GROSS FINDINGS

The great majority of the tumors are unifocal with rare cases reported to be multifocal.[33,35] The tumor size varied from 1 to 30 cm. The tumor can involve any areas of the kidney, including the cortex, medulla, or renal pelvis.[33] Most cases present as encapsulated solid mass but cystic masses also have been reported.[40] The cut surface is solid yellow-tan and focally lobulated. Hemorrhage and necrosis have been reported as well, although they are rare.[44] Compression of the renal pelvis has been reported with consequential pelvis dilatation and infection.[44] Extrarenal extension into the perirenal fat is present in roughly 50% of the cases.[33]

MICROSCOPIC FINDINGS

The most common architectural histologic pattern is tightly packed cords of tumor cells without a significant amount of stroma, followed by trabecular growth pattern, solid nests and sheets of tumor cells, and pseudoglandular structures.[33] The nuclei could be rounded or elongated, most commonly with their long axis perpendicular to the long axis of the cord or trabeculae. The chromatin shows the fine stippled appearance ("salt and pepper") with inconspicuous nucleoli characteristic of neuroendocrine tumors. Calcifications were noted in a subset of cases including psammomatous calcifications[33,40] (Fig. 3). Mitotic activity can be seen and range from 0/10 high-power fields (HPF) to 4/10 HPF.[33] By immunohistochemistry, the tumor is frequently positive for neuroendocrine markers synaptophysin (most commonly positive), chromogranin, and CD56.[33] Cytokeratin Cam5.2 is frequently positive but other cytokeratins, including CK7 and CK20, are usually negative. TTF-1 is also negative in renal carcinoid tumors,[45] but this is similar to lung carcinoid tumors[46] and, therefore, to exclude a metastasis, a careful clinical correlation is necessary. PAX2 and PAX8, which are considered reliable markers of kidney origin, are usually negative in renal carcinoids.[40]

DIFFERENTIAL DIAGNOSIS

The differential diagnosis includes tumors with neuroendocrine features and tumors with architectural patterns similar to those of carcinoid tumors. The main differential diagnoses include papillary renal cell carcinoma, metanephric adenoma, neuroblastoma, paraganglioma, Ewing sarcoma/primitive

neuroectodermal tumor (EWS/PNET), and metastatic neuroendocrine tumor. Solid or trabecular patterns of carcinoid tumor could resemble papillary renal cell carcinoma or metanephric adenoma, especially in small needle biopsies, but the nuclear features should point in the right direction. If in question, immunohistochemistry markers could be helpful, as WT1, which is a reliable marker of metanephric adenoma or PAX8 as a marker of renal origin, are consistently negative in renal carcinoid tumors and neuroendocrine markers synaptophysin and chromogranin are not positive for metanephric adenomas or papillary renal cell carcinomas.[33] EWS/PNET and neuroblastomas are high-grade tumors with frequent mitoses and are negative for chromogranin/synaptophysin. CD99 would not help in this differential diagnosis because it can be positive in both.[40] Paragangliomas could show very similar morphologic features, but the sustentacular pattern highlighted by S100 immunostain characteristic of paragangliomas has not been reported in carcinoid tumors. Neuroblastomas show a neurofibrillary background and Homer-Wright rosettes that are not seen in carcinoid tumors.

DIAGNOSIS

By immunohistochemistry, tumor cells are positive for neuroendocrine markers synaptophysin, chromogranin, and CD56.[45] CD99 is also frequently positive and could lead to misinterpretation as EWS/PNET. Kidney-specific markers PAX2 and PAX8 are usually negative in carcinoid tumors.[40]

PROGNOSIS

Approximately 50% of renal carcinoids present with metastasis or develop metastasis following a resection of the primary tumor, despite low mitotic rate.[45] The most common sites of metastasis include lymph nodes, liver, lung, bone, and soft tissue but usually have a prolonged clinical course despite distant metastasis.[33,35,40,45]

EPITHELIOID ANGIOSARCOMA

Angiosarcoma is a malignant tumor that recapitulates the morphologic and functional features of endothelium to a variable degree. Epithelioid angiosarcoma is a morphologic variant of angiosarcoma in which the great majority of the tumor cells have an epithelioid morphology mimicking a carcinoma.[47,48] Angiosarcomas can occasionally involve the urinary tract and when the epithelioid morphology predominates, they can be misdiagnosed as

---

Pathologic Key Features
OF CARCINOID TUMORS
OF THE KIDNEY

1. The most common architectural histologic pattern is tightly packed cords of tumor cells without significant amount of stroma.

2. The nuclei could be rounded or elongated, most commonly with their long axis perpendicular to the long axis of the cord or trabeculae.

3. Mitotic activity can be seen and range from 0/10 high-power fields (HPF) to 4/10 HPF.

4. Usually positive for neuroendocrine markers synaptophysin, chromogranin, and neurone specific enolase, but negative for PAX8.

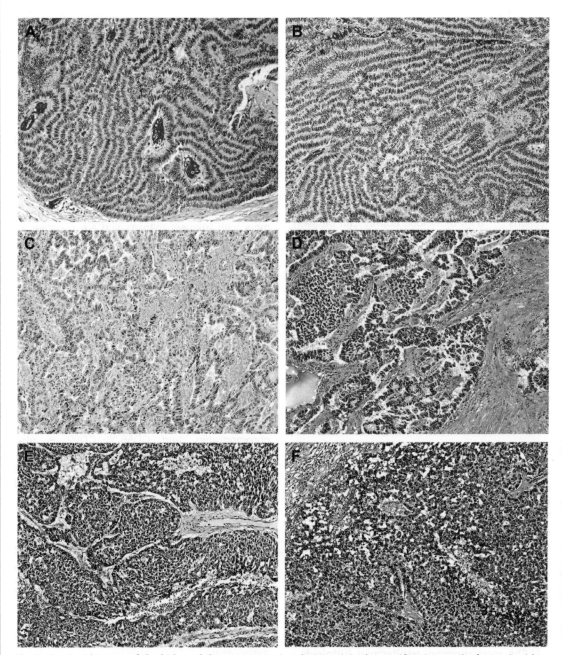

Fig. 3. Carcinoid tumor of the kidney. (A) Low-power view (H&E, original magnification ×40) of a carcinoid tumor of the kidney showing tightly packed cords of cells, the most common pattern observed in this location. (B) Higher magnification (H&E, original magnification ×100) of (A) showing the vesicular chromatin in contrast to the usual "salt and pepper appearance." The architectural pattern is key to recognize the tumor as carcinoid. (C, D) Carcinoid tumor of the kidney showing a trabecular pattern with microcystic spaces in between cords of tumor cells. (H&E, original magnification ×100) (E, F) Solid variant of carcinoid tumor of the kidney. Note that the tumor cells have very scant cytoplasm mimicking Ewing sarcoma/PNET.

carcinoma.[49,50] There is a male predominance of approximately 5:1. The ages at presentation varied from 39 to 83 years.[49,50] A proportion, but not all cases, present with clinical history of radiation therapy to the pelvis meeting diagnostic criteria of radiation-induced sarcoma.[49,51–53] The clinical presentation is invariably gross hematuria and mass. Additional symptoms include irritative lower urinary tract symptoms.[49,51]

Pitfalls
IN THE DIAGNOSIS OF CARCINOID TUMORS OF THE KIDNEY

! Carcinoid tumors are frequently positive for CD99, which could be a diagnostic pitfall with Ewing sarcoma/primitive neuroectodermal tumor (PNET). Ewing/PNETs are usually more mitotically active and show high-grade nuclear features that are not characteristic of carcinoid tumors.

! Paragangliomas could show similar morphologic and immunophenotypic findings but renal carcinoids do not show the sustentacular cell pattern seen with S100 in paragangliomas.

GROSS FINDINGS

Cystoscopically, the tumors show a hemorrhagic appearance and could be located anywhere within the bladder. One tumor is reported to have originated from the ureter.[54] The size of the tumor varied from <1 cm to 10 cm.[49,50] One case was reported to show a papillary appearance.[51]

MICROSCOPIC FINDINGS

Histologically, the tumors are composed of sheets of tumor cells with highly atypical nuclear features and scant to moderate amount of eosinophilic or amphophilic cytoplasm. Some tumors show prominent large nucleoli with excentric nuclei giving a rhabdoid appearance. Intracytoplasmic lumens or vacuoles could occasionally be seen and may contain red blood cell fragments. A hemorrhagic

Pathologic Key Features
OF EPITHELIOID ANGIOSARCOMA OF THE BLADDER

1. Epithelioid angiosarcoma is a morphologic variant of angiosarcoma in which the great majority of the tumor cells have an epithelioid morphology.

2. Tumors are composed of sheets of tumor cells with highly atypical nuclear features and scant to moderate amount of eosinophilic or amphophilic cytoplasm.

3. A hemorrhagic background is commonly seen and fragments of erythrocytes between tumor cells are a consistent finding.

background is commonly seen and fragments of erythrocytes between tumor cells are a consistent finding. Hemosiderin deposition can also be seen.[49] Although the epithelioid morphology predominates in order to be considered "epithelioid" angiosarcoma, some cases also show foci with spindle-shaped cell morphology, or classic morphology with anastomosing blood-filled channels lined by atypical cells.[49,50] Involvement of muscularis propria is frequent and some cases can involve the prostate[49] (Fig. 4).

DIFFERENTIAL DIAGNOSIS

Given the epithelioid morphology of tumor cells and the high-grade features, the main differential diagnosis is with invasive high-grade urothelial carcinoma. Positive immunohistochemistry for vascular markers, including CD31, CD34, ERG, and factor VIII should lead toward the right diagnosis. Most cases are negative for cytokeratin stains but focal positive cytokeratin stain is commonly seen and should not be interpreted as sufficient evidence of epithelial origin. The other main differential diagnosis is epithelioid hemangioendothelioma. However, the high-grade morphology and frequent mitoses seen in epithelioid angiosarcoma are not features of epithelioid hemangioendothelioma.

DIAGNOSIS

By immunohistochemistry, tumor cells are frequently positive for at least one endothelial marker, including CD31, CD34, ERG, or factor VIII.[49] The key to arrive at the correct diagnosis is to identify the high-grade nuclear features, the hemorrhagic background, and fragments of erythrocytes between tumor cells. Cytokeratins may be focally positive.

Pitfalls
IN THE DIAGNOSIS OF EPITHELIOID ANGIOSARCOMA OF THE BLADDER

! Given the epithelioid morphology, the main diagnostic pitfall is with urothelial carcinoma. Positive immunostaining for cytokeratin in epithelioid angiosarcoma could be misleading.

! Epithelioid morphology and positive immunohistochemistry for vascular markers could make epithelioid hemangioendothelioma a potential pitfall; however, epithelioid hemangioendothelioma lacks the high-grade nuclear features of epithelioid angiosarcoma.

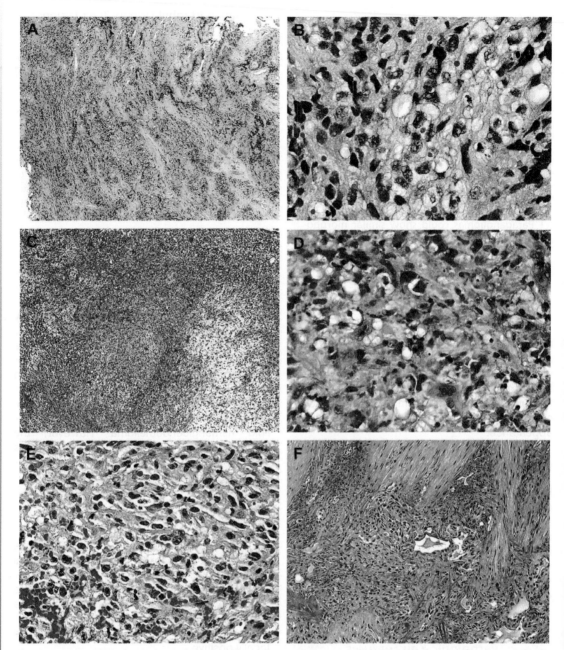

Fig. 4. Epithelioid angiosarcoma of the bladder. (*A*) Low-power view (H&E, original magnification ×20) of a TURBT specimen showing a cellular tumor with marked thermal and mechanical artifact. (*B*) Higher power view (H&E, original magnification ×400) of (*A*) shows tumor cells with highly atypical nuclei and cytoplasmic vacuoles with red blood cell fragments. (*C*) Low-power view (H&E, original magnification ×40) of another bladder tumor showing a diffuse expansion of tumor cells with foci of stromal edema. (*D*) Higher power (H&E, original magnification ×400) of (*C*) showing highly pleomorphic cells with focal cytoplasmic vacuoles and red blood cell fragments. (*E*) Another example of epithelioid angiosarcoma of the bladder showing tumor cells with nuclei with prominent nucleoli and eosinophilic cytoplasm. The interstitium shows inflammatory cells, red blood cells, and hemosiderin pigment. (H&E, original magnification ×200) (*F*) Muscle invasive epithelioid angiosarcoma with pseudoglandular formation, mimicking adenocarcinoma.

PROGNOSIS

Most patients diagnosed with epithelioid angiosarcoma of the bladder have a dismal prognosis, with an average survival of less than 2 years for most patients.[49]

REFERENCES

1. Rosai J. Introduction: Dr Lauren V. Ackerman and his man from Istanbul. Semin Diagn Pathol 2003;20(4): 247–8.

2. McComiskey M, Iavazzo C, Datta M, et al. Balloon cell urethral melanoma: differential diagnosis and management. Case Rep Obstet Gynecol 2015; 2015:919584.

3. DeSimone RA, Hoda RS. Primary malignant melanoma of the urethra detected by urine cytology in a male patient. Diagn Cytopathol 2015;43(8):680–2.

4. Dasgupta T, Grabstald H. Melanoma of the genitourinary tract. J Urol 1965;93:607–14.

5. Bhutani N, Kajal P, Pawar D. Primary malignant melanoma of the female urethra: report of a rare neoplasm of the urinary tract. Int J Surg Case Rep 2017;41:319–22.

6. Oliva E, Quinn TR, Amin MB, et al. Primary malignant melanoma of the urethra: a clinicopathologic analysis of 15 cases. Am J Surg Pathol 2000;24(6): 785–96.

7. Heslinga JM, Lycklama à Nijeholt GA, Ruiter DJ. Primary melanoma in the female distal urethra. Eur Urol 1986;12(6):446–7.

8. Morita T, Suzuki H, Goto K, et al. Primary malignant melanoma of male urethra with fistula formation. Urol Int 1991;46(1):114–5.

9. Ehara H, Takahashi Y, Saitoh A, et al. Clear cell melanoma of the renal pelvis presenting as a primary tumor. J Urol 1997;157(2):634.

10. Venyo AK. Melanoma of the urinary bladder: a review of the literature. Surg Res Pract 2014;2014: 605802.

11. Truong H, Sundi D, Sopko N, et al. A case report of primary recurrent malignant melanoma of the urinary bladder. Urol Case Rep 2013;1(1):2–4.

12. Li Y, Yuan H, Wang A, et al. Malignant melanoma of the penis and urethra: one case report. World J Surg Oncol 2014;12:340.

13. Safadi A, Schwalb S, Ben-Shachar I, et al. Primary malignant urethral melanoma resembling a urethral caruncle. Urol Case Rep 2017;15:28–9.

14. Lemanska A, Banach P, Magnowska M, et al. Vulvar melanoma with urethral invasion and bladder metastases—a case report and review of the literature. Arch Med Sci 2015;11(1):240–52.

15. Nakamoto T, Inoue Y, Ueki T, et al. Primary amelanotic malignant melanoma of the female urethra. Int J Urol 2007;14(2):153–5.

16. Karaman H, Yesil Y. Primary melanoma of the male urethra. Turk J Urol 2013;39(3):201–3.

17. Ha Lan TT, Chen SJ, Arps DP, et al. Expression of the p40 isoform of p63 has high specificity for cutaneous sarcomatoid squamous cell carcinoma. J Cutan Pathol 2014;41(11):831–8.

18. Sugiyama VE, Chan JK, Kapp DS. Management of melanomas of the female genital tract. Curr Opin Oncol 2008;20(5):565–9.

19. Akbas A, Akman T, Erdem MR, et al. Female urethral malignant melanoma with vesical invasion: a case report. Kaohsiung J Med Sci 2010;26(2):96–8.

20. Broussard AP, Chaudoir C, Gomelsky A. Urethral melanoma in an elderly woman. Int Urogynecol J 2015;26(1):149–50.

21. van Engen-van Grunsven AC, Kusters-Vandevelde HV, De Hullu J, et al. NRAS mutations are more prevalent than KIT mutations in melanoma of the female urogenital tract–a study of 24 cases from the Netherlands. Gynecol Oncol 2014;134(1): 10–4.

22. Taube JM, Galon J, Sholl LM, et al. Implications of the tumor immune microenvironment for staging and therapeutics. Mod Pathol 2018;31(2):214–34.

23. Chen YB, Epstein JI. Primary carcinoid tumors of the urinary bladder and prostatic urethra: a clinicopathologic study of 6 cases. Am J Surg Pathol 2011; 35(3):442–6.

24. Martignoni G, Eble JN. Carcinoid tumors of the urinary bladder. Immunohistochemical study of 2 cases and review of the literature. Arch Pathol Lab Med 2003;127(1):e22–4.

25. Burgess NA, Lewis DC, Matthews PN. Primary carcinoid of the bladder. Br J Urol 1992;69(2):213–4.

26. Colby TV. Carcinoid tumor of the bladder. A case report. Arch Pathol Lab Med 1980;104(4): 199–200.

27. Mascolo M, Altieri V, Mignogna C, et al. Calcitonin-producing well-differentiated neuroendocrine carcinoma (carcinoid tumor) of the urinary bladder: case report. BMC Cancer 2005;5:88.

28. Walker BF, Someren A, Kennedy JC, et al. Primary carcinoid tumor of the urinary bladder. Arch Pathol Lab Med 1992;116(11):1217–20.

29. Stanfield BL, Grimes MM, Kay S. Primary carcinoid tumor of the bladder arising beneath an inverted papilloma. Arch Pathol Lab Med 1994;118(6):666–7.

30. Baydar DE, Tasar C. Carcinoid tumor in the urinary bladder: unreported features. Am J Surg Pathol 2011;35(11):1754–7.

31. Epstein JI, Amin MB, Beltran H, et al. Proposed morphologic classification of prostate cancer with neuroendocrine differentiation. Am J Surg Pathol 2014;38(6):756–67.

32. Chin NW, Marinescu AM, Fani K. Composite adenocarcinoma and carcinoid tumor of urinary bladder. Urology 1992;40(3):249–52.

33. Hansel DE, Epstein JI, Berbescu E, et al. Renal carcinoid tumor: a clinicopathologic study of 21 cases. Am J Surg Pathol 2007;31(10):1539–44.

34. Raslan WF, Ro JY, Ordonez NG, et al. Primary carcinoid of the kidney. Immunohistochemical and ultrastructural studies of five patients. Cancer 1993; 72(9):2660–6.

35. Kuba MG, Wasserman A, Vnencak-Jones CL, et al. Primary carcinoid tumor of the renal pelvis arising from intestinal metaplasia: an unusual histogenetic pathway? Appl Immunohistochem Mol Morphol 2017;25(7):e49–57.

36. Begin LR, Guy L, Jacobson SA, et al. Renal carcinoid and horseshoe kidney: a frequent association of two rare entities–a case report and review of the literature. J Surg Oncol 1998;68(2):113–9.

37. Buntley D. Malignancy associated with horseshoe kidney. Urology 1976;8(2):146–8.

38. Fetissof F, Benatre A, Dubois MP, et al. Carcinoid tumor occurring in a teratoid malformation of the kidney. An immunohistochemical study. Cancer 1984; 54(10):2305–8.

39. Faucompret S, Farthouat P, Deligne E, et al. [Kidney cancer in horseshoe kidney. A case report of an unexpected diagnosis]. Ann Urol (Paris) 2002;36(2): 81–6.

40. Jeung JA, Cao D, Selli BW, et al. Primary renal carcinoid tumors: clinicopathologic features of 9 cases with emphasis on novel immunohistochemical findings. Hum Pathol 2011;42(10):1554–61.

41. Shibata R, Okita H, Shimoda M, et al. Primary carcinoid tumor in a polycystic kidney. Pathol Int 2003; 53(5):317–22.

42. Kojiro M, Ohishi H, Isobe H. Carcinoid tumor occurring in cystic teratoma of the kidney: a case report. Cancer 1976;38(4):1636–40.

43. Yoo J, Park S, Jung Lee H, et al. Primary carcinoid tumor arising in a mature teratoma of the kidney: a case report and review of the literature. Arch Pathol Lab Med 2002;126(8):979–81.

44. Kim SS, Choi C, Kang TW, et al. Carcinoid tumor associated with adjacent dysplastic columnar epithelium in the renal pelvis: a case report and literature review. Pathol Int 2016;66(1):42–6.

45. Aung PP, Killian K, Poropatich CO, et al. Primary neuroendocrine tumors of the kidney: morphological and molecular alterations of an uncommon malignancy. Hum Pathol 2013;44(5):873–80.

46. Matoso A, Singh K, Jacob R, et al. Comparison of thyroid transcription factor-1 expression by 2 monoclonal antibodies in pulmonary and nonpulmonary primary tumors. Appl Immunohistochem Mol Morphol 2010;18(2):142–9.

47. Hart J, Mandavilli S. Epithelioid angiosarcoma: a brief diagnostic review and differential diagnosis. Arch Pathol Lab Med 2011;135(2):268–72.

48. Fletcher CD, Beham A, Bekir S, et al. Epithelioid angiosarcoma of deep soft tissue: a distinctive tumor readily mistaken for an epithelial neoplasm. Am J Surg Pathol 1991;15(10):915–24.

49. Matoso A, Epstein JI. Epithelioid angiosarcoma of the bladder: a series of 9 cases. Am J Surg Pathol 2015;39(10):1377–82.

50. Abbasov B, Munguia G, Mazal PR, et al. Epithelioid angiosarcoma of the bladder: report of a new case with immunohistochemical profile and review of the literature. Pathology 2011;43(3):290–3.

51. Wang G, Black PC, Skinnider BF, et al. Post-radiation epithelioid angiosarcoma of the urinary bladder and prostate. Can Urol Assoc J 2016;10(5–6):E197–200.

52. Kulaga A, Yilmaz A, Wilkin RP, et al. Epithelioid angiosarcoma of the bladder after irradiation for endometrioid adenocarcinoma. Virchows Arch 2007; 450(2):245–6.

53. Gerbaud F, Ingels A, Ferlicot S, et al. Angiosarcoma of the bladder: review of the literature and discussion about a clinical case. Urol Case Rep 2017;13:97–100.

54. Padaki P, Hutton R, Amer T, et al. A rare case of primary epithelioid angiosarcoma of the ureter. Ann R Coll Surg Engl 2016;98(8):e184–5.

Mesenchymal Neoplasms of the Genitourinary System
A Selected Review with Recent Advances in Clinical, Diagnostic, and Molecular Findings

Bryce Shawn Hatfield, MD[a], Mark Cameron Mochel, MD[a],
Steven Christopher Smith, MD, PhD[b],*

KEYWORDS

- Soft tissue tumors • Genitourinary pathology • Mesenchymal neoplasms

---

Key points

- Mesenchymal soft tissue tumors involving the genitourinary (GU) tract cover much of the range of such tumors in somatic soft tissues, though organ system–specific pearls and pitfalls apply.

- Lipomatous neoplasms are the most common, including both benign spindle cell and lipomatous tumors related to chromosome 13q/*RB1* loss, and tumors in the atypical lipomatous tumor–dedifferentiated liposarcoma sequence related to *MDM2* amplification.

- New molecular insights have further characterized perivascular epithelioid cell tumors (PEComa), and established pathognomonic, diagnostically useful molecular features in solitary fibrous tumors.

- Emerging data suggest that pseudosarcomatous myofibroblastic proliferations of the GU tract are likely different from both classic inflammatory myofibroblastic tumors of other viscera and nodular fasciitides of soft tissues.

- Pericytic tumors of the kidney appear to show a more indolent course, even for large, deep lesions, compared with their soft tissue counterparts.

ABSTRACT

Mesenchymal neoplasms of the genitourinary (GU) tract often pose considerable diagnostic challenges due to their wide morphologic spectrum, relative rarity, and unexpected incidence at GU sites. Soft tissue tumors arise throughout the GU tract, whether from adventitia surrounding or connective tissues within the kidneys, urinary bladder, and male and female genital organs. This selected article focuses on a subset of these lesions, ranging from benign to malignant and encompassing a range of patterns of mesenchymal differentiation, where recent scholarship has lent greater insight into their clinical, molecular, or diagnostic features.

OVERVIEW

Mesenchymal neoplasms pose a unique challenge to surgical pathologists in general, a

---

Disclosure Statement: Dr S.C. Smith discloses royalty/consulting income for textbook authorship with Amirsys/Elsevier Publishing.
[a] Department of Pathology, VCU School of Medicine, 1200 East Marshall Street, PO Box 980662, Richmond, VA 23298, USA; [b] Departments of Pathology and Urology, VCU School of Medicine, 1200 East Marshall Street, PO Box 980662, Richmond, VA 23298, USA
* Corresponding author.
E-mail address: steven.c.smith@vcuhealth.org

1875-9181/18/© 2018 Elsevier Inc. All rights reserved.

surgpath.theclinics.com

challenge facilitated by the sheer number of entities, the range of patterns of differentiation evident histologically, the histologic similarity of lesions with varying biologic potential, and the relative rarity of these tumors compared with epithelial neoplasms. Contemporary classifications of mesenchymal (specifically, soft tissue and bone) tumors use pathologic assessment of the pattern of differentiation to establish categories of lesions, which may range from benign to intermediate to malignant. Immunophenotypic and molecular testing have taken key roles as ancillary studies for tumors in which the pattern of differentiation is not always evident by routine histopathology. The fourth edition of the World Health Organization (WHO) Classification of Tumors of Soft Tissue and Bone recognizes more than 100 separate entities, each with unique morphologic, immunophenotypic, and/or molecular characteristics.[1] Although the sheer range of these tumors is dazzling, surgical pathologists can narrow the field of possibilities, for any given case, through recognition that a great many of these tumors show characteristic age, sex, and anatomic site predilection.

Unfortunately for the surgical pathologist encountering a soft tissue lesion in an unusual location, such as the genitourinary (GU) tract, the epidemiologic, anatomic, and clinical clues used for diagnosis of mesenchymal tumors at other somatic soft tissue sites may not be applicable due to the rarity of the presentation. In this setting, diagnostic collaboration among surgeon, radiologist, and pathologist becomes *de rigueur*. Consultation within surgical pathology subspecialty areas including among urologic, gynecologic, and even dermatopathology may prove necessary, the latter given the distinctive cutaneous soft tissue tumors that arise about the genital region. Although within the space of a single article a comprehensive review of current developments, even restricted to the GU areas, remains untenable, herein, we have endeavored to cover a number of interesting and salient observations regarding mesenchymal neoplasms that occur in the GU tract. In each case, we cover the clinical and histologic features of each entity, as described for classic soft tissue examples but also with consideration of those that have been described in the GU tract. We further address what newer insights have come in recent years to change our understanding of each tumor, and last, we address recommendations for the recognition and avoidance of diagnostic pitfalls.

SPINDLE CELL/LIPOMATOUS LESIONS RELATED TO 13Q/RB1 LOSS: A HISTOLOGIC AND ANATOMIC SPECTRUM

INTRODUCTION

Recent studies have documented a remarkable, convergent molecular finding that unifies a spectrum of low-grade lipomatous and spindle cell neoplasms that arise in various sites.[2] In addition to the *spindle cell/pleomorphic lipoma* (**Fig. 1**), recognized as the founding entity of this spectrum of tumors, this group now includes 2 additional lesions that are distinctly salient in the GU area, especially cutaneous soft tissues about the genitals and perineum: *cellular angiofibroma* (**Fig. 2**) and *mammary-type myofibroblastoma* (**Fig. 3**). For context, spindle cell/pleomorphic lipomas are an uncommon variant of lipoma that occurs primarily in older individuals, most commonly men 45 to 70 years of age, and have a predilection for the posterior neck, shoulder, and back.[3,4] Recent findings confirm that they arise in women, although less frequently and at younger average age, and at sites beyond the classic head/neck "shawl" distribution, including in viscera and about the groin/labia.[5] Cytogenetic studies have consistently shown deletions of the long arm of chromosome 13, which contains the retinoblastoma (*RB1*) locus as 13q14.[6,7]

Recently, however, mammary-type myofibroblastoma, a neoplasm with overlapping histologic features with spindle cell/pleomorphic lipoma and a predilection for the inguinal region of men and the breast of women, has been shown to have similar, consistent deletions at 13q.[8–10] Finally, cellular angiofibroma, which typically arises in the vulvar, inguinal, and scrotal regions, also has been found to harbor deletions at 13q.[11–13] This cytogenetic similarity has substantiated the concept that these entities represent a spectrum of morphologically and molecularly related lesions, characterized by the variable prominence of different histologic patterns and components, in the context of differing anatomic sites. We regard these as a family of tumors exhibiting a spectrum of variably prominent bland spindle cell, lipomatous, and hyalinized vascular patterns, defined by unifying molecular feature of 13q/*RB1* loss.

Although none of these entities is common in the GU tract, there are reported examples of each lesion affecting GU viscera, including the prostate, urinary bladder, and kidney,[14–17] beyond the cutaneous soft tissues in the inguinoscrotal region where these tumors are best described.[11–13,18–20] As such, careful examination of any GU fatty specimen with an unusual spindle cell proliferation is

Fig. 1. Spindle cell lipoma involving the GU tract. (*A*) A T1-weighted MRI showing a well-circumscribed tumor with variable adipose content arising in deep pelvic fascia inferior to and displacing the penis, and protruding outward into the perineal area (*arrow*). (*B*) Grossly (*inset*) the morphology was consistent with a lipoma, with a well-encapsulated yellow tumor. Histologically (main panel), this tumor showed a variable edematous and fibrous areas, the latter composed of bland, hypocellular CD34-positive (not pictured) spindle cells coursing through a ropey collagen matrix (H&E, 200×).

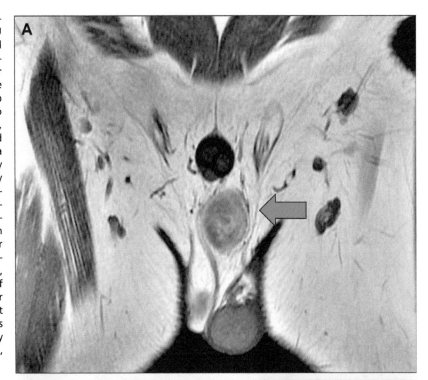

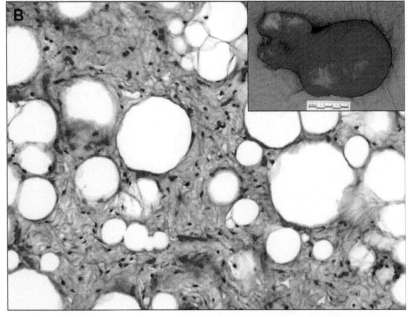

warranted, availing as necessary to the immunohistochemical markers described as follows to support differential diagnostic considerations.

GROSS FEATURES

Spindle cell/pleomorphic lipomas are typically well-circumscribed ovoid masses with variably yellow to gray-white cut surfaces, depending on the relative amounts of fatty and spindle cell components, respectively.[21] Generally, these lesions are firmer than usual lipomas, with a variably gelatinous texture. Scattered cases have been described in GU sites as parts of larger series, although particular details were limited. In one well-described case report, a spindle cell/pleomorphic lipoma in an end-stage renal allograft in a 60-year-old man appeared unencapsulated

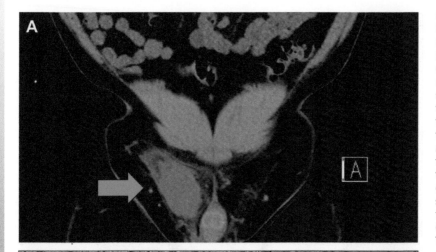

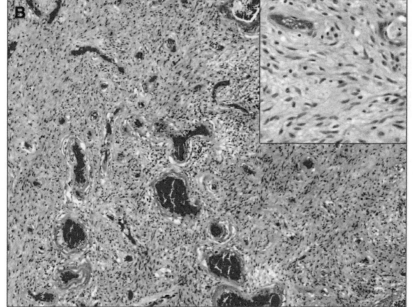

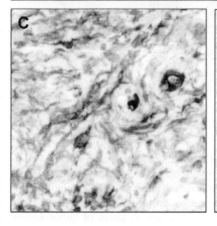

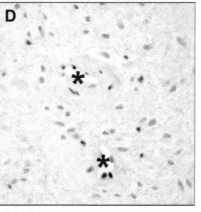

Fig. *2.* Cellular angiofibroma involving the spermatic cord and deep inguinal soft tissues. (*A*) A coronal computed tomography (CT) scan demonstrates an oblong soft tissue density involving the proximal aspect of the spermatic cord (*arrow*). (*B*) Histologically the tumor was characterized by numerous, gaping, hyalinized vessels surrounded by a bland fibrous spindle cell stroma (H&E, 100×) (*inset*, 400×). The tumor was diffusely positive for CD34 (*C*, 400×), with only focal SMA and desmin expression (not pictured). RB protein demonstrated loss in the spindle cell component (*D*, 400×), with internal positive control expression in endothelial cells within the vasculature (*asterisks*). (RB micrograph *Courtesy of* Dr Vickie Jo, Brigham and Women's Hospital, Boston, MA; with permission.)

Printed and bound by CPI Group (UK) Ltd, Croydon, CR0 4YY

03/10/2024

01040298-0018

Fig. *3.* Mammary-type myofibroblastoma. (*A*) At low power, a mammary-type myofibroblastoma shows well-circumscribed growth with limited adipose component, H&E, 100×. (*B*) At higher power the lesional cells are seen to be blind spindle cells coursing in trabeculae and nests through broader and denser, more hyalinized collagen bundles, H&E, 200×. Similar to spindle cell lipoma and cellular angiofibroma, CD34 is diffusely positive (*C*, 200×), whereas relatively extensive desmin positivity (*D*, 400×) is distinctive and more characteristic of mammary-type myofibroblastoma than other tumors in this group.

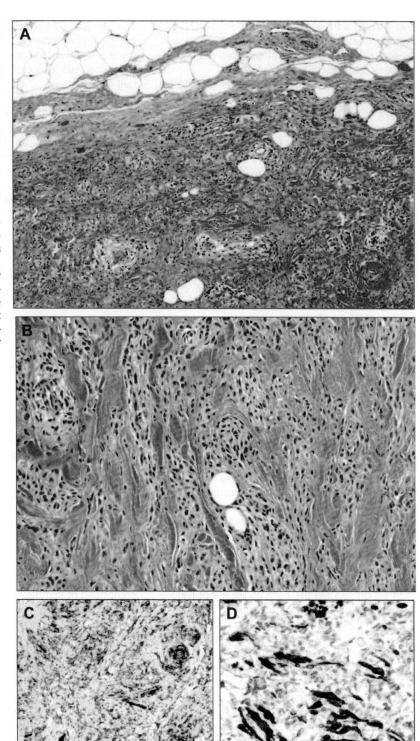

and round with a tan-white to yellowish and partially mucinous cut surface.[17] The lesion was present in the renal sinus fat and showed no evidence of necrosis or hemorrhage.

Mammary-type myofibroblastomas tend to be well circumscribed with a rubbery consistency.[9,18,22] The cut surface has a semifatty appearance with variable mottling or nodularity and varies from yellow to tan-white or gray. Myxoid changes within the tumor can result in a mucinous appearance. The mean tumor size is approximately 5.5 cm to 6.5 cm, with frequently positive margins at excision.[18] Of interest to GU sites, a case of a myofibroblastoma involving the prostate of a 51-year-old man showed a 12-cm multinodular white mass replacing and distorting the prostatic tissue,[14] whereas another involving a kidney in a 16-year-old girl showed a reddish, fleshy surface, distending the organ to 16 cm.[15] Cellular angiofibromas,[20] described primarily as tumors of GU soft tissue sites, often vulvar or inguinoscrotal,[19] grossly appear well circumscribed with round to oval nodules that vary from soft to rubbery. The cut surfaces are solid and tan-pink to yellow-brown or gray in color without hemorrhage or necrosis.

Microscopic Features

The histologic appearances of spindle cell/pleomorphic lipoma, mammary-type myofibroblastomas, and cellular angiofibromas show considerable overlap, with variable proportions of lipomatous, vascular, and spindle cell components described as most characteristic for each type as follows. All display a proliferation of spindled cells within a collagenous background with a variably abundant adipocytic component. Despite this overlap, characteristics specific to each lesion can aid the pathologist in applying a diagnostic label to any given lesion.

Spindle cell/pleomorphic lipomas are characterized by diverse appearances ranging from fat-predominant tumors with limited spindle cell components to lesions composed predominantly of spindle cells with rare adipocytes.[2,3,21,23] In fact, multiple recent series have focused on pauci adipose examples.[24,25] The spindle cells are bland and closely associated with thick, so-called "ropey" collagen bundles, which are arrayed in a variably myxoid to collagenized matrix. Multinucleated giant cells and floret-type giant cells, typical of the "pleomorphic" variant, are commonly seen.[21,26] Mast cells are frequently identified, particularly in areas of stromal edema. Mitotic activity is rare. The background can be extensively myxoid in some examples. CD34 is diffusely positive in the spindle cell component, and desmin and smooth muscle actin (SMA) are expressed in a minority of cases. RB expression is lost in the spindle cell component.[27] Occasionally, mild atypia, including stromal hyperchromasia, variation in the size and differentiation of adipocytes, or even lipoblasts may be identified, raising the possibility of an atypical lipomatous tumor (ALT). True cytologic atypia, most especially enlarged, hyperchromatic stromal cells, should engender consideration of ALT or an emerging spectrum of tumors, which have been termed "atypical spindle cell lipomatous tumor,"[28] as mentioned as follows.

> **Key Features**
> SPINDLE CELL/PLEOMORPHIC LIPOMAS
>
> - Spindle cells with variable adipocytic component
> - Thick, refractile "ropey" collagen bundles are characteristic
> - Multinucleated "floret"-type stromal cells
> - Rare mitotic activity
> - Diffuse CD34 positivity with loss of RB expression in spindle component
> - Lack of true nuclear atypia/hyperchromasia
> - Lack of MDM2/CDK4 expression by immunohistochemistry (IHC) or amplification by fluorescence in situ hybridization (FISH)

Mammary-type myofibroblastomas are composed of spindled cells arranged in long fascicles separated by bands of hyalinized collagen.[9,18] The spindle cells show oval to tapered nuclei, usually somewhat shorter or "stubbier" than in spindle cell lipomas, with inconspicuous nucleoli, and fine chromatin. Similar to spindle cell/pleomorphic lipomas, mast cells are frequently seen in the stromal matrix, which may be myxoid. However, the collagen in myofibroblastomas tends to appear more dense, broad/confluent, and hyalinized than in spindle cell/pleomorphic lipomas, a distinguishing factor. Less frequent patterns include infiltrative growth, seen sometimes between peripheral skeletal muscle fibers, and a Schwannoma-like palisading pattern.[18] Diffuse coexpression of CD34 and desmin is characteristic,[18] and RB expression is lost in most cases.[27]

Key Features
MAMMARY-TYPE MYOFIBROBLASTOMAS

- Spindle cells arranged in long fascicles

- Hyalinized bands of collagen separate fascicles

- Collagen is denser and more hyalinized than spindle cell/pleomorphic lipomas

- Adipose component often less conspicuous than spindle cell/pleomorphic lipomas

- Coexpression of CD34 and desmin with loss of RB expression in most cases

Cellular angiofibromas consist generally of 2 histologic components: a spindle cell proliferation and vascular proliferation. The first component is a proliferation of uniform, short spindle cells with oval to fusiform nuclei and inconspicuous nucleoli. The spindled areas are moderately to highly cellular, and arranged randomly with an occasional fascicular pattern or vague palisading. The surrounding stroma is composed of short bundles of collagen fibers, often finer and wispier than other tumors in this class. The second component is a proliferation of small to medium-sized vessels with mural hyalinization, which contrast the cellularity of the bland spindle cell component. The stroma contains collagen bundles that vary from short and thick to more commonly delicate and fine. Most cases express CD34, although a lower proportion than the other lesions in this class, whereas desmin and SMA are usually negative.[11,20] However, RB expression is lost in all examples studied.[27]

Key Features
CELLULAR ANGIOFIBROMAS

- Spindle cell and vascular proliferation

- Spindle cells are randomly arranged with occasional fascicular growth or palisading

- Less conspicuous, short collagen bundles that are "fine" and "wispy"

- Vascular proliferation of small to medium-sized vessels with often prominent mural hyalinization

- Most are CD34 positive, desmin and SMA negative, with loss of RB expression

DIFFERENTIAL DIAGNOSIS

The differential diagnosis for these 3 entities is highly dependent on the relative proportions of adipose tissue to spindle cell proliferation present, and, in our opinion, the location where the lesion is described. Given the significant overlap among these lesions, differentiating between them can be difficult on histologic grounds. For that matter, the shared cytogenetic findings make ancillary testing unhelpful in terms of their separation. IHC staining, combined with careful morphologic review, remains useful in narrowing the differential diagnosis (Table 1).

Operationally, we tend to use the diagnosis of spindle cell/pleomorphic lipoma most frequently by far, and especially to tumors demonstrating any significant fatty component (which is often apparent by pre-resection MRI). This supports clinicopathologic correlation with radiologic features, and uses a diagnostic term with which, in our experience, many clinicians are more familiar. For tumors in which the spindle cell component shows a more "packeted" or fascicular growth pattern with denser hyalinized stroma, especially if the adipose component was not a defining clinical feature, we use mammary-type myofibroblastoma as the diagnostic term of choice. When vascularity and perivascular hyalinization predominate and the lesion is in the inguinal, gonadal, or groin area, cellular angiofibroma is our favored term. Without being too provocative, we note that given the essentially identical prognostic profile and therapeutic recommendations, distinguishing among these often-overlapping entities is often rather arbitrary.

In fact, we argue that the most useful undertaking in this differential diagnostic area is exclusion of ALT[29] and lesions in the emerging, locally aggressive category of so-called "atypical spindle cell lipomatous tumors."[28] In the case of the differential diagnosis with ALT, we emphasize that tumors in the 13q/RB1 loss family of spindle cell/pleomorphic lipoma, mammary-type myofibroblastoma, and cellular angiofibroma lack true cytologic atypia; that is, they lack the marked and often bizarre stromal hyperchromasia, nucleomegaly, and pleomorphism of the type that is diagnostic of ALT. Immunopositivity for MDM2 and CDK4, diffusely present in ALT (see later in this article), is not seen in the pleomorphic cells of a spindle cell/pleomorphic lipoma or the foci of similar-looking degenerative atypia infrequently seen in mammary-type myofibroblastomas and cellular angiofibromas. For that matter, RB loss is specific to this latter group of tumors, whereas RB is retained in ALT. Cytogenetic studies of spindle

Table 1
Immunophenotypic features of spindle cell and lipomatous lesions with 13q/*RB1* loss

Entity	CD34	SMA	Desmin	RB
Spindle cell/pleomorphic lipoma	+	−	−	Lost
Mammary-type myofibroblastoma	+	+/−	+	Lost, vast majority
Cellular angiofibroma	+/−	−/+	−	Lost

Abbreviations: RB, retinoblastoma; SMA, smooth muscle actin; +, positive immunostaining; -, negative immunostaining; +/-, variable but frequently positive or patchy immunostaining; -/+, variable but frequently negative immunostaining.

cell lipomas and related tumors, whether by FISH or array-based technologies, do not demonstrate the chromosome 12 *MDM2/CDK4* amplifications that are characteristic of ALT, and instead demonstrate chromosome 13q losses involving the *RB1* locus.

An emerging entity, the so-called *atypical spindle cell lipomatous tumor*, which includes lesions that have been reported as "spindle cell liposarcoma"[30] or "fibrosarcoma-like lipomatous neoplasm,"[31] imparts a much greater differential diagnostic challenge. These tumors show many histologic features within the spectrum of spindle cell/pleomorphic lipoma or potentially mammary-type myofibroblastoma, but, in contrast to these entities, demonstrate mild nuclear atypia. The possibility of ALT can be excluded by demonstrating the absence of MDM2/CDK4 expression by IHC or amplification by FISH. Similar to 13q/*RB1*-loss tumors, CD34 is positive in most atypical spindle cell lipomatous tumors,[28,32,33] with S100 expression in a minority, and infrequent desmin expression. Most confusingly, RB expression seems to be lost in most, but not all of these tumors, depending on what diagnostic criteria are used.[2,28,32,33] Although we suspect that molecular studies in coming years will be of great use in clarifying the true relationship between these tumor types, we note that in the largest series of atypical spindle cell lipomatous tumors, no metastasis was observed. Moreover, local recurrence was noted in only 12% of the tumors with follow-up information.[28] For this reason, we would argue that efforts be made primarily to exclude diagnosis of ALT, which shows, depending on whether located in an extremity or in the retroperitoneum, between 50% and 100% risk of recurrence, and approximately 5% to 15% risk of dedifferentiation to a sarcoma with metastatic potential.[34]

Rarely, a spindle cell lipoma/pleomorphic lipoma, mammary-type myofibroblastoma, and cellular angiofibroma could demonstrate exuberant edema and myxoid change, prompting the differential diagnosis with myxoid liposarcoma. However, those entities do not possess the thin, branching "chicken-wire" vasculature of myxoid liposarcoma. Additionally, and most importantly, they lack the t(12;16) *FUS-DDIT3* gene fusion that is characteristic of myxoid liposarcoma.[35]

Angiomyofibroblastoma and cellular angiofibroma have similar gross appearances and well-circumscribed rubbery to fatty nodules. However, angiomyofibroblastoma is a histologically distinctive tumor that shows nests of epithelioid cells, often in clusters, arranged around blood vessels, the latter thin walled and prominent against the often edematous and hypocellular background of the lesion. Cellular angiofibroma, in contrast, shows more uniform cellularity, lacks plump epithelioid cells, and lacks the predilection for the neoplastic cells to aggregate in clumps and nests around prominent hyalinized vessels. Angiomyofibroblastoma tends to be CD34 negative, and diffusely desmin positive, whereas cellular angiofibroma is more often CD34 positive and desmin negative.

△△ **Differential Diagnosis**
TUMORS WITH
CHROMOSOME 13Q/*RB1* LOSS

- Atypical lipomatous tumor/well-differentiated liposarcoma
- Atypical spindle cell lipomatous tumor
- Myxoid liposarcoma
- Angiomyofibroblastoma

DIAGNOSIS

The diagnosis of spindle cell/pleomorphic lipoma at a GU site is based primarily on histologic features, including fibrous bands composed of bland, spindle cells arrayed in variably myxoid stroma with prominent ropey collagen. The well-differentiated adipocytic component may be abundant or represent a minority of the lesion. Furthermore, the multinucleated, floret-like giant cells, which define the pleomorphic variant of this tumor, may be apparent, and given their degenerated look may help raise consideration of this tumor type. Mitotic activity is low, and no atypical mitotic figures are present. A case report of a spindle cell lipoma/pleomorphic lipoma in the kidney revealed a lipomatous mass composed of variably sized adipocytes.[17] Areas with increased cellularity contained the typical bland spindle cells, in a stroma with focal myxoid change, characteristic ropey collagen bundles, and slender blood vessels. Similarly, characteristic histologic features are used to recognize a case in the inguinal area.[36] Among the lesional spindle cells, there is strong positivity for CD34 and variable positivity for S100 and desmin. MDM2 and CDK4 are negative by IHC, *MDM2* amplification is negative by FISH, and RB expression is lost. Correlating with the radiographic impression may be helpful, as fatty tumors in the GU area are sufficiently unusual that imaging of a circumscribed, fat-containing lesion is often available.

Likewise, diagnosis of cellular angiofibroma and mammary-type myofibroblastoma depends mostly on morphologic features. Both tumors are composed of spindle cells in a fibrous, collagenized stroma. However, the configuration of mammary-type myofibroblastomas tends to show long, broad fascicles composed of bland spindle cells, with varying amounts of adipose tissue, and dense, hyalinized collagen bundles interspersed throughout the lesion. The adipose component is less prominent than most spindle cell lipomas, and the vascular pattern, which sometimes shows perivascular hyalinization like cellular angiofibroma, is less conspicuous. Cellular angiofibromas show prominent hyalinized vessels, often reminiscent of a schwannoma, in combination with a perivascular whorling or fascicular growth pattern of the characteristic bland spindle cells. Both lesions share RB loss and CD34 positivity; mammary-type myofibroblastoma often shows diffuse desmin positivity (see **Table 1**).

PROGNOSIS

All 3 of the histologically overlapping entities in the 13q/RB loss family of spindle cell and lipomatous neoplasms are benign and typically cured by local excision. Local recurrence is distinctly rare, and metastases have not been reported.

> **Key Points**
> TUMORS WITH CHROMOSOME
> 13Q/*RB1* LOSS
>
> - Spindle cell/pleomorphic lipoma, mammary-type myofibroblastoma, and cellular angiofibroma show overlapping microscopic features
> - Proliferation of bland spindle cells within variably collagenous and lipomatous background
> - Spindle cell component is unifying, shows CD34 expression and loss of RB by IHC
> - Collagen texture varies between entities, fine fibrillar to dense bandlike
> - Variable adipocytic component from predominant to invisible
> - Vascular component ranges from inconspicuous to hyalinized and gaping

THE ATYPICAL LIPOMATOUS TUMOR–DEDIFFERENTIATED LIPOSARCOMA SPECTRUM OF TUMORS

INTRODUCTION

Liposarcomas are the most common soft tissue sarcomas and most frequently involve the deep soft tissue of the limbs, retroperitoneum, head and neck, and mediastinum. Within the GU tract, liposarcomas most frequently involve the paratestis, spermatic cord, and kidney.[37–40] However, cases involving the renal sinus and bladder also have been reported.[41–43]

With regard to involvement of the GU tract, we focus on the spectrum of tumors that unites ALT (previously, well-differentiated liposarcoma) (**Fig. 4**) and dedifferentiated liposarcoma (DDLPS) (**Fig. 5**). The former often quite closely resembles mature adipose tissue, whereas the latter, by definition shows lack of mature lipomatous differentiation. Given that the kidneys and ureters are retroperitoneal, a key area involved by ALT and DDLPS, these represent common sites of involvement. Similarly, as the testis migrates inferiorly from a retroperitoneal origin into the scrotal sac during development, a herniating abdominopelvic lipomatous neoplasm may also extend downward to involve the processus vaginalis through an indirect hernia. In either case, neoplasms involving the spermatic cord may present as slowly growing, painless masses in the inguinal region that can be mistaken for inguinal hernias.[38] Within the

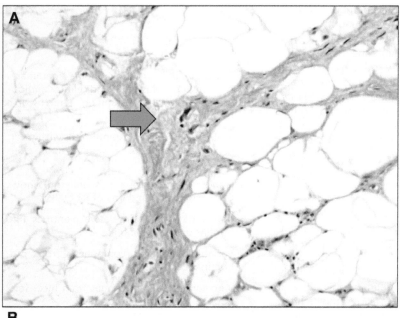

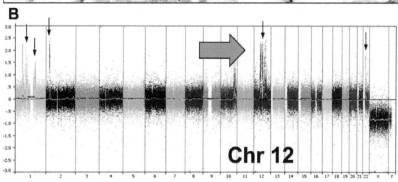

Fig. 4. ALT. (*A*) ALT shows a characteristic pattern of adipose tissue with atypical variation in lipid vacuole size and more prominent septation than benign lipomas or mature fatty tissue. Diagnosis of this tumor type, especially in its lipomalike form (pictured) hinges on identification of enlarged, hyperchromatic, often bizarre atypical stromal cells, frequently present in fibrous septa. In examples in which the stromal atypia is present but not entirely convincing (*arrow*), molecular testing, such as FISH to detect amplification of the *MDM2* locus, or (*B*) single nucleotide polymorphism array profiling for genomic copy number alterations (including the *MDM2* locus on chromosome 12, *arrow*) has an important diagnostic role.

paratesticular soft tissues, painless swelling is the most common presentation for an ALT or DDLPS.[40]

GROSS FEATURES

Liposarcomas may show a diverse gross appearance, relative to the prominence of the well-differentiated lipomatous component compared with dedifferentiated nonadipose patterns. ALTs are well-circumscribed and lobulated, although the borders may occasionally show infiltrative growth. The cut surface is yellow to white, often with thick fibrous bands, gelatinous areas, or focal hemorrhage. Fat necrosis can be apparent if the lesion has been traumatized. Diagnostic areas can be quite focal, and generous sampling is required for adequate characterization.[44,45]

DDLPSs present similarly as large, multinodular masses; however, in nonlipomatous dedifferentiated areas, solid, nonfatty gross appearances

predominate, sometimes with a sarcomatous "fish flesh" or overtly necrotic appearance (see **Fig. 5**). Within the spermatic cord, tumors ranging from 3 cm to 30 cm have been reported.[38] Cut sections show solid, tan-gray areas with frequent necrosis and hemorrhage that correspond to areas of dedifferentiation, admixed with fatty, yellow tissue, corresponding to the well-differentiated adipocytic component. The better differentiated lipomatous component can be mistaken for normal adipose tissue, and generous sampling of all areas, especially transitions, is prudent to confirm the lipomatous origin of dedifferentiated tumors, given that the stromal atypia proving origin from an ALT can be focal.[38]

MICROSCOPIC FEATURES

Characteristically, ALTs show 1 of 3 patterns: lipomalike, sclerosing, and inflammatory, often coexisting within the same tumor. By definition, ALTs

Fig. 5. DDLPS. (*A*) A non-contrast coronal CT scan performed to evaluate a palpable renal mass demonstrated a large mass seemingly replacing the upper pole of the right kidney (*arrow*). (*B*) Grossly, a variably necrotic tumor with a white/gray "fish flesh" appearance was seen arising adjacent to but not invading the upper pole of the kidney (indicated by *arrow*). A significant surrounding adipose component was noted grossly. (*C*) Histologic sections demonstrated a tumor with multiple patterns, H&E 200×, with zoom, predominantly with undifferentiated pleomorphic sarcomatous pattern H&E 200×, with zoom, whereas diagnostic atypical stromal cells of a precursor ALT (*inset*, 400×, *zoomed*) were noted in the surrounding adipose tissue, confirming the impression of DDLPS.

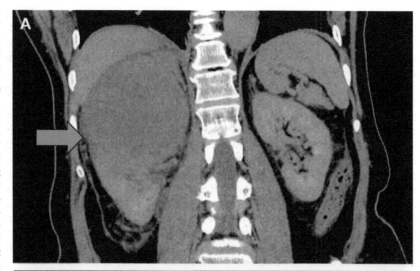

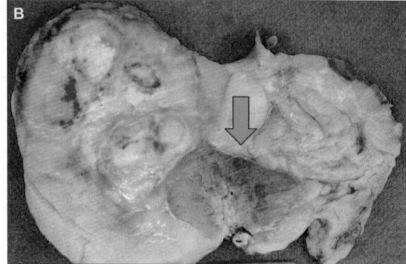

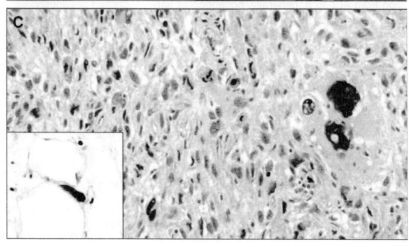

must show at least partial mature lipomatous differentiation, paired with stromal cytologic atypia, adipocyte atypia in terms of variability in cell/fat vacuole size, and scattered lipoblasts. The presence of atypical, markedly enlarged, hyperchromatic, stromal cells, often scattered and sometimes quite rare (see **Fig. 4**), combined with the aforementioned atypical but well-differentiated adipose component, firmly establishes the diagnosis. Lipomalike ALTs, in particular, may show many sections with only marginal atypia, largely attributable to increased variability in size of adipocytes, with rare identification of diagnostic enlarged bizarre, hyperchromatic stromal cells. Such diagnostic areas may be concentrated around lesional vasculature or in areas of fibrous septation. Sclerosing ALTs show scattered areas of mature tissue admixed with a densely collagenized stroma with scattered bizarre, hyperchromatic atypical stromal cells. In the GU tract, sclerosing ALT/well-differentiated liposarcoma is relatively common, particularly in the paratesticular region.[40] These tumors are composed of dense fibrotic regions with a fibrillary collagenous background. The fibrous areas alternate with lipogenic zones containing mature adipocytes. Embedded within the fibrotic regions are the scattered atypical stromal cells with hyperchromatic nuclei. The inflammatory type of ALT shows a dense, often mixed, chronic lymphoplasmacytic and lymphohistiocytic inflammatory component that may obscure the lipomatous nature of the tumor and prompt consideration of lesions such as inflammatory myofibroblastic tumor (see later in this article).[46]

The key histologic feature of DDLPS is the transition from ALT to a, generally, nonlipogenic sarcoma of varying grade. This is typically represented by a grossly apparent nodule within an otherwise recognizable ALT. The transition between the 2 components is typically abrupt and the proportions of each component vary widely by case. Dedifferentiation has been defined as a region devoid of lipogenic differentiation in at least one low-power field.[38,47] In most cases, the dedifferentiated component has the pattern of a high-grade fibrosarcoma, undifferentiated pleomorphic sarcoma, or myxofibrosarcoma.[34,48] Recently, a subset of cases showing so-called "homologous" dedifferentiation in which the high-grade dedifferentiated component shows a pleomorphic liposarcomalike pattern have been described.[49] Low-grade dedifferentiation also may occur and shows features reminiscent of fibromatosis or low-grade fibrosarcoma with concomitant low mitotic activity and less marked nuclear atypia.[47,50] These low-grade areas consist of bland spindle cells arranged in short or long fascicles, with lower cellularity than high-grade dedifferentiated liposarcoma, but increased cellularity when compared with the sclerosing pattern of ALT.[47]

DIFFERENTIAL DIAGNOSIS

There are several important histologic mimics of ALT that must be distinguished, with particular relevance in the GU tract. In the benign category, fat necrosis is composed of injured fat, with decreased cell size and infiltrating lipid-laden macrophages. The macrophages have granular to vacuolated cytoplasm and can mimic lipoblasts. Unlike lipoblasts, the vacuoles do not indent the nuclei, and there is no nuclear hyperchromasia.

Brown fat, or tumoral brown fat (hibernoma), may also show heavily vacuolated cells that can mimic lipoblasts. Nodular rests of brown fat may be seen in perinephric adipose tissue and should be distinguished by the conspicuous lack of atypia or bizarre atypical stromal cells of ALT.[51,52] Finally, the benign pediatric tumor, lipoblastoma, which may occur in the retroperitoneum and pelvic region, is defined by an unusual septate fatty lesion with myxoid stroma and copious lipoblasts at varying points of differentiation. In our experience, myxoid liposarcoma represents a closer differential diagnosis, although a myxoid ALT could be considered. The vast majority of lipoblastomas occur in early childhood, well before most cases of ALT, and harbor PLAG1 rearrangements,[53] which recent scholarship demonstrates may be of diagnostic utility even in small samples.[54] The differential diagnosis with tumors in the spindle cell/pleomorphic lipoma tumor group was discussed previously.

Another interesting differential diagnosis of ALT, particularly the sclerosing variant, is massive localized lymphedema.[55] This uncommon reactive pseudotumor is strongly associated with obesity and often represents a chronic process in dependent areas, where cutaneous soft tissue in the GU tract may be involved. Cases reported in the male external genitalia show dermal expansion by fibrosis and edema with stromal multinucleated fibroblasts.[56] The fibrous septa are composed of an edematous stroma with mildly atypical fibroblasts and loosely fibrillar collagen, which may show some morphologic overlap with sclerosing liposarcoma, albeit without convincing stromal atypia. The clinical history and morphologic findings are often sufficient to establish a diagnosis, but MDM2 and CDK4 IHC or FISH may be used in especially difficult cases.

DDLPS, as well as ALT with significant myxoid or myxofibrosarcomalike areas, can mimic a myxoid liposarcoma, and likely accounts for cases previously diagnosed as "mixed type" liposarcomas.[57] However, myxoid liposarcoma characteristically has a plexiform, "chicken-wire" vasculature with decreased cellularity and limited cytologic atypia. The lipoblasts in myxoid liposarcoma are, most frequently, signet ring in configuration with a single large cytoplasmic vacuole indenting the nucleus. Moreover, there is a degree of monomorphism across the tumor such that even in areas of varying cellularity the constituent cells show similar features, a feature strikingly different from ALT and DDLPS, where cytologic heterogeneity and variability of pattern of differentiation is actually quite characteristic. Additionally, myxoid liposarcoma does not express MDM2 and CDK4,[58,59] and harbors rearrangements of *FUS* or *EWSR1* with *DDIT3*.

Distinguishing undifferentiated pleomorphic sarcoma, fibrosarcoma, and high-grade leiomyosarcoma from DDLPS can be challenging. In particular, small biopsies of deep retroperitoneal GU organs or excisions from the spermatic cord may lack recognizable areas of ALT. However, prior work has shown that a retroperitoneal biopsy yielding the undifferentiated pleomorphic sarcoma pattern is highly likely to be indicative of dedifferentiated liposarcoma.[60] Indeed, it is our routine practice to describe such biopsies, as well as those with myxofibrosarcomatous pattern, as a high-grade sarcoma with "X" pattern, noting the significant frequency with which they represent DDLPS, and recommending correlation with imaging to determine whether an adjacent adipose component is apparent. In such a scenario, MDM2 and CDK4 IHC and FISH[61,62] have proven utility. In current practice, this finding may have direct therapeutic relevance given recent favorable findings with the CDK4 inhibitor, palbociclib, in these tumors.[63]

△△ *Differential Diagnosis*

- Fat necrosis
- Hibernoma
- Lipoblastoma
- Spindle cell/pleomorphic lipoma
- Atypical spindle cell lipomatous tumor
- Massive localized lymphedema

DIAGNOSIS

Diagnosis of ALT is based on documentation of a lipomatous tumor showing significant variability of adipocyte size and morphology and atypia of the adipocytes and stromal cells. The diagnosis is clinched by observation of scattered atypical stromal cells with markedly enlarged and hyper-chromatic nuclei. Although lipoblasts may be observed, they are neither an obligate diagnostic criterion nor a specific feature. Morphologically unusual vessels are often apparent and atypical stromal cells may be seen closely apposed to such structures. The background of these findings is that of a (usually large) grossly multilobulated tumor with prominent septation and fibrous stroma. Diagnosis of a DDLPS is secured when an ALT is observed that shows progression to a usually grossly apparent tumor showing a non–well-differentiated lipomatous pattern of sarcoma of varying grade, usually losing lipomatous differentiation altogether, and representing at least 1 low-power field (although usually at least 1 cm). In any scenario in which the differential diagnosis of an ALT or DDLPS is rendered challenging by location, sample limitations, or morphologic pattern, IHC for MDM2 and CDK4,[61,64–66] with or without the addition of p16,[58,67–69] has use. FISH-based studies for amplification at the *MDM2* locus[32,61,62,70] have become well-established confirmatory tests in equivocal cases.

PROGNOSIS

Overall, studies of the prognosis of ALT and DDLPS have reported highly variable rates of local recurrence and death of disease, partly due to disparate behavior of these tumors based on the primary site, especially for ALT. Retroperitoneal ALT is associated with a rate of recurrence that, depending on follow-up time, has reportedly varied between 31% and 100%.[34,71] In particular, tumors involving the groin have been associated with a high rate of recurrence (11/14 cases in a classic series).[34] The risk of dedifferentiation is thought to be at least 20%. In contrast, in the extremities, the local recurrence rate is approximately 10%, with higher rates of re-recurrence after first recurrence (as much as >50%) and a rate of dedifferentiation in the range of less than 10%.[34,72]

DDLPSs have a significantly worse prognosis, with significant risk of metastatic disease and decreased overall survival.[38,40,47] A recent study by Dantey and colleagues[73] found that the histologic grade of DDLPS correlated with overall survival with a median survival of 113 months for low-grade DDLPS and 48 months for high-grade DDLPS. Metastatic disease was present only in cases with high-grade tumors. Specific to recent experience with DDLPS of the spermatic cord, 6 of 42 cases were low grade, the remainder high grade or mixed. Of patients with follow-up data, 23% recurred and 6% developed metastasis and died of disease.[38]

Key Features
ATYPICAL LIPOMATOUS TUMOR

- Well-circumscribed and lobulated with occasional infiltrative growth

- Yellow to white cut surfaces with thick fibrous bands

- Partial mature lipomatous differentiation with stromal cytologic atypia

- Lipoblasts are not required for diagnosis

- Three characteristic patterns: lipomalike, sclerosing, and inflammatory

  ○ Lipomalike: marginal atypia with rare hyperchromatic, bizarre stromal cells and variably sized adipocytes

  ○ Sclerosing: mature tissue admixed with dense collagenized stroma and scattered bizarre/atypical stromal cells

  ○ Inflammatory: dense mixed chronic lymphoplasmacytic and lymphohistiocytic inflammatory component

- S100 positive with typical MDM2 and CDK4 overexpression

- Amplification at the MDM2 locus by FISH is characteristic

PSEUDOSARCOMATOUS MYOFIBROBLASTIC PROLIFERATIONS VERSUS INFLAMMATORY MYOFIBROBLASTIC TUMOR

INTRODUCTION

Recent scholarship has begun to clarify the controversial relationship between the infrequent pseudosarcomatous myofibroblastic proliferations (PMPs)[74–76] that arise in the GU tract, sometimes related to prior procedures, and a group of increasingly better understood tumors recognized as inflammatory myofibroblastic tumors (IMTs). Classically, IMT has been described as a rare, histologically distinct proliferation of myofibroblastic

spindle cells. IMT has a predilection for children and adolescents and most commonly involves the abdominopelvic region, lung, and retroperitoneum; however, almost any site may be involved by IMT.[77–80] Involvement of the GU tract by classic IMT is rare, with the bladder reported as the most common site of occurrence.[81–83] IMT has also been reported in the kidney, renal pelvis, and perirenal soft tissue.[84] Again, because the diagnostic criteria for IMT versus PMP have differed over time, the nosologic relationship between the 2 entities has been unclear, and much of the literature has conflated the 2.

Focusing on IMT, first, contemporary studies find that approximately 50% IMTs harbor rearrangements of the ALK (anaplastic lymphoma kinase) gene, which is rearranged to result in fusion with multiple partners, including TPM3, TPM4, CARS, CLTC1, ATIC, RANBP2, SEC31L1, and PPFIBP1.[85,86] IHC for ALK generally shows positive staining in IMTs with an ALK rearrangement, especially with more sensitive antibodies.[87] Given that tyrosine kinase inhibitors have shown benefit in patients with ALK rearrangements,[88] ALK IHC is a helpful ancillary study for diagnostic and even predictive purposes.[88–90] Recent scholarship has also identified a number of additional oncogenic kinase fusions, including ROS1, RET, PDGFRB, and ETV6[85,91–93] in ALK-rearrangement-negative classic IMTs, although not specifically in the GU tract.

Somewhat in contrast to IMTs, PMPs of the GU tract (**Fig. 6**) show less predilection for children and the young, a less dense inflammatory background, and greater resemblance to reactive or neoplastic myofibroblastic proliferations like fasciitis.[74,76] They have been denoted variously as PMP, IMT, or even fibromyxoid pseudotumor and postoperative spindle cell nodule, the latter indicative of the association with prior procedures noted in approximately 20%.[74] Given that the pattern of these tumors is quite often fasciitislike, a relationship between the self-limited somatic soft tissue neoplasm related to USP6 rearrangements,[94] nodular fasciitis, has been contemplated as well. We recently contributed to clarification among these 3 entities by using FISH for USP6, ROS1, and ETV6, finding that most PMPs of the GU tract seem to be a distinct lesion without the genetic findings associated with classic IMT or nodular fasciitis.

GROSS FEATURES

The gross appearance of tumors in the IMP/PMP group tends to be lobular and multinodular with hard to rubbery cut surfaces. The tumor is typically

Fig. 6. PMP. (*A*) A coronal CT scan showed an incidental, several centimeter, heterogeneous tumor arising in association with a cortical cyst (*arrow*) in the mid to upper pole of the left kidney. (*B*) Morphologically the tumor showed a "tissue culture"–like pattern of reactive spindle cells with nuclei with open chromatin and tails of amphophilic cytoplasm, coursing through a myxocollagenous stroma with scattered inflammatory cells and extravasated erythrocytes, H&E, 200×, zoomed. Confirmatory of the impression of a myofibroblastic lesion, SMA was positive in a so-called "tram track" pattern highlighting the loose fascicular pattern of the spindle cells (*C*), while pancytokeratin AE1/AE3 aberrantly highlighted many the spindle cells as often seen in reactive myofibroblastic lesions (*D*). Desmin was only focally positive (*E*). Panels C–E photographed at 200×.

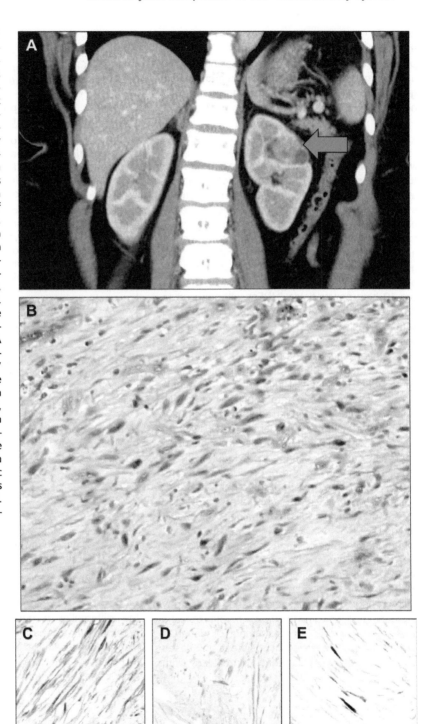

white to tan-yellow to gray. The nodules tend to be solitary; however, multiple nodules restricted to the same anatomic location.[74,77,95] The tumors usually measure 1 to 10 cm in diameter or larger.

Specifically in the GU tract, IMT/PMPs have been identified in the renal pelvis, hilar soft tissue, renal parenchyma, perirenal soft tissue, bladder, ureter, urethra, prostate, and paratesticular tissue.[82,84,96–98] The gross appearance is similar to those found in the soft tissue as firm, tan-white polypoid or nodular masses. Occasionally, the masses may have a myxoid appearance with gelatinous, glistening surfaces and areas of hemorrhage.[84]

MICROSCOPIC FEATURES

Microscopically, these tumors appear as admixtures of spindled, fibroblastic-myofibroblastic, and inflammatory cells in varying proportions, even within the same tumor. In examples in the urinary bladder, often arising in the dome, greater myxoid change tends to be seen at the mucosal aspect, with greater cellularity and fascicular growth deeper in the lesion.[74] Mitotic rate has been quantified on average in the 1 to 2 mitoses per 10 high-power fields (HPFs), although up to 20 have been seen. Atypical mitoses should be absent. Necrosis may be seen in as many as half of cases[74,95] and is associated with ulcer formation.[81] Involvement of the muscularis propria and perivesical fat has been noted in significant subsets of cases. A case of inflammatory myofibroblastic tumor of the prostate consisted of spindle cells in a broad fascicular arrangement with pushing, but not infiltrative, borders.[97] A study of 12 cases of IMT of the kidney revealed the 3 histologic growth patterns described previously with tumors showing one pattern predominating and smaller foci of one or both of the other patterns.[84] Cases of IMT involving the urethra and ureter did not show any additional unique histologic findings.[81,96,98]

Immunophenotypically, a high proportion of these tumors has shown pancytokeratin expression (>70%), Fig. 6, similar to reactive myofibroblastic lesions of diverse sites.[76,95] Furthermore, a high proportion of cases show variable or patchy expression of smooth muscle or myofibroblastic markers such as SMA, caldesmon, or demin.[76] Expression of ALK is inconsistent in cases harboring ALK rearrangements, particularly with respect to specific antibody clones.[87]

DIFFERENTIAL DIAGNOSIS

The differential diagnosis of IMTs is broad and highly dependent on the clinicopathologic setting. The most significant entities in the bladder and other GU tract primary sites include sarcomatoid (usually urothelial) carcinoma, leiomyosarcoma, dedifferentiated liposarcoma, and fibromatosis (Table 2).

In the renal collecting system, ureter, and bladder, sarcomatoid urothelial carcinoma frequently enters

Table 2
Differential diagnosis: inflammatory myofibroblastic tumor/pseudosarcomatous myofibroblastic proliferations

IMT/PMP Versus	Helpful Distinguishing Features
Sarcomatoid urothelial carcinoma	• Positive p63 (focal or patchy), HMWCK, and CK5/6 • Negative staining for SMA, desmin, and ALK
Leiomyosarcoma	• Long, stubby nuclei, prominent eosinophilic cytoplasm, and less collagenization and myxoid change • May have significant nuclear atypia • Atypical mitoses • Stronger and more diffuse SMA and desmin • Weaker keratin expression
Dedifferentiated liposarcoma	• Significant nuclear atypia • MDM2 and/or CDK4 IHC positivity • Positive MDM2 amplification by FISH
Fibromatosis	• Long, sweeping fascicles • Scant inflammatory component • Plump arterioles and periarteriolar edema • Nuclear expression of β-catenin

Abbreviations: ALK, anaplastic lymphoma kinase; FISH, fluorescence in situ hybridization; IHC, immunohistochemistry; IMT, inflammatory myofibroblastic tumor; PMP, pseudosarcomatous myofibroblastic proliferation; SMA, smooth muscle actin.

the differential diagnosis, occurs much more commonly than bona fide IMT, and presents a significant diagnostic challenge, given that cases of PMP/IMT have been reported in association with a separate urothelial carcinoma.[95] In this context, the International Society of Urologic Pathology (ISUP) best practices recommendations for IHC for spindle cell tumors of the bladder may assist the pathologist encountering this differential diagnosis: a panel of ALK, SMA, desmin, pancytokeratin AE1/AE3, and p63, with either of high molecular weight cytokeratin (HMWCK) or CK5/6, is recommended.[99] Sarcomatoid urothelial carcinoma is expected to have positive but focal or patchy staining for p63, HMWCK, and/or CK5/6, particularly among scattered cells with greater epithelioid morphology, and generally negative staining for SMA, desmin, and ALK.[76]

Leiomyosarcoma and IMT are both spindle cell tumors that often contain a fascicular architecture. However, conventional leiomyosarcoma tends to have longer, stubbier nuclei, more prominent eosinophilic cytoplasm, and less interstitial collagenization or myxoid change than IMT/PMP tumors. Many leiomyosarcomas demonstrate a degree of nuclear atypia that is beyond that allowable in an IMT/PMP, if well sampled, and close inspection will demonstrate atypical mitoses. The inflammatory variant of leiomyosarcoma can be particularly histologically challenging to differentiate from IMT. Whereas IHC of these entities shows significant overlap, with respect to SMA, desmin, and, less frequently, keratin, stronger, diffuser SMA and desmin and weaker keratin favor leiomyosarcoma. Rhabdomyosarcoma, which may enter the diagnosis in a subset of cases, demonstrates desmin expression, with more specific MyoD1 and MYF4/myogenin nuclear expression.

Either an ALT or low-grade DDLPS with inflammatory and sclerosing pattern could show histology overlapping with an IMT/PMP, and involve perinephric, periureteral, or perivesical sites. Moreover, ALT and DDLPS with inflammatory patterns have been seen in the paratestis[40] or spermatic cord.[38] Tumors in the ALT-DDLPS spectrum tend to affect older individuals than classic IMTs and do not share the relatively frequent history of antecedent procedures or instrumentation that is characteristic of a significant number of PMPs. However, a DDLPS could bear some morphologic resemblance to an IMT/PMP, particularly the fasciitislike pseudosarcomatous myofibroblastic proliferations of the paratestis and spermatic cord that have been called "proliferative funiculitis."[100] Of utility in distinguishing these entities, many DDLPS in either retroperitoneal or inguinal sites demonstrate a variability of histologic patterns beyond that expected of an IMT/PMP, and certainly any high-grade DDLPS would have atypia beyond that of an IMT/PMP. FISH or IHC for MDM2, with positive immunostaining for CDK4, would establish the ALT or DDLPS diagnosis definitively in any challenging case.[64]

Last, although desmoid-type fibromatosis grows in a uniformly, densely collagenized, often long, sweeping fascicular pattern, without a prominent inflammatory component, one could envisage a scenario rendering a challenging differential diagnosis, especially in the myxoid or edematous examples sometimes presenting in the retroperitoneum or mesentery. Importantly, the vascular pattern of desmoids, with well-developed, plump arterioles and periarteriolar edema, is not characteristic of IMT/PMP. Although lymphocytes may be present sometimes in fibromatosis, the infiltrate is not prominent, and plasma cells are usually absent. Consistent with the high rates of mutation of CTNNB (β-catenin) in desmoids, positive IHC staining showing nuclear accumulation of β-catenin can help confirm the diagnosis.[101]

DIAGNOSIS

Presently, we regard the diagnosis of IMT or PMP in the GU tract as one of systematic exclusion, followed by assessment of actionable therapeutic aspects. First, we endeavor to exclude sarcomatoid carcinoma, usually urothelial, of whichever site is involved, as representing the most likely simulant. This means using broad-spectrum and high molecular weight cytokeratins and p63 as markers for sarcomatoid carcinoma, which are helpfully not expressed in an IMT or PMP. Second, we endeavor to exclude by immunophenotype or molecular studies, sampling, and imaging, as appropriate, a primary spindle cell sarcoma, especially leiomyosarcoma or inflammatory liposarcoma, involving a GU organ or adventitial soft tissue.

Once simulants are excluded, the final distinction regarding whether there is any utility in diagnosing any given tumor as PMP versus IMT. Overall, our approach is to designate most tumors as PMP, especially if the histology is more in the fasciitislike category, if there is any antecedent history of instrumentation, and if the patient is an adult. If the tumor shows an inflammatory pattern classic for IMT, occurs in a child, shows clinically suggestive systemic features of IMT (eg, fever, weight loss), the term IMT is favored. If there is any clinical management decision (eg, large size, recurrence), an IMT designation becomes our more serious consideration due to consideration of kinase inhibitors of ALK and related kinases.[88] In such scenarios, we have ordered additional workup with ancillary studies, including assessment by IHC with newer, sensitive antibodies (or FISH) for ALK (and, if negative, perhaps ROS1).[86,87,92]

Our anecdotal experience has been that relatively few tumors in the IMT/PMP group in adults, whether at GU sites or elsewhere, show ALK expression or rearrangements. Moreover, we have recently studied tumors with the PMP pattern in the GU tract, assaying for both ROS1 and ETV6 rearrangements, as seen in ALK-negative IMTs,[91,93] and USP6 rearrangements, as seen in fasciitis.[94,102] In keeping with the idea that many of the lesions in the GU tract represent reactive proliferations genetically unrelated to the aforementioned tumors, none of the PMPs showed rearrangements at these loci.[103]

PROGNOSIS

Classic IMT is considered a tumor of borderline malignancy, or intermediate (rarely metastasizing) by the WHO.[1] It has a tendency for local recurrence and can rarely metastasize (<5%).[80,104] The local recurrence risk is particularly high for intra-abdominal and retroperitoneal tumors (approximately 25%),[77,78,104,105] which would include examples involving GU organs from those locations. Of the series of these tumors involving the bladder, the recurrence rates have ranged between 0%[106] and 11%[74] to 31%.[95] One metastasis was noted in a post-radiation inflammatory fibrosarcoma with an ALK rearrangement.[95]

SOLITARY FIBROUS TUMOR

INTRODUCTION

One of the most remarkable developments in soft tissue pathology in the past decade has been the nosologic unification of solitary fibrous tumor (SFT) and tumors previously designated as "hemangiopericytoma." This occurred first on histologic grounds in the third edition of the WHO classification of soft tissue tumors,[107] then on molecular grounds when NAB2-STAT6 gene fusions were observed by several groups.[108–110] Originally, hemangiopericytomas were thought to originate from the pericytes (or "perivascular myoid cells") surrounding blood vessels,[111–113] and characterized at diverse sites. In contrast, SFTs were first described as distinctive tumors of the pleura,[114] even earlier than descriptions of hemangiopericytomas. Eventually, increasing experience allowed their recognition at diverse extrapleural sites in soft tissue and viscera. Their shared patternless histopathology and staghorn vasculature and characteristic CD34-positive immunophenotype,[115] enabled the realization that they represented the same entity presenting variable classic to cellular cell density, with less frequent myxoid,[116] epithelioid,[117,118] and lipomatous variants.[119–121] Smaller subsets show atypical features[116,122,123] and sarcomatous dedifferentiation.[117,124,125] Generally, SFTs are tumors of middle-aged adults between 20 and 70 years of age, without significant gender predilection.

SFTs are typically located in the deep soft tissue, including the thigh, pelvis, retroperitoneum, and serosa.[126] With regard to the GU tract (Fig. 7), SFTs have been found in the prostate, bladder, kidney, vulva, vagina, and even the penis.[127–135] They most often present as slowly growing, painless masses. Symptoms are typically the result of mass effect of the tumor encroaching on adjacent structures.

Interestingly, SFTs sometimes may produce insulin-like growth factor 2, in approximately 20% of cases, which can result in a reactive hypoglycemia, and is termed Doege-Potter syndrome.[136–138]

GROSS FEATURES

SFTs tend to grossly appear as circumscribed, solid, and indurated masses that are white-tan to gray in color. The cut surfaces are firm and may have myxoid or hemorrhagic areas. Tumor necrosis and infiltrative borders are associated with locally aggressive or malignant tumors.[139,140] Most tend to be circumscribed, solid, indurated with white-tan to gray coloration; tumors with myxoid or lipomatous differentiation may appear more gelatinous.[141] When present on the pleural surfaces, they are often exophytic. Most measure between 4 cm and 15 cm in greatest dimension, with a mean of approximately 10 cm.[141,142]

Within the bladder, SFTs are well-circumscribed solid masses that are mural-based and protrude into the bladder lumen.[131,143] Reported cases of SFTs involving the kidney reveal variably encapsulated, well-circumscribed parenchymal masses with tan-gray cut surfaces composed of fascicles of fibrous tissue.[135] Prostatic SFTs are white-tan, thinly encapsulated large masses with multinodular growth.[127,143]

MICROSCOPIC FEATURES

The microscopic appearance of SFTs is varied and appears on a spectrum ranging from strikingly cellular neoplasms reminiscent of the originally described "hemangiopericytoma" to neoplasms with decreased cellularity and hyalinized stroma, corresponding to classic SFT. The classic appearance of SFTs is a "patternless pattern" of the cells themselves, superimposed on zones of hypocellularity and hypercellularity. The intervening stroma is composed of thick bands of hyalinized collagen and angulated, thin-walled, branching vessels that are often termed "hemangiopericytomalike" or "staghorn" in appearance. The lesional cells are spindled to ovoid with pale cytoplasm, and indistinct cell borders, excepting cases with so-called "epithelioid" cytomorphology. The nuclei are often tapered to carrot shaped, with even chromatin and pinpoint to inconspicuous nucleoli. On the other end of the spectrum, cellular SFTs consist of dense, hypercellular round to spindle cell tumors with ill-defined cytoplasmic borders arranged around a ramifying network of staghorn vessels.

Within the GU tract, SFTs have a similar histologic appearance to other anatomic sites. In the bladder, SFTs are usually based in the wall and

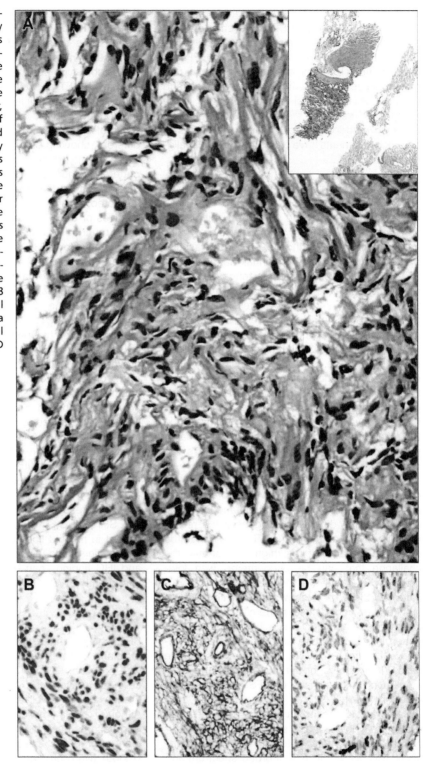

Fig. 7. SFT. (*A*) A core biopsy of an incidentally detected kidney mass demonstrated extensively fragmented tissue with myxoid change (*inset*, H&E 20×). While crushed, at higher power, a tumor composed of patternless small bland spindle cells closely apposed to collagen was apparent, 400×. In this setting, strong/diffuse nuclear positivity for STAT6 (*B*) and diffuse CD34 positivity (*C*) was helpful confirming the diagnosis of SFT. However, a subset of these tumors can demonstrate convincing, diffuse PAX8 positivity (*D*), a pitfall for interpretation as a sarcomatoid renal cell carcinoma. Panels B–D photographed at 400×.

covered by a layer of normal appearing urothelium and lamina propria.[131,143] In addition to features typical of SFTs in other sites, storiform, epithelioid, multinucleated giant cell, and angiosarcomatous patterns have also been described in SFTs of the prostate.[127]

Histologic criteria for malignant SFTs have not been well established, and tumors without worrisome features are well known to metastasize unpredictably. Malignant SFTs are characterized by an area of markedly increased cellularity with greater than 4 mitotic figures per 10 HPFs.[144] Large tumor size, patient age, and mitotic rate have been associated with risk of metastasis and disease-specific survival (discussed further in the "Prognosis" section).[142] Heterologous elements, including rhabdomyosarcomatous and osteosarcomatous elements have been described in malignant cases[125]

DIFFERENTIAL DIAGNOSIS

At the cellular end of the spectrum, spindle cell sarcomas, such as leiomyosarcoma and synovial sarcoma (the latter sharing the "staghorn" vascular pattern), can enter the differential diagnosis with SFT. Helpfully, leiomyosarcoma tends to express much more intense SMA and desmin positivity than the weak, infrequent expression of these markers in SFTs. In any case, neither leiomyosarcoma nor synovial sarcoma shows the convincing diffuse pattern of CD34 that is most characteristic of SFTs. We note, however, that although SFTs certainly do not show intrinsic epithelial elements like biphasic synovial sarcoma, SFTs can entrap glandular structures and simulate biphasic patterns in several anatomic sites.[141] Similarly, in the differential diagnosis with benign and malignant peripheral nerve sheath tumors, SFTs are negative for S100 and SOX10.

Dermatofibrosarcoma protuberans (DFSP), a cellular, diffusely CD34-positive tumor that may arise in the dermis at genital cutaneous sites, also enters the differential diagnosis; the recent description of superficial SFTs involving the dermis in the area of the thigh[145] illustrates the challenge that can be encountered with low-grade CD34-positive spindle cell tumors. Fortunately, DFSP tends to show an exquisite storiform architecture and diffuse pattern of honeycomb infiltration of adipose tissue that contrasts the patternless architecture and broader, less insidious infiltration of SFTs. In any questionable case, FISH studies for the COL1A1-PDGFB rearrangement characteristic of DFSP may be used for confirmation.[146]

Sarcomatoid carcinoma, particularly cases with cytologically lower grade spindle cell "fibromatosislike" patterns, may enter the differential diagnosis. IHC, especially use of broad-spectrum and high molecular weight cytokeratins as well as p63 can provide important assistance. One particular word of caution exists in the differential with sarcomatoid renal cell carcinoma: we[147] and others[129] have recently reported that a subset of

SFTs at diverse sites show expression of PAX8 (and even PAX2) by IHC (see **Fig. 7**). CD34 expression in SFTs, thus, provides a helpful confirmation of mesenchymal origin.

Desmoid-type fibromatosis can enter the differential with SFT as well. Desmoids tend to show sweeping, long fascicles of cells with nuclei that are longer, wavier, and better organized than those of SFTs. The vascular pattern, too, is quite different, showing plump arterioles with periarteriolar edema rather than staghorn branching pattern. Furthermore, fibromatosis tends to show grossly differing features with characteristically indurated, infiltrative, oblong processes between muscles or deep fascial layers, in contrast to the often-rounded gross contours of SFT. Desmoids are negative for CD34, and show nuclear accumulation of β-catenin.[148]

Myxoid liposarcoma can occasionally enter the differential diagnosis of SFT when a lesion has significant myxoid and lipomatous change, and we have reviewed SFTs at non-GU sites where myxoid liposarcoma has been misdiagnosed.[141] Myxoid liposarcomas tend to show multinodular growth with peripheral hypercellularity and plexiform "chicken-wire" vasculature, contrasting the staghorn pattern of SFTs. Signet ring lipoblasts are readily identified in most myxoid liposarcomas, whereas the fatty components of lipomatous SFTs are typically limited to banal adipocytes. SFTs are characterized by thin-walled vessels and at least focal areas of interstitial hyalinization, more than that typical of myxoid liposarcoma. By immunohistochemistry, myxoid liposarcoma expresses S100, whereas SFTs are S100-negative. Additionally, SFTs are positive for CD34, which is typically absent in myxoid liposarcoma. Furthermore, any challenging case with ambiguous morphologic and IHC findings can be tested for the *FUS* (or infrequently *EWSR1*)-*DDIT3* translocations.[149]

DIAGNOSIS

SFTs show a variably cellular, patternless pattern of bland fibroblastic cells, intimately admixed with collagenized, often hyalinized, stroma; these cells are arrayed in juxtaposition with prominent, branching, thin-walled staghorn vasculature. Although cellular, myxoid, lipomatous, and epithelioid variants have been described, the cytologic feature of bland, ovoid to spindled cells with smooth, even chromatin, transcends these varying patterns. For that matter, CD34 expression is apparent in the vast majority of cases.[115,140] Other markers, such as vimentin, CD99, BCL2, and, most recently, GRIA2,[109,150] have been proposed as useful adjuncts for diagnosis. However, we routinely rely on STAT6 IHC,[151-153] which shows a high degree of sensitivity (>90%) and specificity for SFT, given this lesion's association with pathognomonic *NAB2-STAT6* fusions[108-110] and the reliability of the stain as a strong and distinct nuclear marker.

Of note, rare STAT6 immunoreactivity has been identified in a subset of other tumors. Perhaps most challengingly, we[153] and others[154] have found STAT6 expression in dedifferentiated liposarcomas, which may reflect the vicinity of *STAT6* to the *MDM2* and *CDK4* loci amplified in ALT/DDLPS. Other unexpectedly STAT6-positive tumors, including deep fibrous histiocytomas, and, more oriented to the GU tract, prostatic stromal tumors have been described as well.[151,153,155] As always, the morphology and immunophenotype observed must be interpreted in an appropriate clinical and radiographic context.

Key Features
SOLITARY FIBROUS TUMOR

- Can occur almost anywhere in the GU tract with reported cases in the prostate, bladder, kidney, vulva, vagina, and penis

- Slow-growing, rounded, painless mass-forming lesion

- Circumscribed and solid white-tan to gray masses with variably myxoid and hemorrhagic areas

- Typically 4 cm to 15 cm in greatest dimension

- Patternless pattern of cells with zones of hypocellularity and hypercellularity

- Intervening thick bands of collagen and "staghorn" vessels

- CD34, vimentin, CD99, BCL2, STAT6, and GRIA2 are often positive

- Features associated with malignant SFTs include large size (≥15 cm), increased mitotic activity (≥4 mitotic figures per 10 HPFs), age ≥55 years, and necrosis

---

PROGNOSIS

Most SFTs follow a benign course, despite the formal classification of SFT as an intermediate (rarely metastasizing) entity by the WHO. However, approximately 10% of SFTs behave in an aggressive manner, with local recurrences or metastases, prediction of which represents one of the enduring enigmas of surgical pathology. Older criteria of Enzinger and Smith[156] noted that size >5 cm,

mitosis greater than 4 per 10 HPFs, markedly cellular histology, anaplastic or pleormorphic cells, hemorrhage, and necrosis were most suggestive of malignancy. Although other prognostic stratification models have been proposed, in 2012, Demicco and colleagues[142] created a risk stratification model based on 110 SFTs of varying sites and encompassing tumors with both classic and cellular SFT patterns. Their multivariate analysis revealed that small tumors with low mitotic rates were unlikely to metastasize or lead to disease-specific death. However, older patients (≥55 years of age) with large tumors (≥15 cm) showing ≥4 mitotic figures per 10 HPFs were at significantly increased risk of metastasis and death from disease. Recently, Demicco and colleagues[157] updated their model to include the presence or absence of necrosis as an additional risk factor for metastasis and death. Of note, neither of these models focuses on local recurrence as a salient outcome; however, our recent experience with SFTs of head and neck sites (which could be analogous to GU sites given similar challenges of endoscopic surgical management and for functional preservation), found that similar parameters, specifically size and mitotic rate, were associated with local recurrence.[141]

PERIVASCULAR EPITHELIOID CELL TUMOR

INTRODUCTION

Perivascular epithelioid cell tumors (PEComa) encompass a spectrum of lesions with unique histologic and immunohistochemical characteristics occurring at diverse sites.[158] This large family of neoplasms includes angiomyolipoma, clear cell "sugar" tumor (CCST) of the lung, and lymphangioleiomyomatosis. Additionally, there are several other morphologically and immunohistochemically similar neoplasms included under the spectrum of PEComa that arise in various body sites with site-specific names. These tumors demonstrate a unique pattern of differentiation that includes expression of both melanocytic and smooth muscle–associated immunophenotypic markers. Initial descriptions emphasized the epithelioid cytology of the lesional cells, with clear to pale pink cytoplasm, in addition to their perivascular orientation, appearing to radiate from vessel walls (hence the designation of "perivascular epithelioid cells"). In addition, PEComas are associated with tuberous sclerosis (TS), a complex multiorgan syndrome related to constitutional mutation of TSC2 (majority) or TSC1 (subset), resulting in dysregulated mammalian target of rapamycin (mTOR) signaling and diverse, variably penetrant manifestations.[159]

Within the GU tract, PEComas most commonly involve the kidney, as classic angiomyolipomas (AMLs), where they represent the overall most common tumor type in the PEComa family. The vast majority of renal PEComas are sporadic and unrelated to TS, unless multifocal. Most commonly, these tumors show the classic triphasic pattern of adipose, smooth muscle, and vascular differentiation. However, due to characteristic and reproducible imaging features lending these tumors to confident radiologic diagnosis and avoidance of resection, surgical pathologists may encounter classic AMLs less and less frequently. Sporadic AMLs are more common in women and occur in the fifth decade of life. Cases resulting in resection are often symptomatic with abdominal pain, hematuria, fever, or chills. In patients with TS, AMLs are more likely to be asymptomatic, bilateral, multifocal, and smaller than sporadic tumors. Epithelioid AML is a rare variant of AML, which has demonstrated potential for destructive invasion and metastasis,[160] and is characterized morphologically by a pattern of extensive to pure epithelioid morphology with a minor component of adipocytic or myoid differentiation.

Recent studies of the molecular genetics of PEComas have yielded additional insights. Among PEComas negative for TSC1 or TSC2 mutations, a subset harbor rearrangements at the TFE3 locus. These tumors were first described in 2010, where they were described in younger patients without TS.[161] Subsequent studies have found that the partner gene for fusion with TFE3 is most commonly SFPQ/PSF, whereas fusions to DVL2 comprise a smaller subset.[162,163]

With regard to the GU tract, PEComas outside of the kidney are uncommon. The urinary bladder is thought to be the second most common site of involvement[164–171] (exclusive of the uterus). Additionally, rare cases of PEComas involving the prostate, testis, and urethra have been reported.[172–174] In particular, the aforementioned TFE3-rearranged PEComas have been described in the kidney,[162,163,175] urinary bladder,[162,176–178] and prostate,[179] confirming the relevance of this subgroup to GU diagnosis.

GROSS FEATURES

Grossly, AMLs are tan-gray to yellow, well-circumscribed firm masses. The cut surfaces are fleshy to fibrous with foci of hemorrhage. Within soft tissues, AMLs have a broad range in size with averages from 5 to 9 cm. AMLs of the kidney have mean tumor sizes of 1 cm to 4 cm in sporadic cases and 3.5 cm to 19.3 cm in patients with TS.[180–182] Occasionally, cysts may be present and are typical of AML with epithelial cysts (AMLECs, Fig. 8), which may present as suspicious for renal cell carcinoma given complex solid and cystic imaging findings. The cysts often range from 2 cm to 6 cm with a mean diameter of 4 cm.[183,184] Regarding epithelioid AML, the gross morphology reported in the literature has been quite variable[185–187]: generally, these tumors have been mostly solid with areas of hemorrhage and possible necrosis. PEComas of the bladder have ranged from 3 to 9 cm with variably infiltrative borders and patchy necrosis.[160]

MICROSCOPIC FEATURES

Microscopically, classic AML is composed of 3 main elements: blood vessels, smooth muscle, and adipose tissue. The vascular component consists of thick-walled tortuous vessels with medial hyalinization and loss of the internal elastic lamina. The adipocytic component, often predominant, is characterized by mature adipocytes. The smooth muscle cells are spindled to plump and may show nuclear atypia and occasional mitotic figures. In one classic series of nearly 200 AMLs, 77% showed the classic triphasic pattern (each component present >5%), 11% showed a myoid-predominant (>95%) pattern, 4% showed adipose-predominant (>95%) pattern, and 8% showed a significant (>10%) epithelioid pattern.[182] Interestingly, comparing histologic features between sporadic and TS-associated cases, the epithelioid component, presence of epithelial cysts, and any coincident microscopic AML foci were associated with TS.

The histologic features of epithelioid angiomyolipomas deserve particular comment, given their distinctive histomorphology and their mimicry of other neoplasms (as later in this article, see Fig. 8). Depending on criteria used for diagnosis, these tumors are composed purely,[187] predominantly,[188] or variably[186] of polygonal epithelioid cells with eosinophilic cytoplasm and nuclei with vesicular chromatin and prominent nucleoli. Occasional cells will have abundant amphophilic cytoplasm and eccentric nuclei with prominent nucleoli, imparting a ganglion cell–like or even rhabdoidlike pattern. Although often admixed with cells with granular eosinophilic cytoplasm, some cases may demonstrate extensive clear cell cytology, recapitulating the clear cell "sugar tumor" of the lungs. The epithelioid cells are arranged in broad, cohesive sheets or nests with an alveolar arrangement. Densely collagenized

Fig. 8. Morphologic variations of PEComa. (*A*) Recent scholarship has identified a group of AMLs of the kidney with entrapped renal tubules undergoing cystic change, so-called AMLECs, H&E 40×. AMLECs, similar to other PEComas, show diffuse expression of the emerging marker cathepsin K (*inset*, 200×). (*B*) Some PEComas show such extensive patterns of plump round polygonal cells with variably eosinophilic to clear cytoplasm that a differential diagnosis of epithelial malignancy such as renal cell carcinoma may be considered, 400×. Historically, HMB45 (*inset*, 200×) has been proven the most sensitive marker of PEComas. (*C*) A malignant PEComa arising in the kidney, metastatic to the liver at presentation, shows markedly atypical cells with coarse chromatin swirling off dysmorphic vasculature (pictured, 200× with zoom). Atypical mitoses and necrosis were apparent. Among multiple melanocytic markers expressed, MITF expression was strong and diffuse (*inset*, 400×).

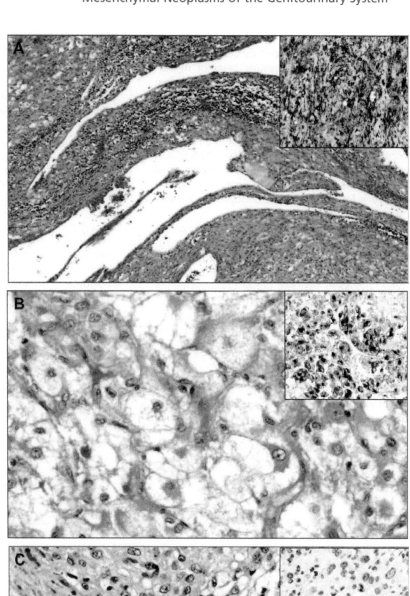

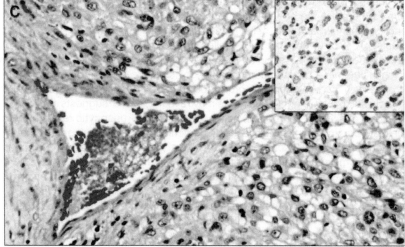

stroma with or without perivascular hyalinization and cordlike or trabecular cellular growth also may be present. PEComas with *TFE3* rearrangements reportedly show nested or alveolar architecture with plump epithelioid cytology. Furthermore, these tumors tend to show decreased positivity for markers of myogenic differentiation.[161,162,175,189]

Finally, AMLECs show a striking pattern of multi-loculated epithelial cysts lined by cuboidal or hob-nailed cells overlying a cellular layer of myoid-predominant spindle cell stroma. The stroma often has an admixed chronic inflammatory infiltrate. AMLECs tend to show a pauciadipose pattern, which may cause diagnostic confusion with other tumors, including mixed epithelial and stromal tu-mors of the kidney. The cyst lining of AMLECs is PAX8 positive, consistent with entrapped renal tubular epithelium, whereas the solid component is positive for myoid and melanocytic markers by immunostaining.

PEComas, including AMLs, may demonstrate histologic features typically indicative of malig-nancy in more common tumor types. Degenerative "bizarre" or smudgy neuroendocrinelike nuclear atypia, cytologic features rather common in the epithelioid PEComas,[182] may prompt consider-ation of a malignant diagnosis. Even classic AMLs may extend to appear to invade renal sinus soft tissues and into lymphatics or even large ves-sels. Unless other worrisome features (predomi-nant epithelioid cytomorphology, significant mitosis, necrosis, see later in this article) are pre-sent, these do not denote a poor prognosis. By that same token, apparent involvement of regional lymph nodes in tumors with otherwise typical fea-tures tends to be considered evidence of multicen-tric disease rather than metastasis.[160,190,191]

DIFFERENTIAL DIAGNOSIS

The differential diagnosis of AMLs (Table 3) with a predominant adipocytic component can be confused with well-differentiated liposarcoma due to the presence of variably sized adipocytes and sometimes atypical cells resembling lipo-blasts. The presence of thick-walled tortuous and maldeveloped vessels in an AML is a key his-tologic clue to help differentiate these neoplasms. In our experience, revisiting the gross specimen to sample solid or heterogeneous areas may reveal a myoid or epithelioid component helping to secure the diagnosis in essentially all cases. In particularly ambiguous cases, IHC can be helpful. AMLs are positive for melanocytic markers and smooth mus-cle markers, whereas liposarcomas are negative. Unexpected MDM2 and p16 expression, consid-ered aberrant, by IHC have been identified in both AMLs, similar to ALT and DDLPS.[64,192,193] Therefore, a panel of immunostains including markers of melanocytic differentiation is recom-mended. Furthermore, in this context, FISH for MDM2 amplification acts as the gold standard test, which can substantiate or eliminate a diag-nosis of ALT (and DDLPS).

Table 3 Differential diagnosis: perivascular epithelioid cell tumor (PEComa)	
PEComa Versus	**Helpful Distinguishing Features**
Atypical lipomatous tumor	• Lacks thick-walled tortuous and maldeveloped vessels • Negative for Melan A, HMB45, and SMA • FISH is positive for *MDM2* amplification
Oncocytic renal cell carcinoma	• Positive expression for PAX8 • May show Melan A and HMB45 expression
Melanoma	• Lacks lipomatous and smooth muscle differentiation • S100 diffusely positive in nuclear and cytoplasmic distribution • Usually SOX10 positive • *BRAF* mutation excludes PEComa
Leiomyosarcoma	• Greater nuclear atypia, coagulative tumor cell necrosis, brisk mitotic activity • Usually negative for melanocytic markers (rare HMB45 expression) • Negative staining for Melan A

Abbreviations: FISH, fluorescence in situ hybridization; SMA, smooth muscle actin.

Oncocytic renal cell carcinoma and oncocytoma may enter the differential diagnosis for epithelioid AML. Indeed, contemporary descriptions of the spectrum of renal cell neoplasia in the setting of TS suggests that prior reports of "oncocytoma," oncocytic renal cell carcinoma, and clear cell renal cell carcinoma in that syndromal setting may have actually been PEComas misdiagnosed in the pre-IHC era.[194] Contemporary series confirm that renal cell carcinoma, even rare translocation-associated renal cell carcinomas that demonstrate melano-cytic differentiation,[195,196] demonstrate diffuse expression of the renal tubular-associated marker, PAX8, which remains negative in the PEComas that show overlapping histology (and even *TFE3* rearrangements)[175] with renal cell carcinoma.

Epithelioid PEComas may demonstrate several features, including variably clear and granular cyto-plasm, prompting consideration of adrenocortical neoplasms. Although these lesions share Melan A and HMB45 expression, adrenocortical neoplasms may show focal keratin positivity and are SMA negative.[197] Expression of the marker SF1 is also characteristic of adrenal cortical neoplasms.[198]

Melanoma and epithelioid AML share histologic features and immunohistochemical expression of melanocytic differentiation, findings that may create diagnostic confusion. A clinical history of melanoma and the presence of multifocal lesions should raise suspicion for metastatic melanoma. Evidence of lipomatous or smooth muscular differentiation establishes the tumor as an AML, and smooth muscle markers are typically negative in melanoma. Of great utility, S100 is typically diffusely positive in a nuclear and cytoplasmic distribution in melanoma, whereas S100 is either negative or weakly and focally positive in PEComa. Although epithelioid PEComa may show S100 positivity, it tends to be weaker, patchier, and more restricted to the cytoplasm than that seen in melanoma. For that matter, SOX10, which is diffusely positive in more than 95% of melanomas, is negative in the PEComa family.[199] Finally, identification of a lesional *BRAF* mutation would support a melanoma diagnosis within this differential diagnosis.

Leiomyosarcoma, the most common primary sarcoma of the kidney, may morphologically mimic myoid-predominant AML. On the balance, leiomyosarcoma tends to have greater nuclear atypia, coagulative tumor cell necrosis, and more frequent mitotic figures than a myoid-predominant AML. Additionally, leiomyosarcoma tends to be negative for melanocytic markers, although we note that prior reports have described HMB45 expression, usually focal, in leiomyosarcomas of both genital stroma (eg, uterine type)[200] and somatic soft tissues.[201] Similarly, cathepsin K, a marker used increasingly to support diagnoses of PEComa and melanoma, has demonstrated positive expression in most leiomyosarcomas within one large cohort of tumors.[202] In contrast to HMB-45 and cathepsin K, Melan A lacks this pitfall and shows typical positivity in PEComa and predictable negativity in leiomyosarcoma.

DIAGNOSIS

Classic angiomyolipomas can be diagnosed solely based on histologic features. The finding of a triphasic neoplasm containing thick-walled, tortuous blood vessels, spindle cells, and adipose tissue is sufficient for diagnosis in most cases. However, when one of the components predominates, the diagnosis becomes more challenging and IHC gains utility. The histomorphology of epithelioid

PEComa, especially in its pure form, prompts a broad differential diagnosis, which may be resolved through the use of a panel of immunohistochemical markers selected based on the site of involvement and the corresponding primary neoplasms under consideration. We note that truly "pure" epithelioid PEComa occurs with exceptional rarity, and that most resection cases in which the epithelioid pattern is encountered can be resolved by more extensive gross sampling. However, small biopsy specimens may limit pathologic examination to the epithelioid component.

IHC may aid diagnosis in cases with unusual histologic patterns and cases with limited biopsy tissue. One of the larger studies of reactivity for a panel of immunostains in uterine and extrauterine PEComas found that the most prevalent immunophenotypic marker expressed was HMB45 (92%), followed by SMA (86%), Melan A (72%), MiTF (50%), desmin (36%), S100 (33%), and TFE3 (29%),[203] findings that are consistent with numerous other studies.[204–207] IHC for cathepsin K is diffusely positive in the vast majority of PEComas, negative in the vast majority of epithelial neoplasms, and occasionally positive in mesenchymal tumors beyond PEComa.[202,208] Given this profile, cathepsin K may be useful in the differential diagnosis, particularly with epithelial neoplasms.

PROGNOSIS

Sporadic AMLs are benign neoplasms that can be managed with active surveillance, surgical excision, or arterial embolization.[209] In patients with TS or unresectable tumors, mTOR inhibitors are an emerging option for therapy.[210,211] Recently, PPARγ has been implicated as having a possible regulator of AML growth and may be an option for targeted therapy.[212]

Histopathologic criteria for malignancy of PEComas have been investigated. In the examination of PEComas with non-AML, non-lymphangioleiomyomatosis, non–clear cell sugar tumor histology, arising at diverse gynecologic and soft tissue sites, Folpe and colleagues[203] proposed a prognostic classification system for PEComas based on the criteria of presence or absence of worrisome features, including large size (>5 cm), infiltrative growth pattern, high nuclear grade and cellularity, mitotic rate of greater than 1 per 50 HPFs, necrosis, or vascular invasion. Based on consideration of these criteria, tumors with none of these features were considered benign and associated with no clinical aggression (recurrence and/or metastasis). Tumors with either >5 cm size or nuclear pleomorphism and/or multinucleate giant cells only were considered uncertain malignant potential and associated with rare aggression (up to 12% for the tumors >5 cm). Finally, tumors with 2 or more worrisome features were considered malignant with most showing aggression.

With respect to the GU tract, 2 prognostic studies have investigated PEComas of the kidney with variable epithelioid morphology.[186,187] Among 41 pure epithelioid PEComas, significantly enriched with consultation cases, Nese and colleagues[187] demonstrated metastatic disease at presentation in 29%. Of 33 patients with follow-up data, local recurrence and metastasis was seen in 17% and 49%, respectively, including 33% of patients who died of disease. Adverse prognostic parameters associated with these aggressive outcomes in univariate analyses included syndromal TS or another AML lesion, size >7 cm, extrarenal disease, and infiltrative growth pattern. They proposed stratifying pure epithelioid PEComas with less than 2 adverse parameters as low risk, tumors with 2 to 3 adverse parameters as intermediate risk, and tumors with 4 or more adverse factors as high risk.

One additional heavily consultation-based series of 34 cases of AML with variable epithelioid proportion and nuclear atypia (defined as polygonal cells with abundant cytoplasm, vesicular nuclei, prominent nucleoli, and at least twofold variation in nuclear size) revealed clinical malignancy (local recurrence or metastasis) in just more than a quarter of cases. PEComas showing malignant behavior tended to occur in older patients, with larger tumors, and with higher proportions of epithelioid cytology and atypical cells. Malignancy was further associated with higher mitotic count, necrosis, vascular invasion, and invasion of the renal vein. The authors proposed their own prognostic classification based on 4 features, including greater than 70% atypical epithelioid cells, ≥ 2 mitoses/10 HPF, presence of atypical mitoses, and necrosis, such that if 3 or more of these parameters were present, the model was highly predictive of malignant behavior.[186]

A remarkably less aggressive course was noted in a study of the outcomes of a multi-institutional series of consecutive, resected PEComas harboring more than 80% epithelioid morphology from 3 referral centers (consultation cases excluded). He and colleagues[188] identified that less than 5% of all PEComas resected met this 80% epithelioid criterion, and of the 20 consecutive cases, many of which showed large size and half of which showed necrosis, only a single metastasis was seen during follow-up. Although this latter finding requires further study prospectively, we interpret it as signifying that the true rate of malignancy in these tumors is probably significantly lower than the aforementioned consultation series.[186,187] Nonetheless, when we diagnose a PEComa with significant proportion of epithelioid features, we note that a significant subset can show evolution of metastasis and discuss the aforementioned prognostic findings and parameters.

PERICYTIC (PERIVASCULAR MYOID CELL) TUMORS

INTRODUCTION

Within the fourth edition of the WHO classification, the category of pericytic (perivascular myoid cell) tumors includes glomus tumors, myopericytoma, myofibroma, and angioleiomyoma.[1,213–215] These entities are morphologically related and characteristically demonstrate a pattern of differentiation related to the perivascular myoid cells. The glomus tumor, which was first described in detail in 1942 by Stout and Murray[113] is derived from modified perivascular smooth muscle cells in the wall of arteriovenous shunts (Sucquet-Hoyer canals) that are involved in thermoregulation. These sporadic glomus tumors tend to occur as solitary tumors on the distal extremities of adults, whereas glomuvenous malformations, a heritable condition, occur as multifocal lesions on the extremities of children. Variants of glomus tumor include glomangiomas and glomangiomyomas.[215,216] Based on overlapping morphologic features with glomus tumor, myopericytoma, and myofibroma have been organized under the umbrella of pericytic tumors. Furthermore, even angioleiomyoma, given its perivascular growth of smooth muscle cells and increasingly recognized overlapping features with myopericytoma, has been included in the pericytic (perivascular) category of neoplasms rather than the smooth muscle group.[217]

Within the GU tract, pericytic tumors have been described most frequently involving the kidney. Glomus tumors[218–229] and myopericytomas[230–234] have been rarely reported in the kidney (**Fig. 9**). Angioleiomyomas have been observed in the kidney, but only in single case reports or as single cases in a series.[228,235–237] The penis is an additional site of involvement, including glomus tumors,[238,239] myopericytoma,[240] and myofibroma.[241,242] The urinary bladder has been involved by glomus tumors,[243,244] myofibroma,[245] and myopericytoma.[234,246] Thus, occurrence of these tumors in the GU tract represents a rare phenomenon, and exclusion of much more common lesions in the histologic differential diagnosis is the most important undertaking when evaluating these neoplasms. Recent scholarship in this realm

Fig. 9. Pericytic tumors. (*A*) A renal glomus tumor shows a predominantly solid pattern of small, monotonous round cells without atypia (*inset*, H&E, 400×), arrayed around hyalinized vessels with focal stromal myxoid change (main panel 40×). (*B*) A renal myopericytoma shows glomoid and more spindled myoid cells whirling around small vessels in an edematous stroma (400×). Reflective of its myoid nature, SMA is diffusely positive (*inset*, 200×).

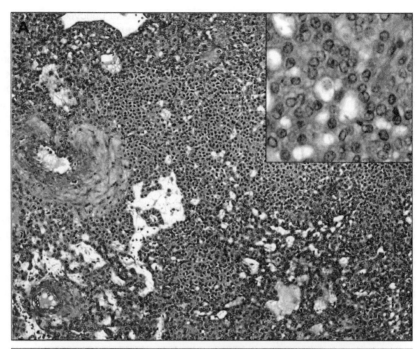

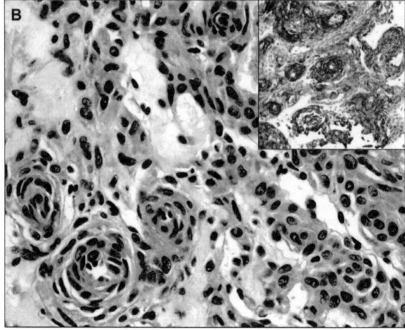

prompted the inclusion of this category of tumors in this review, particularly our recent work on the largest reported cohort of renal pericytic tumors.[228]

GROSS FEATURES

Across all sites, pericytic tumors have been described as firm and variably gray-white to red-brown in appearance, depending on the proportion of solid glomoid (classic round cell/epithelioid glomus tumor–like) and solid myoid (vascular smooth muscle–like) versus vascular space; these tumors are not surprisingly often described as hemorrhagic. Most tend to arise in superficial cutaneous soft tissues.[247,248] Focusing on visceral examples in the GU tract, the tumors have ranged from 1.1 cm to 20 cm with a mean of approximately 4.5 cm.[228,229,233] The tumors tend to be well-circumscribed; however, focally infiltrative borders are not uncommon. In the kidney, pericytic tumors tend to have a nonspecific appearance, with cut surfaces appearing gray-white to red-brown with variable hemorrhage and gelatinous changes.[218]

MICROSCOPIC FEATURES

Pericytic (perivascular) tumors of the kidney most commonly display the morphology of glomus tumors, with identical features to those described at other sites. Glomus tumors characteristically present as circumscribed lobules of monotonous cells with round to ovoid, centrally located nuclei and amphophilic to eosinophilic cytoplasm with well-defined cell borders. Solid glomus tumors are composed of nests of glomus cells with admixed small blood vessels; the stromal background varies from scant (in cellular/solid examples) to myxoid, edematous, or hyalinized. Cases within the kidney show prominent vasculature with variably sized blood vessels, stromal hyalinization, and focal myxoid change. Symplastic, degenerative-type cytologic atypia was present in a subset of cases.[228]

Myopericytomas of the kidney demonstrate morphologic features similar to the spectrum of those seen in soft tissue. These tumors are defined by concentric growth of lesional cells around thin-walled vascular lumina. Tumor cells are small with round to ovoid to spindled nuclei and eosinophilic cytoplasm. These cells are less densely packed than in glomus tumor, with a distinctly myoid (smooth muscle–like) appearance and syncytial arrangement, lacking the defined cell membranes of glomus tumors.[232] There is a predilection for perivascular, concentric growth, as described in somatic soft tissue cases. The background vasculature can have a glomangiopericytomalike growth with dilated, thin-walled vessels.

A rare subset of renal pericytic tumors demonstrate perivascular concentric growth, although with more smooth muscle–like cytologic features, more reminiscent of angioleiomyoma. The vascular components of these lesions have been described as predominantly venous[235] or venous with a cavernous hemangiomalike pattern.[228] The dense solid pattern of angioleiomyoma that is so often seen in peripheral soft tissues (as well as adipocytic metaplasia) has not been described in the kidney to date.

Intratumoral histomorphologic heterogeneity, with juxtaposition of patterns characteristic of different types of pericytic neoplasms, is a frequent feature of renal pericytic tumors. In all but one of the

renal pericytic tumors that we studied (other than pure/classic glomus tumors or glomus tumor variants), there were multiple patterns of pericytic tumors, with tumors demonstrating solid glomuslike areas, myopericytomalike areas, and angioleiomyomalike areas. Although myopericytomas of soft tissues often show areas that are angioleiomyomalike or myofibromalike,[216] the amount of variation seen in these renal examples was remarkable among several GU and soft tissue pathologists reviewing the cases.[228]

DIFFERENTIAL DIAGNOSIS

The primary differential diagnosis (Table 4) of pericytic (perivascular) tumors in the kidney is juxtaglomerular cell tumor (JGCT).[249] The gross appearance of JGCTs shows some overlap with glomus tumors. Specifically, JGCTs present as small, well-circumscribed masses in the kidney with tan to yellow cut surfaces. Microscopically, JGCTs are composed of uniform polygonal cells with distinct cell borders and eosinophilic cytoplasm. The architecture can be sheetlike or trabecular and associated with hemangiopericytomalike vessels with focal myxoid stromal changes. The tumor cell nuclei are bland, and mitotic activity is typically limited. In summary, the characteristic histologic features of JGCT closely resemble those of the classic renal glomus tumors described previously.

The differential between glomus tumors and JGCTs is one in which clinicopathologic correlation can be quite helpful. The classic history of a younger patient with poorly controlled hypertension, hyperkalemia, and plasma renin activity, resolving after resection, is quite characteristic of JGCT but not always present.[250] In contrast, we have seen renal glomus tumors that are associated with hypertension, but without postoperative resolution.[228] Ultimately, observation of rhomboid renin crystals by electron microscopy remains the gold standard for JGCT diagnosis.[249] Although renin IHC has been used in this differential, we have seen focal, strong renin staining in renal glomus tumors,[251] leading us to question the prospective utility of this marker in diagnostic scenarios with unknown or ambiguous clinical features. More traditional IHC markers may have a role: on the balance, stronger positivity for myoid markers, including SMA, caldesmon, and calponin favors diagnosis of a pericytic neoplasm, whereas stronger CD34 and CD117 positivity favors JGCT.

Given the prominent vascularity of renal pericytic tumors at the glomus tumor or myopericytoma end of the spectrum, a primary vascular neoplasm could enter the differential diagnosis.

Table 4
Differential diagnosis: pericytic (perivascular) tumors

Pericytic (Perivascular) Tumors Versus	Helpful Distinguishing Features
Juxtaglomerular cell tumor (JGCT)	• History of a (usually young) patient with poorly controlled hypertension and hyperkalemia • Elevated plasma renin activity • Rhomboid renin crystals identified on electron microscopy (gold standard) • Strong CD34 and CD117 positivity with relatively weaker SMA, caldesmon, and calponin • Emerging use of renin IHC
Hemangioma, including anastomosing hemangioma	• Anastomosing capillary-sized vessels with fibrin thrombi and occasional endothelial hobnailing • Absent mitosis and cytologic atypia • ERG positivity, lack of SMA positive myoid stroma
Myoid-predominant AML/PEComa	• Adipose tissue component may be present • Expresses melanocytic markers • Tortuous dysplastic vessels
Leiomyoma	• Densely packed fascicles lacking prominent vascular component • Elongated smooth muscle cells
Solitary fibrous tumor	• Stronger, diffuse expression of CD34 • STAT6 nuclear expression • Greater prominence of collagenous stroma • Staghorn vascular pattern

Abbreviations: AML, angiomyolipoma; IHC, immunohistochemistry; PEComa, perivascular epithelioid cell tumor; SMA, smooth muscle actin.

In fact, we have recently reported a series of hemangiomas in kidneys, usually end-stage, showing the pattern of so-called "anastomosing hemangioma"[252] as described in the GU tract[253] and elsewhere.[254] These tumors show a network of anastomosing capillary-sized vessels, lined by endothelial cells, often with hobnail growth, and associated with fibrin thrombi. The striking interstitial proliferation of nonendothelial stromal cells can impart an almost "splenic" look to the background. Mitoses are generally absent and cytologic atypia nonexistent to mild. Although expression of CD34 as seen in hemangiomas could overlap with a pericytic (especially a glomus) tumor, more specific vascular markers, such as ERG, are positive in endothelial neoplasms and negative in pericytic tumors other than in the vascular component.

At the angioleiomyoma end of the spectrum, the differential diagnosis includes smooth muscle tumors. Certainly, an angioleiomyoma could provoke consideration of a myoid-predominant AML/PEComa (as previously), although the presence of any adipose component or expression of melanocytic markers would serve to establish the diagnosis as an AML. Although after exclusion of myoid-predominant or monophasic myoid AML/

PEComa, true leiomyomas of the kidney are quite rare (and likely in most cases represent displaced genital stroma-type leiomyomas[255]), such leiomyomas occur in the urinary bladder, prostate, and other sites in the GU tract where distinction based on morphologic grounds, specifically the pericytic orientation and concentric proliferation of the myoid cells of pericytic lesions, is distinctive. In contrast, true smooth muscle tumors tend to show more densely packed and compact fascicles of more elongated smooth muscle cells lacking a prominent and intrinsic vascular component. For that matter, SFT could enter the differential diagnosis as well, especially given the shared expression of CD34. However, the extent of CD34 expression tends to be much more diffuse and strong in SFTs, and STAT6 nuclear expression is expected.

DIAGNOSIS

Pericytic neoplasms demonstrate the differentiation pattern of perivascular myoid cells, including expression of SMA and often CD34. These lesions comprise a spectrum from solid and epithelioid forms (glomus tumors) showing glomoid cytomorphology to spindled myoid forms (angioleiomyoma), with the many tumors falling between these extremes ending up classified as myopericytomas, a term that we favor for many. Tumors showing this pattern in children are often termed myofibroma, whereas we tend to label lesions even with a myofibromatous pattern in adults as myopericytoma. Variants have been described, based on the underlying architecture of the vasculature, which may show a staghorn and ramifying pattern or cavernous pattern. As examples, cases with glomoid cells of the vascular media are termed glomangiomas, whereas those with spindled myoid cells are termed glomangiomyoma. For our part, when encountering a renal tumor with glomus tumor pattern, we actively seek clarification as to whether there is any history of (and especially, change in) hypertensive status vis à vis exclusion of JGCT (as previously). On an occasion in consultation where these data were not available, we have used diagnostic terminology, such as pericytic (perivascular myoid cell) tumor with glomus tumor–like pattern, adding a comment recommending need for clarification of any presence, nature, and sequence of hypertension in association with the tumor and its resection.

Recent studies have characterized novel markers for pericytic tumors, including CD146 and RGS5, which are diffusely positive in pericytic tumors but not in simulants.[256,257] These markers may add diagnostic value beyond the less specific expression of SMA. However, these markers have not been studied in the pericytic tumors of the GU tract. Interestingly, a recent study by Meguro and colleagues[258] has evaluated myosin 1B (MYO1B), a novel pericyte marker, and h-caldesmon expression in glomus tumors and angioleiomyomas. In contrast to the aforementioned newer markers, angioleiomyomas were MYO1B negative, whereas glomus tumors were MYO1B positive. Last, we note that a recent study has linked glomus tumors to neurofibromatosis, especially involvement of multiple digits.[259] To our knowledge, GU tract involvement has not been described in this syndromal scenario, although we recommend awareness of the association.

PROGNOSIS

Pericytic (perivascular) tumors of the soft tissue are usually benign and are cured by simple excision; however, a subset of glomus tumors has demonstrated a high rate of metastatic disease and death. Prognostication of the behavior of these tumors remains an area in which recent data call into question the application of criteria developed for soft tissue pericytic tumors to visceral GU examples. Much of the traditional concept of pericytic tumor prognosis was driven by a study of atypical glomus tumors by Folpe and colleagues.[260] This study, which evaluated 52 glomus tumors, most all of soft tissue, resulted in the proposition that pathologists classify as malignant any deep tumor measuring >2 cm, or showing atypical mitotic figures, or demonstrating moderate to high nuclear grade and mitotic activity ($\geq$5 mitotic figures/50 HPF). An uncertain malignant potential category was proposed for glomus tumors that were superficial with increased mitosis, or were large without other worrisome criteria, or were at a deep location. These criteria would render, operationally, essentially all renal examples large enough to come to light clinically as either malignant by these aforementioned criteria,[260] or perhaps as uncertain malignant potential as suggested by the WHO classification.[1]

Considering our recent experience with renal pericytic tumors, and our review of all known published cases, we would question the appropriateness of application of any of these prognostic criteria to renal examples. In fact, save for the persistence of hypertension in scattered cases within our cohort, no negative or aggressive sequelae were noted in the 17 cases we studied. Additionally, to our knowledge only a single case of metastasis of a malignant glomus tumor of the kidney has been described[222] (although other reports describe "malignant" glomus tumors of the kidney without metastasis labeled "malignant" based on the aforementioned soft tissue criteria[225,261–263]). Overall, our assessment is that these tumors tend to be more indolent than soft tissue pericytic tumors. Furthermore, given that we have observed no worse risk than a typical renal cell carcinoma of similar size, nephron-sparing partial nephrectomy or even surveillance could be considered in an appropriate clinical setting.

REFERENCES

1. Fletcher CDM, Bridge JA, Hogendoorn PCW, et al, editors. World Health Organization classification of tumours of soft tissue and bone. 4th edition. Lyon (France): International Agency for Research on Cancer (IARC); 2013.
2. McCarthy AJ, Chetty R. Tumours composed of fat are no longer a simple diagnosis: an overview of fatty tumours with a spindle cell component. J Clin Pathol 2018;71(6):483–92.
3. Enzinger FM, Harvey DA. Spindle cell lipoma. Cancer 1975;36(5):1852–9.
4. Shmookler BM, Enzinger FM. Pleomorphic lipoma: a benign tumor simulating liposarcoma. A clinicopathologic analysis of 48 cases. Cancer 1981; 47(1):126–33.

5. Ko JS, Daniels B, Emanuel PO, et al. Spindle cell lipomas in women: a report of 53 cases. Am J Surg Pathol 2017;41(9):1267–74.

6. Dal Cin P, Sciot R, Polito P, et al. Lesions of 13q may occur independently of deletion of 16q in spindle cell/pleomorphic lipomas. Histopathology 1997; 31(3):222–5.

7. Fletcher CD, Akerman M, Dal Cin P, et al. Correlation between clinicopathological features and karyotype in lipomatous tumors. A report of 178 cases from the chromosomes and morphology (CHAMP) collaborative study group. Am J Pathol 1996;148(2):623–30.

8. Maggiani F, Debiec-Rychter M, Verbeeck G, et al. Extramammary myofibroblastoma is genetically related to spindle cell lipoma. Virchows Arch 2006;449(2):244–7.

9. McMenamin ME, Fletcher CD. Mammary-type myofibroblastoma of soft tissue: a tumor closely related to spindle cell lipoma. Am J Surg Pathol 2001; 25(8):1022–9.

10. Pauwels P, Sciot R, Croiset F, et al. Myofibroblastoma of the breast: genetic link with spindle cell lipoma. J Pathol 2000;191(3):282–5.

11. Flucke U, van Krieken JH, Mentzel T. Cellular angiofibroma: analysis of 25 cases emphasizing its relationship to spindle cell lipoma and mammary-type myofibroblastoma. Mod Pathol 2011;24(1):82–9.

12. Maggiani F, Debiec-Rychter M, Vanbockrijck M, et al. Cellular angiofibroma: another mesenchymal tumour with 13q14 involvement, suggesting a link with spindle cell lipoma and (extra)-mammary myofibroblastoma. Histopathology 2007;51(3):410–2.

13. Panagopoulos I, Gorunova L, Bjerkehagen B, et al. Loss of chromosome 13 material in cellular angiofibromas indicates pathogenetic similarity with spindle cell lipomas. Diagn Pathol 2017;12(1):17.

14. Cohen AJ, Steele GS. A mammary-type myofibroblastoma of the prostate: a case report. Urol Case Rep 2016;8:44–6.

15. Datta B, Giri A, Halder B. Histopathological evaluation of surgically treated adult renal tumors: report from a tertiary care center in India. Indian J Cancer 2016;53(1):124–6.

16. Sabah M, Mohan P, Kay E. Para-testicular cellular angiofibroma: a rare tumour in a male renal transplant patient. Virchows Arch 2006;449(4):489–92.

17. Zhao Z, Selvarajan S, Tiong AL, et al. Spindle cell lipoma in an end-stage renal allograft: case report. Transplant Proc 2016;48(9):3145–8.

18. Howitt BE, Fletcher CD. Mammary-type myofibroblastoma: clinicopathologic characterization in a series of 143 cases. Am J Surg Pathol 2016; 40(3):361–7.

19. Iwasa Y, Fletcher CD. Cellular angiofibroma: clinicopathologic and immunohistochemical analysis of 51 cases. Am J Surg Pathol 2004;28(11):1426–35.

20. Nucci MR, Granter SR, Fletcher CD. Cellular angiofibroma: a benign neoplasm distinct from angiomyofibroblastoma and spindle cell lipoma. Am J Surg Pathol 1997;21(6):636–44.

21. Fletcher CD, Martin-Bates E. Spindle cell lipoma: a clinicopathological study with some original observations. Histopathology 1987;11(8):803–17.

22. Magro G, Caltabiano R, Di Cataldo A, et al. CD10 is expressed by mammary myofibroblastoma and spindle cell lipoma of soft tissue: an additional evidence of their histogenetic linking. Virchows Arch 2007;450(6):727–8.

23. Miettinen M, Mandahl N. Spindle cell/pleomorphic lipoma. In: Fletcher CD, Bridge JA, Hogendoorn PCW, et al, editors. WHO classificiation of tumours of soft tissue and bone. 4th edition. Lyon (France): International Agency for Research on Cancer (IARC); 2013. p. 29–30.

24. Sachdeva MP, Goldblum JR, Rubin BP, et al. Low-fat and fat-free pleomorphic lipomas: a diagnostic challenge. Am J Dermatopathol 2009;31(5):423–6.

25. Billings SD, Folpe AL. Diagnostically challenging spindle cell lipomas: a report of 34 "low-fat" and "fat-free" variants. Am J Dermatopathol 2007;29(5):437–42.

26. Beham A, Schmid C, Hodl S, et al. Spindle cell and pleomorphic lipoma: an immunohistochemical study and histogenetic analysis. J Pathol 1989; 158(3):219–22.

27. Chen BJ, Marino-Enriquez A, Fletcher CD, et al. Loss of retinoblastoma protein expression in spindle cell/pleomorphic lipomas and cytogenetically related tumors: an immunohistochemical study with diagnostic implications. Am J Surg Pathol 2012;36(8):1119–28.

28. Marino-Enriquez A, Nascimento AF, Ligon AH, et al. Atypical spindle cell lipomatous tumor: clinicopathologic characterization of 232 cases demonstrating a morphologic spectrum. Am J Surg Pathol 2017; 41(2):234–44.

29. Evans HL. Atypical lipomatous tumor, its variants, and its combined forms: a study of 61 cases, with a minimum follow-up of 10 years. Am J Surg Pathol 2007;31(1):1–14.

30. Dei Tos AP, Mentzel T, Newman PL, et al. Spindle cell liposarcoma, a hitherto unrecognized variant of liposarcoma. Analysis of six cases. Am J Surg Pathol 1994;18(9):913–21.

31. Deyrup AT, Chibon F, Guillou L, et al. Fibrosarcoma-like lipomatous neoplasm: a reappraisal of so-called spindle cell liposarcoma defining a unique lipomatous tumor unrelated to other liposarcomas. Am J Surg Pathol 2013;37(9):1373–8.

32. Creytens D, van Gorp J, Savola S, et al. Atypical spindle cell lipoma: a clinicopathologic, immunohistochemical, and molecular study emphasizing its relationship to classical spindle cell lipoma. Virchows Arch 2014;465(1):97–108.

33. Mentzel T, Palmedo G, Kuhnen C. Well-differentiated spindle cell liposarcoma ('atypical spindle cell lipomatous tumor') does not belong to the spectrum of atypical lipomatous tumor but has a close relationship to spindle cell lipoma: clinicopathologic, immunohistochemical, and molecular analysis of six cases. Mod Pathol 2010;23(5):729–36.

34. Weiss SW, Rao VK. Well-differentiated liposarcoma (atypical lipoma) of deep soft tissue of the extremities, retroperitoneum, and miscellaneous sites. A follow-up study of 92 cases with analysis of the incidence of "dedifferentiation". Am J Surg Pathol 1992;16(11):1051–8.

35. Henske EP, Neumann HP, Scheithauer BW, et al. Loss of heterozygosity in the tuberous sclerosis (TSC2) region of chromosome band 16p13 occurs in sporadic as well as TSC-associated renal angiomyolipomas. Genes Chromosomes Cancer 1995; 13(4):295–8.

36. Takeda T, Ando R, Unno R, et al. A case of spindle cell lipoma in the inguinal region. Hinyokika Kiyo 2016;62(4):205–8, [in Japanese].

37. Farrow GM, Harrison EG, Utz DC, et al. Sarcomas and sarcomatoid and mixed malignant tumors of the kidney in adults - part I. Cancer 1968;22: 545–50.

38. Kryvenko ON, Rosenberg AE, Jorda M, et al. Dedifferentiated liposarcoma of the spermatic cord: a series of 42 cases. Am J Surg Pathol 2015;39(9): 1219–25.

39. Mayes DC, Fechner RE, Gillenwater JY. Renal liposarcoma. Am J Surg Pathol 1990;14(3):268–73.

40. Montgomery E, Fisher C. Paratesticular liposarcoma: a clinicopathologic study. Am J Surg Pathol 2003;27(1):40–7.

41. Biernat W, Salska Z, Biernat S. Myxoid liposarcoma of the urinary bladder. Pol J Pathol 1996;47(1): 41–3.

42. Kobayashi Y, Nakayama M, Matsuzaki K, et al. Liposarcoma arising from the right renal sinus with inferior vena caval involvement. J Solid Tumors 2015;5:69–72.

43. Kunze E, Theuring F, Kruger G. Primary mesenchymal tumors of the urinary bladder. A histological and immunohistochemical study of 30 cases. Pathol Res Pract 1994;190(4):311–32.

44. Dei Tos AP. Liposarcomas: diagnostic pitfalls and new insights. Histopathology 2014;64(1):38–52.

45. Dei Tos AP, Pedeutour F. Atypical lipomatous tumour. In: Fletcher CDMF, Bridge JA, Hogendoorn PCW, et al, editors. WHO classification of tumours of soft tissue and bone. Lyon (France): IARC Press; 2013. p. 33–6.

46. Kraus MD, Guillou L, Fletcher CD. Well-differentiated inflammatory liposarcoma: an uncommon and easily overlooked variant of a common sarcoma. Am J Surg Pathol 1997;21(5):518–27.

47. Henricks WH, Chu YC, Goldblum JR, et al. Dedifferentiated liposarcoma: a clinicopathological analysis of 155 cases with a proposal for an expanded definition of dedifferentiation. Am J Surg Pathol 1997;21(3):271–81.

48. McCormick D, Mentzel T, Beham A, et al. Dedifferentiated liposarcoma. Clinicopathologic analysis of 32 cases suggesting a better prognostic subgroup among pleomorphic sarcomas. Am J Surg Pathol 1994;18(12):1213–23.

49. Marino-Enriquez A, Fletcher CD, Dal Cin P, et al. Dedifferentiated liposarcoma with "homologous" lipoblastic (pleomorphic liposarcoma-like) differentiation: clinicopathologic and molecular analysis of a series suggesting revised diagnostic criteria. Am J Surg Pathol 2010;34(8):1122–31.

50. Elgar F, Goldblum JR. Well-differentiated liposarcoma of the retroperitoneum: a clinicopathologic analysis of 20 cases, with particular attention to the extent of low-grade dedifferentiation. Mod Pathol 1997;10(2):113–20.

51. Val-Bernal JF, Azueta A, Ortiz-Rivas LA, et al. Incidental lipoma-like hibernoma arising from the adrenal gland: a well-differentiated liposarcoma mimicker. Pathol Res Pract 2013;209(12):812–6.

52. Furlong MA, Fanburg-Smith JC, Miettinen M. The morphologic spectrum of hibernoma: a clinicopathologic study of 170 cases. Am J Surg Pathol 2001; 25(6):809–14.

53. Choi J, Bouron Dal Soglio D, Fortier A, et al. Diagnostic utility of molecular and cytogenetic analysis in lipoblastoma: a study of two cases and review of the literature. Histopathology 2014;64(5):731–40.

54. Ferreira J, Esteves G, Fonseca R, et al. Fine-needle aspiration of lipoblastoma: cytological, molecular, and clinical features. Cancer Cytopathol 2017; 125(12):934–9.

55. Kurt H, Arnold CA, Payne JE, et al. Massive localized lymphedema: a clinicopathologic study of 46 patients with an enrichment for multiplicity. Mod Pathol 2016;29(1):75–82.

56. Lee S, Han JS, Ross HM, et al. Massive localized lymphedema of the male external genitalia: a clinicopathologic study of 6 cases. Hum Pathol 2013; 44(2):277–81.

57. Sioletic S, Dal Cin P, Fletcher CD, et al. Well-differentiated and dedifferentiated liposarcomas with prominent myxoid stroma: analysis of 56 cases. Histopathology 2013;62(2):287–93.

58. Thway K, Flora R, Shah C, et al. Diagnostic utility of p16, CDK4, and MDM2 as an immunohistochemical panel in distinguishing well-differentiated and dedifferentiated liposarcomas from other adipocytic tumors. Am J Surg Pathol 2012;36(3):462–9.

59. Wang T, Goodman MA, McGough RL, et al. Immunohistochemical analysis of expressions of RB1, CDK4, HSP90, cPLA2G4A, and CHMP2B is helpful

in distinction between myxofibrosarcoma and myxoid liposarcoma. Int J Surg Pathol 2014;22(7): 589–99.

60. Coindre JM, Mariani O, Chibon F, et al. Most malignant fibrous histiocytomas developed in the retroperitoneum are dedifferentiated liposarcomas: a review of 25 cases initially diagnosed as malignant fibrous histiocytoma. Mod Pathol 2003;16(3): 256–62.

61. Weaver J, Goldblum JR, Turner S, et al. Detection of MDM2 gene amplification or protein expression distinguishes sclerosing mesenteritis and retroperitoneal fibrosis from inflammatory well-differentiated liposarcoma. Mod Pathol 2009; 22(1):66–70.

62. Weaver J, Rao P, Goldblum JR, et al. Can MDM2 analytical tests performed on core needle biopsy be relied upon to diagnose well-differentiated liposarcoma? Mod Pathol 2010;23(10):1301–6.

63. Dickson MA, Schwartz GK, Keohan ML, et al. Progression-free survival among patients with well-differentiated or dedifferentiated liposarcoma treated with CDK4 inhibitor palbociclib: a phase 2 clinical trial. JAMA Oncol 2016;2(7):937–40.

64. Binh MB, Sastre-Garau X, Guillou L, et al. MDM2 and CDK4 immunostainings are useful adjuncts in diagnosing well-differentiated and dedifferentiated liposarcoma subtypes: a comparative analysis of 559 soft tissue neoplasms with genetic data. Am J Surg Pathol 2005;29(10):1340–7.

65. Dei Tos AP, Doglioni C, Piccinin S, et al. Coordinated expression and amplification of the MDM2, CDK4, and HMGI-C genes in atypical lipomatous tumours. J Pathol 2000;190(5):531–6.

66. Italiano A, Bianchini L, Keslair F, et al. HMGA2 is the partner of MDM2 in well-differentiated and dedifferentiated liposarcomas whereas CDK4 belongs to a distinct inconsistent amplicon. Int J Cancer 2008;122(10):2233–41.

67. He M, Aisner S, Benevenia J, et al. p16 immunohistochemistry as an alternative marker to distinguish atypical lipomatous tumor from deep-seated lipoma. Appl Immunohistochem Mol Morphol 2009; 17(1):51–6.

68. Kammerer-Jacquet SF, Thierry S, Cabillic F, et al. Differential diagnosis of atypical lipomatous tumor/well-differentiated liposarcoma and dedifferentiated liposarcoma: utility of p16 in combination with MDM2 and CDK4 immunohistochemistry. Hum Pathol 2017;59:34–40.

69. Kang Y, Horvai AE. p16 immunohistochemistry is less useful than MDM2 and CDK4 to distinguish dedifferentiated liposarcomas from other retroperitoneal mimics. Appl Immunohistochem Mol Morphol 2017;25(1):58–63.

70. Weaver J, Downs-Kelly E, Goldblum JR, et al. Fluorescence in situ hybridization for MDM2 gene

amplification as a diagnostic tool in lipomatous neoplasms. Mod Pathol 2008;21(8):943–9.

71. Singer S, Antonescu CR, Riedel E, et al. Histologic subtype and margin of resection predict pattern of recurrence and survival for retroperitoneal liposarcoma. Ann Surg 2003;238(3):358–70, [discussion: 370–1].

72. Mavrogenis AF, Lesensky J, Romagnoli C, et al. Atypical lipomatous tumors/well-differentiated liposarcomas: clinical outcome of 67 patients. Orthopedics 2011;34(12):e893–8.

73. Dantey K, Schoedel K, Yergiyev O, et al. Correlation of histological grade of dedifferentiation with clinical outcome in 55 patients with dedifferentiated liposarcomas. Hum Pathol 2017;66:86–92.

74. Harik LR, Merino C, Coindre JM, et al. Pseudosarcomatous myofibroblastic proliferations of the bladder: a clinicopathologic study of 42 cases. Am J Surg Pathol 2006;30(7):787–94.

75. Houben CH. Pseudosarcomatous myofibroblastic proliferations of the bladder: a clinicopathologic study of 42 cases. Am J Surg Pathol 2007;31(4): 642, [author reply: 642].

76. Westfall DE, Folpe AL, Paner GP, et al. Utility of a comprehensive immunohistochemical panel in the differential diagnosis of spindle cell lesions of the urinary bladder. Am J Surg Pathol 2009;33(1): 99–105.

77. Coffin CM, Watterson J, Priest JR, et al. Extrapulmonary inflammatory myofibroblastic tumor (inflammatory pseudotumor). A clinicopathologic and immunohistochemical study of 84 cases. Am J Surg Pathol 1995;19(8):859–72.

78. Meis JM, Enzinger FM. Inflammatory fibrosarcoma of the mesentery and retroperitoneum. A tumor closely simulating inflammatory pseudotumor. Am J Surg Pathol 1991;15(12):1146–56.

79. Ramachandra S, Hollowood K, Bisceglia M, et al. Inflammatory pseudotumour of soft tissues: a clinicopathological and immunohistochemical analysis of 18 cases. Histopathology 1995;27(4):313–23.

80. Coffin CM, Fletcher CD. Inflammatory myofibroblastic tumour. In: Fletcher CD, Bridge JA, Hogendoorn PCW, et al, editors. WHO classification of tumours of soft tissue and bone. Lyon (France): International Agency for Research on Cancer (IARC); 2013. p. 83–4.

81. Hojo H, Newton WA Jr, Hamoudi AB, et al. Pseudosarcomatous myofibroblastic tumor of the urinary bladder in children: a study of 11 cases with review of the literature. An intergroup rhabdomyosarcoma study. Am J Surg Pathol 1995;19(11):1224–36.

82. Horn LC, Reuter S, Biesold M. Inflammatory pseudotumor of the ureter and the urinary bladder. Pathol Res Pract 1997;193(9):607–12.

83. Jones EC, Clement PB, Young RH. Inflammatory pseudotumor of the urinary bladder. A

clinicopathological, immunohistochemical, ultra-structural, and flow cytometric study of 13 cases. Am J Surg Pathol 1993;17(3):264–74.

84. Kapusta LR, Weiss MA, Ramsay J, et al. Inflammatory myofibroblastic tumors of the kidney: a clinicopathologic and immunohistochemical study of 12 cases. Am J Surg Pathol 2003;27(5):658–66.

85. Antonescu CR, Suurmeijer AJ, Zhang L, et al. Molecular characterization of inflammatory myofibroblastic tumors with frequent ALK and ROS1 gene fusions and rare novel RET rearrangement. Am J Surg Pathol 2015;39(7):957–67.

86. Lovly CM, Gupta A, Lipson D, et al. Inflammatory myofibroblastic tumors harbor multiple potentially actionable kinase fusions. Cancer Discov 2014; 4(8):889–95.

87. Taheri D, Zahavi DJ, Del Carmen Rodriguez M, et al. For staining of ALK protein, the novel D5F3 antibody demonstrates superior overall performance in terms of intensity and extent of staining in comparison to the currently used ALK1 antibody. Virchows Arch 2016;469(3):345–50.

88. Butrynski JE, D'Adamo DR, Hornick JL, et al. Crizotinib in ALK-rearranged inflammatory myofibroblastic tumor. N Engl J Med 2010;363(18):1727–33.

89. Gambacorti-Passerini C, Orlov S, Zhang L, et al. Long-term effects of crizotinib in ALK-positive tumors (excluding NSCLC): a phase 1b open-label study. Am J Hematol 2018;93(5):607–14.

90. Mosse YP, Voss SD, Lim MS, et al. Targeting ALK with crizotinib in pediatric anaplastic large cell lymphoma and inflammatory myofibroblastic tumor: a children's oncology group study. J Clin Oncol 2017;35(28):3215–21.

91. Alassiri AH, Ali RH, Shen Y, et al. ETV6-NTRK3 is expressed in a subset of ALK-negative inflammatory myofibroblastic tumors. Am J Surg Pathol 2016;40(8):1051–61.

92. Hornick JL, Sholl LM, Dal Cin P, et al. Expression of ROS1 predicts ROS1 gene rearrangement in inflammatory myofibroblastic tumors. Mod Pathol 2015;28(5):732–9.

93. Yamamoto H, Yoshida A, Taguchi K, et al. ALK, ROS1 and NTRK3 gene rearrangements in inflammatory myofibroblastic tumours. Histopathology 2016;69(1):72–83.

94. Erickson-Johnson MR, Chou MM, Evers BR, et al. Nodular fasciitis: a novel model of transient neoplasia induced by MYH9-USP6 gene fusion. Lab Invest 2011;91(10):1427–33.

95. Montgomery EA, Shuster DD, Burkart AL, et al. Inflammatory myofibroblastic tumors of the urinary tract: a clinicopathologic study of 46 cases, including a malignant example inflammatory fibrosarcoma and a subset associated with high-grade urothelial carcinoma. Am J Surg Pathol 2006;30(12):1502–12.

96. Alkan A, Toprak S, Köksoy EB. A paratesticular inflammatory myofibroblastic tumor and review of the literature. J Oncol Sci 2017;3:135–6.

97. Kocer NE, Bal N, Gul U, et al. Inflammatory myofibroblastic tumor of the prostate. Journal of Clinical and Analytical Medicine 2016;7:124–6.

98. Kumar G, Venkateswarly M, Reddy M, et al. Inflammatory myofibroblastic tumor of proximal urethra in a pregnant female: a unique case report. J Case Rep Stud 2016;4:1–5.

99. Amin MB, Trpkov K, Lopez-Beltran A, et al. Members of the IIiDUPG. Best practices recommendations in the application of immunohistochemistry in the bladder lesions: report from the International Society of Urologic Pathology consensus conference. Am J Surg Pathol 2014; 38(8):e20–34.

100. Hollowood K, Fletcher CD. Pseudosarcomatous myofibroblastic proliferations of the spermatic cord ("proliferative funiculitis"). Histologic and immunohistochemical analysis of a distinctive entity. Am J Surg Pathol 1992;16(5):448–54.

101. Montgomery E, Torbenson MS, Kaushal M, et al. Beta-catenin immunohistochemistry separates mesenteric fibromatosis from gastrointestinal stromal tumor and sclerosing mesenteritis. Am J Surg Pathol 2002;26(10):1296–301.

102. Oliveira AM, Perez-Atayde AR, Dal Cin P, et al. Aneurysmal bone cyst variant translocations upregulate USP6 transcription by promoter swapping with the ZNF9, COL1A1, TRAP150, and OMD genes. Oncogene 2005;24(21):3419–26.

103. Jebastin JA, Gupta NS, Carskadon S, et al. Pseudosarcomatous myofibroblastic proliferations of the urinary bladder lack the USP6 gene rearrangement common in nodular fasciitis. Mod Pathol 2017;30:233A.

104. Gleason BC, Hornick JL. Inflammatory myofibroblastic tumours: where are we now? J Clin Pathol 2008;61(4):428–37.

105. Coffin CM, Hornick JL, Fletcher CD. Inflammatory myofibroblastic tumor: comparison of clinicopathologic, histologic, and immunohistochemical features including ALK expression in atypical and aggressive cases. Am J Surg Pathol 2007;31(4): 509–20.

106. Spiess PE, Tuziak T, Tibbs RF, et al. Pseudosarcomatous and sarcomatous proliferations of the bladder. Hum Pathol 2007;38(5):753–61.

107. Fletcher CDM, Unni KK, Mertens F, editors. Pathology and genetics of tumours of soft tissue and bone. 3rd edition. Lyon (France): International Agency for Research on Cancer (IARC); 2002.

108. Chmielecki J, Crago AM, Rosenberg M, et al. Whole-exome sequencing identifies a recurrent NAB2-STAT6 fusion in solitary fibrous tumors. Nat Genet 2013;45(2):131–2.

109. Mohajeri A, Tayebwa J, Collin A, et al. Comprehensive genetic analysis identifies a pathognomonic NAB2/STAT6 fusion gene, nonrandom secondary genomic imbalances, and a characteristic gene expression profile in solitary fibrous tumor. Genes Chromosomes Cancer 2013;52(10):873–86.

110. Robinson DR, Wu YM, Kalyana-Sundaram S, et al. Identification of recurrent NAB2-STAT6 gene fusions in solitary fibrous tumor by integrative sequencing. Nat Genet 2013;45(2):180–5.

111. Stout AP. Tumors featuring pericytes; glomus tumor and hemangiopericytoma. Lab Invest 1956;5(2): 217–23.

112. Stout AP. Hemangiopericytoma; a study of 25 cases. Cancer 1949;2(6):1027–54, illust.

113. Stout AP, Murray MR. Hemangiopericytoma: a vascular tumor featuring Zimmermann's pericytes. Ann Surg 1942;116(1):26–33.

114. Klemperer P, Rabin CB. Primary neoplasm of the pleura: a report of five cases. Arch Pathol 1931; 11:385–412.

115. Flint A, Weiss SW. CD-34 and keratin expression distinguishes solitary fibrous tumor (fibrous mesothelioma) of pleura from desmoplastic mesothelioma. Hum Pathol 1995;26(4):428–31.

116. de Saint Aubain Somerhausen N, Rubin BP, Fletcher CD. Myxoid solitary fibrous tumor: a study of seven cases with emphasis on differential diagnosis. Mod Pathol 1999;12(5):463–71.

117. Mosquera JM, Fletcher CD. Expanding the spectrum of malignant progression in solitary fibrous tumors: a study of 8 cases with a discrete anaplastic component–is this dedifferentiated SFT? Am J Surg Pathol 2009;33(9):1314–21.

118. Wetzel WJ. Solitary fibrous tumor. Hum Pathol 1996;27(5):513–4.

119. Nielsen GP, Dickersin GR, Provenzal JM, et al. Lipomatous hemangiopericytoma. A histologic, ultrastructural and immunohistochemical study of a unique variant of hemangiopericytoma. Am J Surg Pathol 1995;19(7):748–56.

120. Lee JC, Fletcher CD. Malignant fat-forming solitary fibrous tumor (so-called "lipomatous hemangiopericytoma"): clinicopathologic analysis of 14 cases. Am J Surg Pathol 2011;35(8):1177–85.

121. Guillou L, Gebhard S, Coindre JM. Lipomatous hemangiopericytoma: a fat-containing variant of solitary fibrous tumor? Clinicopathologic, immunohistochemical, and ultrastructural analysis of a series in favor of a unifying concept. Hum Pathol 2000;31(9):1108–15.

122. Dantey K, Cooper K. Myxoid solitary fibrous tumor: a study of three cases. Int J Surg Pathol 2013; 21(4):358–62.

123. Nielsen GP, O'Connell JX, Dickersin GR, et al. Solitary fibrous tumor of soft tissue: a report of 15 cases, including 5 malignant examples with light microscopic, immunohistochemical, and ultrastructural data. Mod Pathol 1997;10(10):1028–37.

124. Subramaniam MM, Lim XY, Venkateswaran K, et al. Dedifferentiated solitary fibrous tumour of the nasal cavity: the first case reported with molecular characterization of a TP53 mutation. Histopathology 2011;59(6):1269–74.

125. Thway K, Hayes A, Ieremia E, et al. Heterologous osteosarcomatous and rhabdomyosarcomatous elements in dedifferentiated solitary fibrous tumor: further support for the concept of dedifferentiation in solitary fibrous tumor. Ann Diagn Pathol 2013; 17(5):457–63.

126. Fletcher CD, Bridge JA, Lee JC. Extrapleural solitary fibrous tumour. In: Fletcher CD, Bridge JA, Hogendoorn PCW, et al, editors. WHO classification of tumours of soft tissue and bone. 4th edition. Lyon (France): International Agency for Research on Cancer (IARC); 2013. p. 80–2.

127. Herawi M, Epstein JI. Solitary fibrous tumor on needle biopsy and transurethral resection of the prostate: a clinicopathologic study of 13 cases. Am J Surg Pathol 2007;31(6):870–6.

128. Chen Y, Wang F, Han A. Fat-forming solitary fibrous tumor of the kidney: a case report and literature review. Int J Clin Exp Pathol 2015;8(7):8632–5.

129. Ichiyanagi O, Ito H, Takai S, et al. A GRIA2 and PAX8-positive renal solitary fibrous tumor with NAB2-STAT6 gene fusion. Diagn Pathol 2015;10:155.

130. Castellani D, Sebastiani G, Maurelli S, et al. Solitary fibrous tumor/hemangiopericytoma of the penis: report of the first case. Urologia 2015;82(2):127–9.

131. Bainbridge TC, Singh RR, Mentzel T, et al. Solitary fibrous tumor of urinary bladder: report of two cases. Hum Pathol 1997;28(10):1204–6.

132. Mustafa HJ, Menon S. Solitary fibrous tumor in a female urinary bladder. Urol Case Rep 2016;7: 1–2.

133. Rekhi B, Bapat P, Shetty O. A rare case of a vaginal solitary fibrous tumor, presenting as a cystic mass, showing NAB2ex4-STAT6ex2 fusion and STAT6 immunostaining. Int J Gynecol Pathol 2017;1.

134. Tardio JC, Machado I, Alemany I, et al. Solitary fibrous tumor of the vulva: report of 2 cases, including a de novo dedifferentiated solitary fibrous tumor diagnosed after molecular demonstration of NAB2-STAT6 gene fusion. Int J Gynecol Pathol 2017;1.

135. Wang J, Arber DA, Frankel K, et al. Large solitary fibrous tumor of the kidney: report of two cases and review of the literature. Am J Surg Pathol 2001;25(9):1194–9.

136. Balduyck B, Lauwers P, Govaert K, et al. Solitary fibrous tumor of the pleura with associated hypoglycemia: Doege-Potter syndrome: a case report. J Thorac Oncol 2006;1(6):588–90.

137. Steigen SE, Schaeffer DF, West RB, et al. Expression of insulin-like growth factor 2 in mesenchymal neoplasms. Mod Pathol 2009;22(7):914–21.

138. Zafar H, Takimoto CH, Weiss G. Doege-Potter syndrome: hypoglycemia associated with malignant solitary fibrous tumor. Med Oncol 2003;20(4):403–8.

139. Hasegawa T, Matsuno Y, Shimoda T, et al. Extrathoracic solitary fibrous tumors: their histological variability and potentially aggressive behavior. Hum Pathol 1999;30(12):1464–73.

140. Vallat-Decouvelaere AV, Dry SM, Fletcher CD. Atypical and malignant solitary fibrous tumors in extrathoracic locations: evidence of their comparability to intra-thoracic tumors. Am J Surg Pathol 1998;22(12):1501–11.

141. Smith SC, Gooding WE, Elkins M, et al. Solitary fibrous tumors of the head and neck: a multi-institutional clinicopathologic study. Am J Surg Pathol 2017;41(12):1642–56.

142. Demicco EG, Park MS, Araujo DM, et al. Solitary fibrous tumor: a clinicopathological study of 110 cases and proposed risk assessment model. Mod Pathol 2012;25(9):1298–306.

143. Westra WH, Grenko RT, Epstein J. Solitary fibrous tumor of the lower urogenital tract: a report of five cases involving the seminal vesicles, urinary bladder, and prostate. Hum Pathol 2000;31(1):63–8.

144. Gold JS, Antonescu CR, Hajdu C, et al. Clinicopathologic correlates of solitary fibrous tumors. Cancer 2002;94(4):1057–68.

145. Feasel P, Al-Ibraheemi A, Fritchie K, et al. Superficial solitary fibrous tumor: a series of 26 cases. Am J Surg Pathol 2018;42(6):778–85.

146. Karanian M, Perot G, Coindre JM, et al. Fluorescence in situ hybridization analysis is a helpful test for the diagnosis of dermatofibrosarcoma protuberans. Mod Pathol 2015;28(2):230–7.

147. McDaniel AS, Palanisamy N, Smith SC, et al. A subset of solitary fibrous tumors express nuclear PAX8 and PAX2: a potential diagnostic pitfall. Histol Histopathol 2016;31(2):223–30.

148. Ng TL, Gown AM, Barry TS, et al. Nuclear beta-catenin in mesenchymal tumors. Mod Pathol 2005;18(1):68–74.

149. Gibas Z, Miettinen M, Limon J, et al. Cytogenetic and immunohistochemical profile of myxoid liposarcoma. Am J Clin Pathol 1995;103(1):20–6.

150. Vivero M, Doyle LA, Fletcher CD, et al. GRIA2 is a novel diagnostic marker for solitary fibrous tumour identified through gene expression profiling. Histopathology 2014;65(1):71–80.

151. Doyle LA, Vivero M, Fletcher CD, et al. Nuclear expression of STAT6 distinguishes solitary fibrous tumor from histologic mimics. Mod Pathol 2014;27(3):390–5.

152. Koelsche C, Schweizer L, Renner M, et al. Nuclear relocation of STAT6 reliably predicts NAB2-STAT6 fusion for the diagnosis of solitary fibrous tumour. Histopathology 2014;65(5):613–22.

153. Demicco EG, Harms PW, Patel RM, et al. Extensive survey of STAT6 expression in a large series of mesenchymal tumors. Am J Clin Pathol 2015;143(5):672–82.

154. Doyle LA, Tao D, Marino-Enriquez A. STAT6 is amplified in a subset of dedifferentiated liposarcoma. Mod Pathol 2014;27(9):1231–7.

155. Guner G, Bishop JA, Bezerra SM, et al. The utility of STAT6 and ALDH1 expression in the differential diagnosis of solitary fibrous tumor versus prostate-specific stromal neoplasms. Hum Pathol 2016;54:184–8.

156. Enzinger FM, Smith BH. Hemangiopericytoma. An analysis of 106 cases. Hum Pathol 1976;7(1):61–82.

157. Demicco EG, Wagner MJ, Maki RG, et al. Risk assessment in solitary fibrous tumors: validation and refinement of a risk stratification model. Mod Pathol 2017;30(10):1433–42.

158. Thway K, Fisher C. PEComa: morphology and genetics of a complex tumor family. Ann Diagn Pathol 2015;19(5):359–68.

159. Mochel MC, Smith SC. Kidney tumors associated with hereditary cancer syndromes: an emerging opportunity and responsibility in surgical pathology. AJSP: Reviews & Reports 2017;22(6):313–28.

160. Martignoni G, Pea M, Zampini C, et al. PEComas of the kidney and of the genitourinary tract. Semin Diagn Pathol 2015;32(2):140–59.

161. Argani P, Aulmann S, Illei PB, et al. A distinctive subset of PEComas harbors TFE3 gene fusions. Am J Surg Pathol 2010;34(10):1395–406.

162. Agaram NP, Sung YS, Zhang L, et al. Dichotomy of genetic abnormalities in PEComas with therapeutic implications. Am J Surg Pathol 2015;39(6):813–25.

163. Rao Q, Shen Q, Xia QY, et al. PSF/SFPQ is a very common gene fusion partner in TFE3 rearrangement-associated perivascular epithelioid cell tumors (PEComas) and melanotic Xp11 translocation renal cancers: clinicopathologic, immunohistochemical, and molecular characteristics suggesting classification as a distinct entity. Am J Surg Pathol 2015;39(9):1181–96.

164. Chan AW, Chan CK, Chiu Y, et al. Primary perivascular epithelioid cell tumour (PEComa) of the urinary bladder. Pathology 2011;43(7):746–9.

165. Huang Y, Lu G, Quan J, et al. Primary perivascular epithelioid cell tumor of the bladder. Ann Diagn Pathol 2011;15(6):427–30.

166. Kalyanasundaram K, Parameswaran A, Mani R. Perivascular epithelioid tumor of urinary bladder and vagina. Ann Diagn Pathol 2005;9(5):275–8.

167. Pan CC, Yu IT, Yang AH, et al. Clear cell myomelanocytic tumor of the urinary bladder. Am J Surg Pathol 2003;27(5):689–92.
168. Parfitt JR, Bella AJ, Wehrli BM, et al. Primary PEComa of the bladder treated with primary excision and adjuvant interferon-alpha immunotherapy: a case report. BMC Urol 2006;6:20.
169. Sukov WR, Cheville JC, Amin MB, et al. Perivascular epithelioid cell tumor (PEComa) of the urinary bladder: report of 3 cases and review of the literature. Am J Surg Pathol 2009;33(2):304–8.
170. Weinreb I, Howarth D, Latta E, et al. Perivascular epithelioid cell neoplasms (PEComas): four malignant cases expanding the histopathological spectrum and a description of a unique finding. Virchows Arch 2007;450(4):463–70.
171. Yin L, Bu H, Chen M, et al. Perivascular epithelioid cell neoplasm of the urinary bladder in an adolescent: a case report and review of the literature. Diagn Pathol 2012;7:183.
172. De Dominicis G, Boscaino A, Marsilia GM, et al. Clear cell "sugar" tumors of urethra: a previously undescribed occurrence and review of published data. Urology 2009;74(3):542–3.
173. Lane TM, Masood J, Shah N, et al. Angiomyolipoma of the testis. J Urol 2004;171(2 Pt 1):794.
174. Pan CC, Yang AH, Chiang H. Malignant perivascular epithelioid cell tumor involving the prostate. Arch Pathol Lab Med 2003;127(2):E96–8.
175. Argani P, Zhong M, Reuter VE, et al. TFE3-fusion variant analysis defines specific clinicopathologic associations among Xp11 translocation cancers. Am J Surg Pathol 2016;40(6):723–37.
176. Williamson SR, Bunde PJ, Montironi R, et al. Malignant perivascular epithelioid cell neoplasm (PEComa) of the urinary bladder with TFE3 gene rearrangement: clinicopathologic, immunohistochemical, and molecular features. Am J Surg Pathol 2013;37(10):1619–26.
177. Russell CM, Buethe DD, Dickinson S, et al. Perivascular epithelioid cell tumor (PEComa) of the urinary bladder associated with Xp11 translocation. Ann Clin Lab Sci 2014;44(1):91–8.
178. Chen XF, Yeong J, Chang KTE, et al. TFE3-expressing epithelioid rich perivascular epithelioid cell neoplasm (PEComa) of the bladder with unusual benign course. Ann Clin Lab Sci 2018;48(1):110–5.
179. Wang XT, Xia QY, Ni H, et al. Xp11 neoplasm with melanocytic differentiation of the prostate harbouring the novel NONO-TFE3 gene fusion: report of a unique case expanding the gene fusion spectrum. Histopathology 2016;69(3):450–8.
180. Seyam RM, Bissada NK, Kattan SA, et al. Changing trends in presentation, diagnosis and management of renal angiomyolipoma: comparison of sporadic and tuberous sclerosis complex-associated forms. Urology 2008;72(5):1077–82.
181. Sooriakumaran P, Gibbs P, Coughlin G, et al. Angiomyolipomata: challenges, solutions, and future prospects based on over 100 cases treated. BJU Int 2010;105(1):101–6.
182. Aydin H, Magi-Galluzzi C, Lane BR, et al. Renal angiomyolipoma: clinicopathologic study of 194 cases with emphasis on the epithelioid histology and tuberous sclerosis association. Am J Surg Pathol 2009;33(2):289–97.
183. Davis CJ, Barton JH, Sesterhenn IA. Cystic angiomyolipoma of the kidney: a clinicopathologic description of 11 cases. Mod Pathol 2006;19(5):669–74.
184. Fine SW, Reuter VE, Epstein JI, et al. Angiomyolipoma with epithelial cysts (AMLEC): a distinct cystic variant of angiomyolipoma. Am J Surg Pathol 2006;30(5):593–9.
185. Agaimy A. The expanding family of SMARCB1(INI1)-deficient neoplasia: implications of phenotypic, biological, and molecular heterogeneity. Adv Anat Pathol 2014;21(6):394–410.
186. Brimo F, Robinson B, Guo C, et al. Renal epithelioid angiomyolipoma with atypia: a series of 40 cases with emphasis on clinicopathologic prognostic indicators of malignancy. Am J Surg Pathol 2010;34(5):715–22.
187. Nese N, Martignoni G, Fletcher CD, et al. Pure epithelioid PEComas (so-called epithelioid angiomyolipoma) of the kidney: a clinicopathologic study of 41 cases: detailed assessment of morphology and risk stratification. Am J Surg Pathol 2011;35(2):161–76.
188. He W, Cheville JC, Sadow PM, et al. Epithelioid angiomyolipoma of the kidney: pathological features and clinical outcome in a series of consecutively resected tumors. Mod Pathol 2013;26(10):1355–64.
189. Maloney N, Giannikou K, Lefferts J, et al. Expanding the histomorphologic spectrum of TFE3 rearranged PEComas. Hum Pathol 2018.
190. Hornick JL, Pan CC. PEComa. In: Fletcher CD, Bridge JA, Hogendoorn PCW, et al, editors. WHO classification of tumours of soft tissue and bone. 4th edition. Lyon (France): International Agency for Research on Cancer (IARC); 2013. p. 230–1.
191. Martignoni G, Pea M, Reghellin D, et al. Molecular pathology of lymphangioleiomyomatosis and other perivascular epithelioid cell tumors. Arch Pathol Lab Med 2010;134(1):33–40.
192. Asch-Kendrick RJ, Shetty S, Goldblum JR, et al. A subset of fat-predominant angiomyolipomas label for MDM2: a potential diagnostic pitfall. Hum Pathol 2016;57:7–12.
193. Lin X, Laskin WB, Lu X, et al. Expression of MDM2 and p16 in angiomyolipoma. Hum Pathol 2018;75:34–40.

194. Guo J, Tretiakova MS, Troxell ML, et al. Tuberous sclerosis-associated renal cell carcinoma: a clinicopathologic study of 57 separate carcinomas in 18 patients. Am J Surg Pathol 2014;38(11): 1457–67.

195. Calio A, Brunelli M, Segala D, et al. t(6;11) renal cell carcinoma: a study of seven cases including two with aggressive behavior, and utility of CD68 (PG-M1) in the differential diagnosis with pure epithelioid PEComa/epithelioid angiomyolipoma. Mod Pathol 2018;31(3):474–87.

196. Smith NE, Illei PB, Allaf M, et al. t(6;11) renal cell carcinoma (RCC): expanded immunohistochemical profile emphasizing novel RCC markers and report of 10 new genetically confirmed cases. Am J Surg Pathol 2014;38(5):604–14.

197. Zarineh A, Silverman JF. Adrenal perivascular epithelioid cell tumor: a case report with discussion of differential diagnoses. Arch Pathol Lab Med 2011;135(4):499–502.

198. Duregon E, Volante M, Giorcelli J, et al. Diagnostic and prognostic role of steroidogenic factor 1 in adrenocortical carcinoma: a validation study focusing on clinical and pathologic correlates. Hum Pathol 2013;44(5):822–8.

199. Miettinen M, McCue PA, Sarlomo-Rikala M, et al. Sox10–a marker for not only schwannian and melanocytic neoplasms but also myoepithelial cell tumors of soft tissue: a systematic analysis of 5134 tumors. Am J Surg Pathol 2015;39(6):826–35.

200. Simpson KW, Albores-Saavedra J. HMB-45 reactivity in conventional uterine leiomyosarcomas. Am J Surg Pathol 2007;31(1):95–8.

201. Bonsib SM. HMB-45 reactivity in renal leiomyomas and leiomyosarcomas. Mod Pathol 1996;9(6): 664–9.

202. Zheng G, Martignoni G, Antonescu C, et al. A broad survey of cathepsin K immunoreactivity in human neoplasms. Am J Clin Pathol 2013; 139(2):151–9.

203. Folpe AL, Mentzel T, Lehr HA, et al. Perivascular epithelioid cell neoplasms of soft tissue and gynecologic origin: a clinicopathologic study of 26 cases and review of the literature. Am J Surg Pathol 2005;29(12):1558–75.

204. Jungbluth AA, King R, Fisher DE, et al. Immunohistochemical and reverse transcription-polymerase chain reaction expression analysis of tyrosinase and microphthalmia-associated transcription factor in angiomyolipomas. Appl Immunohistochem Mol Morphol 2001;9(1):29–34.

205. Makhlouf HR, Ishak KG, Shekar R, et al. Melanoma markers in angiomyolipoma of the liver and kidney: a comparative study. Arch Pathol Lab Med 2002; 126(1):49–55.

206. Pea M, Bonetti F, Zamboni G, et al. Melanocyte-marker-HMB-45 is regularly expressed in angiomyolipoma of the kidney. Pathology 1991; 23(3):185–8.

207. Zavala-Pompa A, Folpe AL, Jimenez RE, et al. Immunohistochemical study of microphthalmia transcription factor and tyrosinase in angiomyolipoma of the kidney, renal cell carcinoma, and renal and retroperitoneal sarcomas: comparative evaluation with traditional diagnostic markers. Am J Surg Pathol 2001;25(1):65–70.

208. Martignoni G, Bonetti F, Chilosi M, et al. Cathepsin K expression in the spectrum of perivascular epithelioid cell (PEC) lesions of the kidney. Mod Pathol 2012;25(1):100–11.

209. Flum AS, Hamoui N, Said MA, et al. Update on the diagnosis and management of renal angiomyolipoma. J Urol 2016;195(4 Pt 1):834–46.

210. Brakemeier S, Bachmann F, Budde K. Treatment of renal angiomyolipoma in tuberous sclerosis complex (TSC) patients. Pediatr Nephrol 2017;32(7):1137–44.

211. Gennatas C, Michalaki V, Kairi PV, et al. Successful treatment with the mTOR inhibitor everolimus in a patient with perivascular epithelioid cell tumor. World J Surg Oncol 2012;10:181.

212. Pleniceanu O, Shukrun R, Omer D, et al. Peroxisome proliferator-activated receptor gamma (PPARgamma) is central to the initiation and propagation of human angiomyolipoma, suggesting its potential as a therapeutic target. EMBO Mol Med 2017;9(4):508–30.

213. Folpe AL, Brems H, Legius E. Glomus tumours. In: Fletcher CD, Bridge JA, Hogendoorn PCW, et al, editors. WHO classification of tumours of soft tissue and bone. 4th edition. Lyon (France): International Agency for Research on Cancer (IARC); 2013. p. 116–7.

214. Hisaoka M, Quade BJ. Angioleiomyoma. In: Fletcher CD, Bridge JA, Hogendoorn PCW, et al, editors. WHO classification of tumours of soft tissue and bone. 4th edition. Lyon (France): International Agency for Research on Cancer (IARC); 2013. p. 120–1.

215. Mentzel T, Bridge JA. Myopericytoma, including myofibroma. In: Fletcher CD, Bridge JA, Hogendoorn PCW, et al, editors. WHO classification of tumours of soft tissue and bone. 4th edition. Lyon (France): International Agency for Research on Cancer (IARC); 2013. p. 118–20.

216. Granter SR, Badizadegan K, Fletcher CD. Myofibromatosis in adults, glomangiopericytoma, and myopericytoma: a spectrum of tumors showing perivascular myoid differentiation. Am J Surg Pathol 1998;22(5):513–25.

217. Jo VY, Fletcher CD. WHO classification of soft tissue tumours: an update based on the 2013 (4th) edition. Pathology 2014;46(2):95–104.

218. Al-Ahmadie HA, Yilmaz A, Olgac S, et al. Glomus tumor of the kidney: a report of 3 cases involving

renal parenchyma and review of the literature. Am J Surg Pathol 2007;31(4):585–91.

219. Billard F, Dumollard JM, Cucherousset J, et al. Two benign vascular tumors of the kidney capsule. Ann Pathol 1991;11(4):266–70, [in French].

220. Gravet C, Roquet L, Rioux-Leclercq N, et al. Glomus tumor of kidney: unusual location of a rare mesenchymal tumor. Ann Pathol 2015;35(5): 440–4, [in French].

221. Herawi M, Parwani AV, Edlow D, et al. Glomus tumor of renal pelvis: a case report and review of the literature. Hum Pathol 2005;36(3):299–302.

222. Lamba G, Rafiyath SM, Kaur H, et al. Malignant glomus tumor of kidney: the first reported case and review of literature. Hum Pathol 2011;42(8): 1200–3.

223. Nuwayhid Z, Rodriguez MM, Prescott A, et al. Renal glomus tumor in an adolescent: a conservative approach. J Pediatr Surg 2010;45(6):e23–6.

224. Onishi T, Kato M, Hoshina A. Glomus tumor of the hypoplastic kidney. Int J Urol 2010;17(7):677–8.

225. Sasaki K, Bastacky SI, Hrebinko RL, et al. Glomus tumor of the kidney: case report and literature review. Int J Surg Pathol 2011;19(3):393–7.

226. Schwarz R. A case of renal glomus tumor. Zentralbl Chir 1957;82(35):1516–20, [in German].

227. Siddiqui NH, Rogalska A, Basil IS. Glomangiomyoma (glomus tumor) of the kidney. Arch Pathol Lab Med 2005;129(9):1172–4.

228. Sirohi D, Smith SC, Epstein JI, et al. Pericytic tumors of the kidney—a clinicopathologic analysis of 17 cases. Hum Pathol 2017;64:106–17.

229. Sugimoto K, Yamamoto Y, Hashimoto K, et al. Glomus tumor of the kidney. Int J Urol 2010;17(2): 187–8.

230. Dhingra S, Ayala A, Chai H, et al. Renal myopericytoma: case report and review of literature. Arch Pathol Lab Med 2012;136(5):563–6.

231. Lau SK, Klein R, Jiang Z, et al. Myopericytoma of the kidney. Hum Pathol 2010;41(10):1500–4.

232. Li J, Zhao M, Chen Z, et al. Renal myopericytoma: a clinicopathologic study of six cases and review of the literature. Int J Clin Exp Pathol 2015;8(5):4307–20.

233. Zhang Z, Yu D, Shi H, et al. Renal myopericytoma: a case report with a literature review. Oncol Lett 2014;7(1):285–7.

234. Zhao M, Williamson SR, Sun K, et al. Benign perivascular myoid cell tumor (myopericytoma) of the urinary tract: a report of 2 cases with an emphasis on differential diagnosis. Hum Pathol 2014;45(5):1115–21.

235. Huang Y, Xiong Z. Angioleiomyoma of the kidney parenchyma. Indian J Pathol Microbiol 2013; 56(3):318–9.

236. Kunimatsu N, Kunimatsu A, Kojima K, et al. A case of renal angioleiomyoma with rapid growing: CT findings with histopathological correlation. Radiat Med 2004;22(6):437–41.

237. Vogel J, Harder T, Weissbach L. Aneurysmal hemorrhage of the kidney caused by angioleiomyoma. Eur Urol 1986;12(6):438–40.

238. Park DS, Cho TW, Kang H. Glomus tumor of the glans penis. Urology 2004;64(5):1031.

239. Dagur G, Warren K, Miao Y, et al. Unusual glomus tumor of the penis. Curr Urol 2016;9(3):113–8.

240. Rodriguez D, Cornejo KM, Sadow PM, et al. Myopericytoma tumor of the glans penis. Can J Urol 2015;22(3):7830–3.

241. Val-Bernal JF, Garijo MF. Solitary cutaneous myofibroma of the glans penis. Am J Dermatopathol 1996;18(3):317–21.

242. Rao MV, Polcari I, Barkan GA, et al. Penile myofibroma occurring in a dorsal hood prepuce. Urology 2011;77(3):726–7.

243. Tripodi SA, Rocca BJ, Mourmouras V, et al. Benign glomus tumor of the urinary bladder. Arch Pathol Lab Med 2013;137(7):1005–8.

244. Shim HS, Choi YD, Cho NH. Malignant glomus tumor of the urinary bladder. Arch Pathol Lab Med 2005;129(7):940–2.

245. Pensabene M, Siracusa F, Rodolico V, et al. Solitary myofibroma of the bladder trigone in a 3-month-old patient: first case report. Case Rep Pediatr 2016; 2016:1951840.

246. Nagai T, Kamimura T, Itou K, et al. Myopericytoma in urinary bladder: a case report. J Med Case Rep 2017;11(1):46.

247. Mentzel T, Dei Tos AP, Sapi Z, et al. Myopericytoma of skin and soft tissues: clinicopathologic and immunohistochemical study of 54 cases. Am J Surg Pathol 2006;30(1):104–13.

248. Matsuyama A, Hisaoka M, Hashimoto H. Angioleiomyoma: a clinicopathologic and immunohistochemical reappraisal with special reference to the correlation with myopericytoma. Hum Pathol 2007;38(4):645–51.

249. Kuroda N, Gotoda H, Ohe C, et al. Review of juxtaglomerular cell tumor with focus on pathobiological aspect. Diagn Pathol 2011;6:80.

250. Endoh Y, Motoyama T, Hayami S, et al. Juxtaglomerular cell tumor of the kidney: report of a non-functioning variant. Pathol Int 1997;47(6): 393–6.

251. Kuroda N, Maris S, Monzon FA, et al. Juxtaglomerular cell tumor: a morphological, immunohistochemical and genetic study of six cases. Hum Pathol 2013;44(1):47–54.

252. Kryvenko ON, Haley SL, Smith SC, et al. Haemangiomas in kidneys with end-stage renal disease: a novel clinicopathological association. Histopathology 2014;65(3):309–18.

253. Montgomery E, Epstein JI. Anastomosing hemangioma of the genitourinary tract: a lesion mimicking angiosarcoma. Am J Surg Pathol 2009;33(9): 1364–9.

254. John I, Folpe AL. Anastomosing hemangiomas arising in unusual locations: a clinicopathologic study of 17 soft tissue cases showing a predilection for the paraspinal region. Am J Surg Pathol 2016;40(8):1084–9.

255. Patil PA, McKenney JK, Trpkov K, et al. Renal leiomyoma: a contemporary multi-institution study of an infrequent and frequently misclassified neoplasm. Am J Surg Pathol 2015;39(3):349–56.

256. Shen J, Shrestha S, Yen YH, et al. The pericyte antigen RGS5 in perivascular soft tissue tumors. Hum Pathol 2016;47(1):121–31.

257. Shen J, Shrestha S, Yen YH, et al. Pericyte antigens in perivascular soft tissue tumors. Int J Surg Pathol 2015;23(8):638–48.

258. Meguro S, Akamatsu T, Matsushima S, et al. Phenotypic characterization of perivascular myoid cell neoplasms, using myosin 1B, a newly identified human pericyte marker. Hum Pathol 2017;62: 187–98.

259. Kumar MG, Emnett RJ, Bayliss SJ, et al. Glomus tumors in individuals with neurofibromatosis type 1. J Am Acad Dermatol 2014;71(1):44–8.

260. Folpe AL, Fanburg-Smith JC, Miettinen M, et al. Atypical and malignant glomus tumors: analysis of 52 cases, with a proposal for the reclassification of glomus tumors. Am J Surg Pathol 2001;25(1):1–12.

261. Gill J, Van Vliet C. Infiltrating glomus tumor of uncertain malignant potential arising in the kidney. Hum Pathol 2010;41(1):145–9.

262. Chen YA, Li HN, Wang RC, et al. Malignant glomus tumor of the kidney: a case report and review of the literature. Clin Genitourin Cancer 2017;15(1): e151–3.

263. Lu YY, Wang RC, Wang HY. Malignant glomus tumor of the kidney. Am J Med Sci 2017;353(3):310.

Genitourinary Pathology Reporting Parameters Most Relevant to the Medical Oncologist

Clara Hwang, MD

KEYWORDS

- Pathology • Chemotherapy • Risk assessment • Prostate cancer • Urothelial cancer
- Kidney cancer • Testicular cancer

Key points

- Pathology assessment plays an important role in achieving the goal of identifying disease states with a homogeneous natural history and response to systemic therapy.
- Pathologic variables commonly used for risk assessment in genitourinary oncology include histologic subtype, histologic grade, and pathologic tumor and nodal staging.
- Medical oncologists commonly use these pathologic variables to inform clinical decision making, but the positive and negative predictive values of all classifiers to guide treatment decisions remain suboptimal.
- Next-generation classifiers, including molecular subtyping, may improve our ability to predict clinical treatment outcomes.

ABSTRACT

Pathologic variables play an important role in prognostication in urologic malignancies. Histologic subtype, histologic grade, and anatomic extent of disease (pathologic tumor and nodal staging) influence treatment decisions in both the adjuvant and metastatic settings. This article discusses treatment paradigms for the most common urologic malignancies, followed by the evidence base to support the relationship between pathologic assessment and decision making by the medical oncologist.

OVERVIEW

Medical oncologists traditionally work closely with pathologists to establish a treatment plan, starting with establishment of the oncologic diagnosis. Within any particular diagnosis and stage of disease, heterogeneity is apparent in the risk of disease recurrence, disease progression, and response to therapy. Heterogeneity in clinical outcomes is a known barrier to progress for almost all cancers and motivates the search for more refined categories of disease. This variability and unpredictability of clinical outcome leads to difficulties in treatment recommendations: patients may suffer excess toxicity from treatment that was never needed, or suffer the consequences of disease progression from treatment that is withheld. Advances in the classification of genitourinary malignancies are reflected in recent updates to staging and pathology guidelines. The goal of this review was to provide the reader with a brief summary of decision points for each of the common

---

Disclosure Statement: None.
Department of Internal Medicine, Division of Hematology and Oncology, Henry Ford Cancer Institute, Henry Ford Health System, 2799 West Grand Boulevard, CFP5, Detroit, MI 48202, USA
E-mail address: chwang2@hfhs.org

Surgical Pathology 11 (2018) 877–891
https://doi.org/10.1016/j.path.2018.07.009
1875-9181/18/© 2018 Elsevier Inc. All rights reserved.

genitourinary malignancies, followed by a discussion of how the pathology evaluation informs those decisions. The modern-day pursuit for molecular classifiers to guide precision medicine decisions is seen as a natural evolution of long-standing efforts to correctly categorize neoplastic disease.

PROSTATE CANCER

The typical role of the medical oncologist is to guide systemic therapy recommendations as part of a multidisciplinary team. In general, systemic therapy choices in prostate cancer consist of hormonal therapy, cytotoxic therapy, immunotherapy, and bone-targeting radiopharmaceuticals. Systemic therapy is offered to patients with prostate cancer in two clinical scenarios: (1) established metastatic disease and (2) when there is a significant risk of treatment failure after local therapy. Pathologic parameters are central to risk stratification, and thus, decisions about adjuvant systemic therapy. Pathologic assessment may also influence the specific type of systemic treatment chosen by the medical oncologist.

The evaluation of a patient with prostate cancer typically begins with evaluation of the prostate biopsy. While conventional acinar adenocarcinoma is by far the most common neoplasm of the prostate, the presence of rare histologic subtypes (eg, small cell carcinoma, transitional cell carcinoma, lymphoma, sarcoma, variant histologies) is critical to direct systemic therapy recommendations.[1,2] Chemotherapy agents used in these clinical scenarios follow principles from other disease sites where these histologic subtypes are more commonly encountered.

Although the remainder of the prostate cancer discussion will focus on the management of conventional adenocarcinoma, special mention is made here regarding small cell carcinoma, an uncommon but aggressive prostate cancer variant with poor prognosis.[3,4] Early metastatic spread, including the possibility of intracranial disease, mandates a more extensive imaging evaluation when small cell carcinoma is found. This predilection for early metastases compels the need for medical oncology consultation. Cytotoxic chemotherapy is recommended even for apparently localized disease, using small-cell lung cancer regimens such as cisplatin/carboplatin and etoposide. Small cell carcinoma of the prostate is associated with low prostate-specific antigen (PSA) levels and does not usually respond to hormonal manipulations. Because small cell carcinoma can arise in cases of conventional adenocarcinoma (typically of high grade), biopsy

of metastatic visceral disease should be performed when transformation to small cell carcinoma is suspected.

Key Features
SMALL-CELL PROSTATE CANCER

- Cytotoxic chemotherapy is recommended for small-cell prostate cancer, even for apparently localized disease, using small-cell lung cancer regimens.

- Small cell carcinoma of the prostate is associated with low PSA levels and does not usually respond to hormonal manipulations.

- Biopsy of metastatic visceral disease should be performed when transformation to small cell carcinoma is suspected.

Returning to the management of conventional adenocarcinoma, histologic grade is a key parameter of the prostate biopsy. Both the Gleason score and International Society of Urologic Pathology (ISUP) grade group should be reported. In 2014, the ISUP adopted a new grade grouping system in prostate cancer to refine and simplify stratification by pathologic grade (**Table 1**).[5] These new grade groups made it more clear that Gleason 3 + 3 = 6 cancer belongs to the lowest category of risk (grade group 1). The new groupings also provide more refined risk stratification for intermediate and high-risk prostate cancers. Grade group 2 (Gleason 3 + 4 = 7) is differentiated from grade group 3 (Gleason 4 + 3 = 7), highlighting the effect of a predominant Gleason pattern 4 in defining favorable and unfavorable intermediate-risk prostate cancer. High-risk Gleason 8 to 10 cancers have historically been considered together, but the new grouping system distinguishes Gleason

Table 1
International Society of Urologic Pathology (ISUP) grade groupings

ISUP Grade	Gleason Equivalent
Group 1	Gleason score ≤6 (3 + 3 and below)
Group 2	Gleason 3 + 4 = 7
Group 3	Gleason 4 + 3 = 7
Group 4	Gleason 8 (4 + 4, 3 + 5, 5 + 3)
Group 5	Gleason sum 9 and Gleason sum 10

8 (grade group 4) from Gleason 9 and 10 cancers (grade group 5). These grade groupings have been validated and predict both recurrence and mortality.[6,7] The ISUP grade groupings have been endorsed by multiple updated prostate cancer guidelines, including the World Health Organization and the American Joint Committee on Cancer (AJCC).[8,9]

At the time of initial clinical staging, prostate cancer is broadly grouped into localized disease (no evidence of nodal or distant metastatic disease), regional (pelvic nodal metastases), and metastatic (nodal disease beyond the pelvis, bone, or visceral disease). Localized disease is risk stratified further using clinical T stage, PSA values, and pathologic grade.[10,11] Reflecting the importance of PSA and histologic grade in prostate cancer risk stratification, both of these variables have been added to traditional anatomic criteria in modern staging systems.[9] Initial treatment recommendations for localized disease depend on this risk-stratification system.

Patients with low-risk localized disease (PSA <10 ng/mL, grade group 1, clinical stage T1-T2a) may be offered surveillance, surgery or radiation; systemic therapy is not required or recommended. Systemic therapy for patients with intermediate-risk cancer (PSA ≥10 and <20, grade group 2–3, clinical stage T2b-T2c) depends on the definitive treatment modality that is offered. There is no evidence to support the initial use of systemic therapy if surgery is chosen as definitive treatment; however, a short course of androgen-deprivation therapy (ADT) (4–6 months) is recommended with radiation for unfavorable intermediate-risk prostate cancer.[12] For patients with localized cancer and high recurrence risk (PSA ≥20, grade group 4–5, clinical stage T3a-T4), a longer course of 2 to 3 years of ADT with radiation improves outcomes.[13–15] Patients with clinically apparent nodal metastases are treated in a similar fashion, with more motivation for the use of systemic therapy given the higher risk of systemic recurrence. Adding docetaxel to radiation/ADT benefits some patients with high-risk disease and may be considered in carefully selected patients.[16–18] As an alternative adjuvant therapy with less toxicity, results from a phase III trial of abiraterone plus ADT in hormone-naïve prostate cancer suggest a possible role for adjuvant abiraterone in high-risk nonmetastatic prostate cancer.[19]

For patients with localized disease who undergo surgical resection, pathologic evaluation of the radical prostatectomy specimen again influences adjuvant therapy decisions. The presence of positive margins, extracapsular extension, seminal vesicle invasion, and/or nodal metastases identifies a group of patients in whom adjuvant radiation should be considered.[20–28] If nodal metastases are found, adjuvant androgen deprivation improved survival in a phase III trial.[29] Both radiation therapy and ADT add to treatment toxicity. Avoiding treatment toxicity in men who are not destined to relapse is a high priority for physicians and patients. Unfortunately, the ability to predict relapse and progression is only modest with current risk stratification groups and more accurate models are a significant clinical need. Thirty percent of men with pelvic nodal metastases will not relapse after surgery alone, leading some to propose additional criteria, such as nodal metastatic burden and pathologic grade to further risk stratify patients for adjuvant hormonal therapy.[30,31]

Similar calculations are made in other clinical scenarios, such as patients who relapse after definitive therapy. The prognosis for patients with biochemical (PSA-only) relapse is heterogeneous and thus the timing of systemic therapy is uncertain. Data suggest that early androgen deprivation improves overall survival, but at the cost of excess cardiovascular toxicity.[32] Clinicians often use pathologic parameters (grade, stage) in addition to PSA kinetics to risk stratify patients, but using prognostic models to dictate treatment decisions has not been validated prospectively.

For patients with metastatic prostate cancer, ADT is standard of care. In recent years, the addition of either docetaxel[17,33] or abiraterone[19,34] to ADT was proven to improve survival for patients with metastatic castration-sensitive prostate cancer. Pathologic parameters to assist in patient selection for this type of treatment intensification do not exist; consequently, decisions are based on clinical parameters. Treatment selection for patients with castration-sensitive disease is similarly challenged. Predictive biomarkers represent a promising area in which pathologic features may direct systemic therapy in the future. Examples of such biomarkers include the following: (1) androgen receptor splice variants that predict resistance to hormonal therapies[35]; (2) DNA repair defects that are associated with benefit from PARP-inhibitors and platinum agents in advanced prostate cancer[36,37]; and (3) high microsatellite instability that can be used to select patients for pembrolizumab in a tumor-agnostic fashion.[38]

In summary, the key pathologic features for the medical oncologist in prostate cancer are (1) the histologic subtype, (2) histologic grade, and (3) pathologic T and N staging, especially the presence of nodal metastatic disease. Outcome prediction remains imperfect in all clinical scenarios, leading to inevitable undertreatment and overtreatment. Prospective validation is needed of risk classifiers to guide treatment decisions. Biomarkers that predict systemic therapy response (such as the presence of androgen receptor splice variants) are under active investigation.

Key Features
PROSTATE CANCER

- Key pathologic features for the medical oncologist include histologic subtype, histologic grade, and pathologic staging for prostate cancer.

- Patients with nodal metastatic disease are at high risk of relapse after local therapy and adjuvant androgen deprivation is recommended.

KIDNEY CANCER

Systemic therapy options in renal cell carcinoma (RCC) consist of immunotherapy, vascular endothelial growth factor (VEGF) inhibitors, and mechanistic target of rapamycin (mTOR) inhibitors.[39] Immunotherapy approaches include interferon, interleukin-2, nivolumab, and ipilimumab. VEGF inhibition can be accomplished by bevacizumab and the many VEGF receptor tyrosine kinase inhibitors (eg, sunitinib). Temsirolimus and everolimus together comprise the mTOR inhibitor class. Contemporary decision points for the medical oncologist in the treatment of RCC are the selection of patients for adjuvant therapy and choosing between systemic treatment options for metastatic disease.

Risk stratification of localized RCC can identify high-risk patients with poor overall survival after radical nephrectomy. TNM stage and histologic grade (both primarily derived from the pathology report) are independent predictors of outcome in RCC. When combined with performance status, these variables can be used to stratify patients with localized RCC into low-risk, intermediate-risk, and high-risk groups.[40–42] With 5-year overall survival rates of 67% and 44% for intermediate-risk and high-risk disease, these patients have the potential to benefit substantially from effective adjuvant therapy. Unfortunately, until recently, multiple randomized clinical trials in the adjuvant setting failed to identify any intervention that improved outcomes for patients with poor prognosis.

High-risk patients with RCC in the S-TRAC trial were randomized to receive 1 year of adjuvant sunitinib or placebo after radical nephrectomy. Patients were required to have completely resected nonmetastatic clear-cell RCC (ccRCC), with at least T3 disease or positive lymph nodes. Disease-free survival favored the sunitinib arm (hazard ratio of 0.76, 95% confidence interval 0.59–0.98), but there was no overall survival benefit with a median follow-up of 5.4 years.[43] Although the S-TRAC trial was reported as positive, the lack of a survival benefit along with the toxicity of sunitinib has led many experts to continue to recommend observation. Furthermore, negative results for adjuvant sunitinib (and sorafenib) were reported with the ASSURE trial, a difference some have attributed to different entry criteria (high-grade T1b and non–clear-cell tumors were allowed) and less dose intensity.[44] Medical oncologists may discuss adjuvant sunitinib with patients who meet the pathologic entry criteria for the S-TRAC trial. Clinical trial enrollment (evaluating a novel immunotherapy approach, for example) is another important option for high-risk patients after radical nephrectomy and should be offered when available.

Pathologic factors play a limited role in treatment selection for metastatic RCC. Histologic subtype has a modest impact, but the evidence base for the management of non-ccRCC is extremely limited. In practice, treatment for non-ccRCC mirrors that for ccRCC, with the caveat that sarcomatoid, collecting duct, and medullary subtypes may benefit from the use of cytotoxic therapies that have no role in the treatment of ccRCC.[45–47] Prognosis for metastatic non-ccRCC is generally worse than for ccRCC. Sunitinib and everolimus both have some degree of activity in non-ccRCC, with an advantage for sunitinib in randomized phase II trials.[48–50] MET alterations are frequent in papillary RCC and may identify a subset of patients with response to MET inhibitor therapy.[51,52] Responses to nivolumab have also been reported for non-ccRCC.[53] No predictive biomarkers, including histologic subtype, are currently validated to guide systemic therapy choice in RCC, although laboratory parameters (lactate dehydrogenase [LDH], calcium, hemoglobin, neutrophil count, platelet count) are commonly used for prognostication.[54,55] There is great interest in using molecular subtyping to guide systemic therapy decisions (eg, TSC1/2 or MTOR alteration to predict benefit from mTOR inhibition) but further study is needed before these tests can be recommended for routine clinical use.

> ### Key Features
> #### KIDNEY CANCER
>
> - Pathologic grade and stage are used to stratify patients with kidney cancer into low-risk, intermediate-risk, and high-risk groups.
> - High-risk renal cancer may be considered for clinical trials or adjuvant therapy, although the precise role for adjuvant therapy remains debated.
> - Sarcomatoid, collecting duct, and medullary subtypes are typically treated differently than usual RCC types (with cytotoxic chemotherapy).

BLADDER CANCER

Systemic therapy plays a central role in the management of patients with bladder cancer with nodal and distant metastatic disease. In addition, chemotherapy is routinely offered to select patients at high risk of recurrence with local therapy alone. Chemotherapy can be offered in the perioperative setting or concurrently with radiation for localized disease. Histologic subtype is important to the medical oncologist in all stages of the disease, whereas additional features of the pathologic examination help predict recurrence for apparently localized disease. Urothelial carcinoma is the most common histologic subtype and is addressed first.

LOCALIZED DISEASE

The presence of muscle invasion on transurethral resection of bladder tumor (TUR) is a critical distinction for the oncologist with profound treatment implications. If no muscularis propria is present in the TUR specimen, repeat TUR is recommended to rule out muscle-invasive disease. Patients with bladder cancer with no evidence of muscle invasion are primarily managed by urologists. Patients with localized muscle-invasive bladder cancer may be offered definitive treatment with either radical cystectomy or radiation. For both radiation[56,57] and surgery, the addition of chemotherapy to definitive local treatment improves outcomes, leading to the recommendation for medical oncology consultation for chemotherapy-eligible patients with muscle-invasive disease (at least cT2).

Level 1 evidence[58,59] supports the use of neoadjuvant cisplatin-based combination chemotherapy. In comparison with cystectomy alone, neoadjuvant chemotherapy is associated with an absolute overall survival benefit of ~5% at 5 years in meta-analyses.[60,61] It should be noted that there is no evidence to support the use of non–cisplatin-containing regimens in the neoadjuvant setting. The modest benefit of neoadjuvant chemotherapy and the possible harm of delaying definitive treatment have motivated the field to predict which patients are most likely to benefit from a neoadjuvant approach. For example, there is an interest in using biomarkers to predict chemo-sensitivity and chemo-resistance such that only patients who are predicted to respond to treatment are exposed to the toxicity of chemotherapy.[62–64] Such efforts should be considered investigational. Clinical factors have also been considered: patients at higher risk of relapse have more to gain from neoadjuvant chemotherapy and the absolute survival benefit is more apparent in T3/T4 tumors than in T2 disease.[58] Unfortunately, clinical T staging is prone to error, with frequent upstaging on cystectomy specimens.[65] The most recent iteration of the National Comprehensive Cancer Network guidelines in bladder cancer do not recommend withholding neoadjuvant chemotherapy for patients with cT2 disease except when there is a contraindication to cisplatin and for certain variant histologies.[66]

Although evidence supporting neoadjuvant chemotherapy is changing clinical norms, many patients still do not receive neoadjuvant chemotherapy in routine practice, perhaps in part because of the previously mentioned concerns.[67] After cystectomy, patients with pT3/4 disease or lymph node metastases have a high risk for treatment failure,[68–72] leading to the question of whether adjuvant chemotherapy should be considered. The evidence to support adjuvant chemotherapy in high-risk bladder cancer is not as robust as the evidence for neoadjuvant chemotherapy. Phase III trials failed to show a benefit for adjuvant chemotherapy, but were hampered by low statistical power and poor accrual. Meta-analyses of randomized clinical trial data demonstrated a survival benefit for adjuvant cisplatin-based chemotherapy compared with cystectomy alone.[73,74] An overall survival benefit for adjuvant chemotherapy is also supported by data from a large observational study.[75] Taken together, the evidence suggests that adjuvant chemotherapy may be considered for high-risk patients with adverse pathologic features ($\geq$pT3, lymph node metastases).

METASTATIC DISEASE

Combination chemotherapy with a platinum-based regimen is the standard frontline approach for patients with metastatic urothelial cancer.[76–78] Immunotherapy with atezolizumab[79] or pembrolizumab[80] can be considered for patients who are not candidates for cytotoxic chemotherapy. After platinum failure, multiple immunotherapy agents (atezolizumab,[81,82] avelumab,[83,84] durvalumab,[85] nivolumab,[86,87] and pembrolizumab[88]) have been approved in the second-line setting. Cytotoxic therapies that are commonly used after platinum failure include pemetrexed[89] and the taxanes.[90,91] Gemcitabine and platinum agents can be used in the second-line setting if not previously administered.

With the increasing number of systemic agents known to be active in urothelial cancer, there is a growing need to find predictive biomarkers to aid with treatment selection, especially in the second-line setting, in which response rates are ~20%.[92,93] Although promising, the use of such biomarkers to predict therapeutic benefit is not yet routine clinical practice. PD-L1 status has been studied as a predictive biomarker for all of the immunotherapy agents approved in urothelial cancer, and in some studies PD-L1 positivity is associated with higher response rates to immunotherapy. However, the assessment of PD-L1 status varied significantly between studies (ie, what antibody was used for immunohistochemistry, whether immune cells, tumor cells, or both were evaluated for PD-L1 expression, and what percentage of PD-L1–positive cells was used to assign the PD-L1 expression category). Notably, the benefit of pembrolizumab over cytotoxic chemotherapy was observed regardless of PD-L1 status,[94] and also did not predict for benefit with nivolumab.[87] Because (1) most studies were not designed to assess the power of the biomarker to predict benefit from chemotherapy over immunotherapy and vice versa, and (2) benefit of immunotherapy is still observed in patients with low PD-L1 expression, regulatory bodies have not mandated the use of PD-L1 status with immunotherapy. If the clinician requests it, the particular PD-L1 assay should be clarified and matched to the agent being considered. Higher mutational load was associated with benefit from atezolizumab[82] but similarly has not been rigorously validated as a predictive biomarker for treatment selection. As another example, mutations in *ERCC2* and other genes involved in DNA repair[95] are associated with benefit from platinum-based therapy but their use remains investigational.

THE IMPACT OF VARIANT HISTOLOGY

As with other genitourinary cancers, the histologic subtype of a bladder cancer has a significant impact on prognosis and treatment recommendations. Patients with variant histology appear to have worse prognosis compared with urothelial (transitional cell) carcinoma. Because of their relative rarity, there is a limited evidence base to guide treatment recommendations for non-urothelial carcinoma of the bladder.

Chemotherapy is recommended as initial therapy for small cell carcinoma of the bladder,[96,97] with consolidation surgery or radiation for localized disease. A platinum/etoposide combination is most commonly used, with encouraging results reported in a phase II trial of alternating ifosfamide/doxorubicin and cisplatin/etoposide.[98] As in other disease sites, small cell carcinoma of the bladder is an aggressive malignancy and brain MRI is recommended for advanced disease.

Whether or not to administer neoadjuvant chemotherapy for bladder cancer with variant histology is difficult to answer based on the existing literature. As alluded to previously, neoadjuvant chemotherapy is standard for small cell carcinoma of the bladder on the basis of retrospective data.[96,97,99] Micropapillary[100] and plasmacytoid[101] variants respond to the typical platinum-combination regimens used in urothelial carcinoma when given in the neoadjuvant setting; however, there is an absence of randomized controlled data and a retrospective analysis (potentially confounded by selection bias) did not identify a survival benefit for neoadjuvant chemotherapy.[99] Neoadjuvant chemotherapy is not recommended for patients with pure squamous or pure adenocarcinoma of the bladder because they respond poorly to traditional urothelial carcinoma regimens.

For patients with pure squamous or adenocarcinoma of the bladder and metastatic disease, combination therapy with ifosfamide, paclitaxel, and cisplatin has activity in patients with metastatic adenocarcinoma and squamous cell carcinoma of the bladder.[102] Combination therapy with paclitaxel, carboplatin, and gemcitabine is another option with activity in patients with squamous cell carcinoma of the bladder.[103] Five-fluorouracil combined with either cisplatin or oxaliplatin (such as FOLFOX) has activity in adenocarcinoma of the bladder.[104] There is limited evidence to support the use of immunotherapy in patients with nonurothelial cancer of the bladder although this is an area of investigation.

> ## Key Features
> ### BLADDER CANCER
>
> - Chemotherapy is recommended as initial therapy for small-cell bladder cancer.
>
> - Level 1 evidence supports the use of neoadjuvant cisplatin-based combination chemotherapy for localized muscle-invasive urothelial carcinoma of the bladder.
>
> - Need for neoadjuvant therapy with other variant histology is less clear at present.
>
> - Neoadjuvant therapy is in general not recommended for pure squamous cell carcinoma or pure adenocarcinoma, which appear to respond poorly to traditional urothelial carcinoma regimens.
>
> - If a PD-L1 assay is requested, the antibody used should be documented and matched to the agent being considered.

TESTICULAR CANCER

Testicular cancer is unique in solid tumor oncology because of the curative potential of systemic therapy, even in the setting of advanced disease. The success of cytotoxic chemotherapy for testicular cancer has resulted in cure rates of ~98% overall. Broadly, testicular neoplasms are classified into seminomatous and nonseminomatous germ cell tumors. Nonseminomatous germ cell tumors may contain seminomatous elements but are characterized by the presence of other histologic subtypes (embryonal, yolk sac, choriocarcinoma, or teratoma). Pure seminoma is associated with a better response to chemotherapy and radiotherapy compared with nonseminomatous germ cell tumors. Treatment algorithms for testicular cancer are therefore highly dependent on these 2 pathologic categories.

Classifying a testicular cancer as pure seminoma requires both the absence of nonseminomatous components as well as a normal level of alpha-feto protein (AFP). AFP may be produced by tumors with embryonal, yolk sac, and teratoma elements, but is not produced by seminoma or choriocarcinoma. An elevated AFP therefore leads to a presumption of nonseminomatous components and, therefore, a modest intensification of the treatment approach. Elevation of beta-human chorionic gonadotropic (βHCG) and LDH can be seen in both seminoma and nonseminoma, although the level of βHCG elevation in a pure

seminoma is typically modest, likely attributable to a small component of admixed trophoblastic cells. Very high levels of βHCG elevation would typically imply an unsampled choriocarcinoma component.

As with other genitourinary malignancies, the pathologist plays a key role in providing prognostic information to help guide adjuvant therapy. Standards for pathologic reporting reflect our current understanding of how pathologic risk factors are associated with tumor behavior. Risk-stratification systems are used in all stages of the disease to tailor treatment recommendations for patients with testicular cancer. The goal for patients with good prognosis is to minimize treatment-morbidity while maintaining excellent outcomes. In contrast, new treatment paradigms, and perhaps treatment intensification, are needed for patients with poor prognosis.

In addition to risk stratification, pathologic assessment may influence other management decisions. For example, predominance of choriocarcinoma, especially in conjunction with βHCG levels greater than 100,000 and widespread pulmonary metastases, may raise the suspicion of intracranial metastases. Brain imaging is recommended in this scenario, which is not routine in the staging of testicular germ cell tumors. The unique biology of teratoma also has clinical implications for patients with nonseminomatous germ cell tumors. Teratoma is chemo-resistant and radio-resistant, and has the potential for transformation to secondary, somatic-type malignancy, with poor prognosis. These features drive recommendations for surgical resection of postchemotherapy residual masses in nonseminomatous germ cell tumors.

EARLY-STAGE TUMORS: SEMINOMA

In modern practice, patients with clinical stage I seminoma are commonly offered surveillance after orchiectomy. Pathologic review of the orchiectomy specimen to exclude any evidence of nonseminomatous elements is an important component of the definition of stage I seminoma. Other requirements for classification as stage I seminoma include normal AFP before orchiectomy, normal β-HCG and LDH postorchiectomy, and negative imaging studies (computed tomography [CT] of the abdomen and pelvis; chest radiograph or CT).

The relapse rate for pure seminoma after orchiectomy in the absence of nodal or other metastatic disease is less than 20%.[105] The success of salvage therapy for relapses is associated with a 99.3% 15-year disease-specific survival, rendering surveillance an attractive option for patients with stage I seminoma. If adjuvant therapy is considered, the patient may undergo either radiation or adjuvant chemotherapy with single-agent carboplatin, both of which reduce the relapse rate to 3% to 4%.[106] Adjuvant radiation is overtreatment for most patients with stage I seminoma who are not destined to relapse and there are concerns regarding second malignancies and excess long-term mortality.[107–109] Fully mature data regarding the long-term toxicity from single-agent carboplatin are not available, even if early reports did not identify any excess toxicity from adjuvant single-agent carboplatin.[110] Despite toxicity concerns, adjuvant therapy may still represent less toxicity if compared with salvage treatment. Thus, there is still interest in identifying risk factors to identify patients at higher risk of recurrence.

Tumor diameter larger than 4 cm and infiltration of the rete testis were identified as independent predictors of relapse in a pooled analysis of patients with clinical stage I seminoma managed with active surveillance.[111] Not all studies have confirmed these associations.[112] In contrast to nonseminomatous germ cell tumors, lymphovascular invasion is not an independent prognostic factor for relapse, nor is pathologic T stage.[112] The most consistent finding is the higher risk of relapse in patients with larger tumors. Only a minority of studies have confirmed invasion of the rete testis as an independent risk factor for relapse and reported hazard ratios are more modest compared with tumor size. It has been argued that failure to distinguish stromal invasion from pagetoid spread to the rete testis may explain this discrepancy. After review of the evidence, invasion of the rete testis was not felt to warrant specific T classification in the most recent edition of the AJCC staging manual. In contrast, pure seminoma tumors larger than 3 cm size are now classified as T1b.

Although reporting of tumor size and invasion of the rete testis are a routine part of the pathologic assessment for stage I seminoma, it is still debated whether these risk factors are able to identify a high-risk group in which adjuvant treatment is justified. High-risk patients have a recurrence risk of 25% to 30% compared with ~5% relapse risk for low-risk patients.[113–115] The use of pathologic features to guide adjuvant therapy for stage I seminoma is not uniformly recommended in consensus guidelines, citing this lack of discriminatory ability and the lack of prospective validation of prognostic factors. Risk-adapted strategies using tumor size and rete testis invasion are currently under investigation.[116,117]

Pathologic features do not generally influence treatment of patients with clinical stage II seminoma (involvement of the retroperitoneal lymph nodes). These patients are treated either with radiation or combination platinum-chemotherapy. Standard chemotherapy consists of 3 cycles of BEP (bleomycin, etoposide, and cisplatin) or 4 cycles of EP (etoposide and cisplatin). The recommendation for chemotherapy versus radiation is based primarily on the burden of retroperitoneal disease. Relapse after radiation is more likely with increasing nodal size, as is reflected in the current AJCC staging system.[9,118,119] Patients with IIA disease ($\leq$2 cm) are typically treated with radiation, IIB disease (2–5 cm) may be offered either modality, and IIC (>5 cm) disease is treated with chemotherapy.

EARLY-STAGE TUMORS: NONSEMINOMA

As with pure seminoma, most patients with stage I nonseminomatous germ cell tumors (NSGCT) will not relapse and effective salvage chemotherapy results in high cure rates. Surveillance and adjuvant therapy are both considered acceptable management options in this clinical scenario. In contrast to seminoma, adjuvant treatment options for patients with stage I nonseminoma include either retroperitoneal lymph node dissection or combination chemotherapy with 1 cycle of BEP.[120,121] For patients who relapse, 3 or 4 cycles of BEP are prescribed as salvage treatment, depending on risk stratification at the time of relapse (see later in this article). Four cycles of EP can also be given for good-risk patients. Balancing the risks of adjuvant treatment with the benefits of preventing toxicity from salvage chemotherapy again depends on the risk of relapse for an individual patient. Features of the pathology report are central to risk stratification of stage I NSGCT.

Relapse rates for clinical stage I nonseminoma are slightly higher than for seminoma (approximately 30%). The use of pathologic variables, especially lymphovascular invasion, can stratify patients into groups with relapse rates nearing 50% in high-risk disease and 16% in low-risk patients.[122,123] Lymphovascular invasion has the strongest association with risk of occult metastatic disease for patients with clinical stage I nonseminomatous germ cell tumors. To reflect the importance of this finding, the presence of lymphovascular invasion in an organ-confined tumor changes pT staging from pT1 to pT2. Tumors with a greater percentage of embryonal carcinoma also carry a higher risk of relapse.[124,125] Predominance of choriocarcinoma histology is associated with aggressive clinical behavior,[126,127] whereas yolk sac tumors are less likely to metastasize. Higher T stage is also associated with occult metastases. These well-established prognostic factors have been incorporated into international pathology standards for testicular cancer reporting.[9,128] Recommendations include a thorough assessment of the percentage and classification of histologic subtypes in the specimen, as well as the presence of lymphovascular invasion.

Pathologic lymph node evaluation also plays a role in the management of nonseminomatous germ cell tumors when retroperitoneal lymph node dissection (RPLND) is performed. As outlined previously, RPLND may be performed in the adjuvant setting for clinical stage I NSGCT. The finding of occult nodal disease identifies a pathologic stage II tumor. RPLND may be performed for therapeutic and diagnostic purposes in clinical stage II NSGCT and is mandatory for postchemotherapy masses in more advanced disease. The main question after RPLND is whether adjuvant treatment is recommended. Both the number and size of lymph nodes involved with tumor are incorporated into pathologic nodal staging. The finding of pN2 or pN3 disease in stage II NSGCT is associated with relapse rates in excess of 50%, and generally treated with adjuvant chemotherapy. The presence of viable germ cell tumor in a resected postchemotherapy mass also mandates further chemotherapy, whereas necrosis, fibrosis, or teratoma alone does not require further treatment.

Key Features
TESTICULAR CANCER

- Lymphovascular invasion has the strongest association with risk of occult metastatic disease for patients with clinical stage I nonseminomatous germ cell tumors.

- The relevance of traditional pathologic parameters, such as lymphovascular invasion and rete testis invasion, is less clear in pure seminoma.

- Size has been incorporated into AJCC staging for pure seminoma, based on size larger than 3 cm indicating pT1b.

- Viable non-teratoma germ cell tumor in postchemotherapy mass necessitates further chemotherapy, whereas necrosis, fibrosis, and teratoma do not.

ADVANCED DISEASE

Patients with advanced testicular cancer undergoing initial chemotherapy are assigned to good, intermediate, and poor risk categories based on the International Germ Cell Cancer Collaborative Group (IGCCCG) scoring system.[129] The variables assessed in this scoring system are histologic subtype (seminoma vs nonseminoma), primary site (retroperitoneal/testicular vs mediastinal), sites of visceral metastatic disease (pulmonary vs nonpulmonary), and degree of tumor marker elevation. Histologic subtype has a substantial impact on initial prognosis. No patients with pure seminoma are classified as poor risk, even if other adverse features such as nonpulmonary visceral metastases are present. An area of research is whether molecular classification can further refine clinical prognostic systems.[130,131] Gene expression, gene mutations, epigenetic changes, protein abundance, and posttranslational modifications may all impact cancer prognosis. Our understanding of how molecular changes impact clinical behavior is still evolving. Molecular analysis and reporting have not yet entered routine clinical practice for testicular cancer but may become more important in the future.

For patients requiring salvage therapy, the primary clinical question is when to proceed with high-dose chemotherapy with stem cell rescue over conventional-dose chemotherapy. For the most part, risk-stratification systems for patients undergoing salvage therapy have found greater predictive power from clinical factors such as site of primary, the quality of response to initial chemotherapy, and tumor markers at relapse.[132–135] However, the IGCCCG score, which includes histologic subtype, was retained in 1 prognostic model predicting outcomes with high-dose chemotherapy.[134]

NON–GERM CELL TESTICULAR NEOPLASMS

Although germ cell tumors comprise the vast majority of testicular neoplasms, the genitourinary pathologist will at times be called on to evaluate non–germ cell neoplasms of the testis. Sex cord-stromal tumors (Leydig cell, Sertoli cell, and granulosa cell tumors) make up 4% of testicular neoplasms and have unique clinical characteristics and treatment paradigms.[136,137] As a whole, they are best treated surgically because they are relatively resistant to chemotherapy and radiotherapy. As a result, the prognosis for patients with metastatic disease is relatively grim.[138–140] Gonadoblastomas are tumors with both sex cord and germ cell elements. If malignant germ cell elements are present, treatment of metastatic disease is directed against the germ cell component.[141] Similarly, systemic therapy is tailored to histologic subtype for an intratesticular lymphoma, adenocarcinoma, or mesothelioma.

SUMMARY

Selection of systemic therapy for patients with metastatic genitourinary malignancies remains problematic. Biomarker-driven therapy (such as trastuzumab for *HER2*-amplified breast cancer) is not yet standard in any genitourinary malignancy. Pathologic variables play a larger role in choosing high-risk patients for adjuvant systemic therapy. Common principles of risk assessment are seen across sites of disease: pathologic extent of disease and histologic grade predict outcomes and these variables have been refined in efforts to improve cancer staging. Risk classification systems frequently incorporate clinical variables to improve prognostic performance. Regrettably, overtreatment and undertreatment are still common problems. Further work is needed to improve our ability to identify patients with uniform outcome and treatment response.

ACKNOWLEDGMENTS

The author gratefully acknowledges Dr Elisabeth Heath for her careful and critical reading of this article; her comments and encouragements are deeply appreciated.

REFERENCES

1. Mazzucchelli R, Lopez-Beltran A, Cheng L, et al. Rare and unusual histological variants of prostatic carcinoma: clinical significance. BJU Int 2008; 102(10):1369–74.

2. Humphrey PA. Histological variants of prostatic carcinoma and their significance. Histopathology 2012;60(1):59–74.

3. Spiess PE, Pettaway CA, Vakar-Lopez F, et al. Treatment outcomes of small cell carcinoma of the prostate: a single-center study. Cancer 2007; 110(8):1729–37.

4. Wang W, Epstein JI. Small cell carcinoma of the prostate. A morphologic and immunohistochemical study of 95 cases. Am J Surg Pathol 2008;32(1):65–71.

5. Epstein JI, Egevad L, Amin MB, et al. The 2014 International Society of Urological Pathology (ISUP) Consensus Conference on Gleason Grading of Prostatic Carcinoma: definition of grading patterns and proposal for a new grading system. Am J Surg Pathol 2016;40(2):244–52.

6. Epstein JI, Zelefsky MJ, Sjoberg DD, et al. A contemporary prostate cancer grading system:

a validated alternative to the Gleason score. Eur Urol 2016;69(3):428–35.

7. Berney DM, Beltran L, Fisher G, et al. Validation of a contemporary prostate cancer grading system using prostate cancer death as outcome. Br J Cancer 2016;114(10):1078–83.

8. Moch H, Humphrey P, Ulbright TM, et al. WHO classification of tumours of the urinary system and male genital organs. 4th edition. Lyon (France): International Agency for Research on Cancer; 2016.

9. Amin MB, American Joint Committee on Cancer, American Cancer Society. AJCC cancer staging manual. In: Amin MB, Edge SB, Gress DM, et al, editors. 8th edition. Chicago: American Joint Committee on Cancer, Springer; 2017. p. 723–45.

10. National Comprehensive Cancer Network. Prostate Cancer (Version 2.2018). Available at: https://www.nccn.org/professionals/physician_gls/pdf/prostate.pdf. Accessed April 1, 2018.

11. Sanda MG, Cadeddu JA, Kirkby E, et al. Clinically localized prostate cancer: AUA/ASTRO/SUO guideline. Part I: risk stratification, shared decision making, and care options. J Urol 2018;199(3): 683–90.

12. Pisansky TM, Hunt D, Gomella LG, et al. Duration of androgen suppression before radiotherapy for localized prostate cancer: radiation therapy oncology group randomized clinical trial 9910. J Clin Oncol 2015;33(4):332–9.

13. Bolla M, Van Tienhoven G, Warde P, et al. External irradiation with or without long-term androgen suppression for prostate cancer with high metastatic risk: 10-year results of an EORTC randomised study. Lancet Oncol 2010;11(11):1066–73.

14. Horwitz EM, Bae K, Hanks GE, et al. Ten-year follow-up of radiation therapy oncology group protocol 92-02: a phase III trial of the duration of elective androgen deprivation in locally advanced prostate cancer. J Clin Oncol 2008;26(15):2497–504.

15. Bolla M, de Reijke TM, Van Tienhoven G, et al. Duration of androgen suppression in the treatment of prostate cancer. N Engl J Med 2009;360(24):2516–27.

16. Fizazi K, Faivre L, Lesaunier F, et al. Androgen deprivation therapy plus docetaxel and estramustine versus androgen deprivation therapy alone for high-risk localised prostate cancer (GETUG 12): a phase 3 randomised controlled trial. Lancet Oncol 2015;16(7):787–94.

17. James ND, Sydes MR, Clarke NW, et al. Addition of docetaxel, zoledronic acid, or both to first-line long-term hormone therapy in prostate cancer (STAMPEDE): survival results from an adaptive, multiarm, multistage, platform randomised controlled trial. Lancet 2016;387(10024):1163–77.

18. Sandler HM, Hu C, Rosenthal SA, et al. A phase III protocol of androgen suppression (AS) and 3DCRT/IMRT versus AS and 3DCRT/IMRT followed

by chemotherapy (CT) with docetaxel and prednisone for localized, high-risk prostate cancer (RTOG 0521). J Clin Oncol 2015;33(18_suppl): LBA5002.

19. James ND, de Bono JS, Spears MR, et al. Abiraterone for prostate cancer not previously treated with hormone therapy. N Engl J Med 2017;377(4): 338–51.

20. Van der Kwast TH, Bolla M, Van Poppel H, et al. Identification of patients with prostate cancer who benefit from immediate postoperative radiotherapy: EORTC 22911. J Clin Oncol 2007;25(27):4178–86.

21. Swanson GP, Goldman B, Tangen CM, et al. The prognostic impact of seminal vesicle involvement found at prostatectomy and the effects of adjuvant radiation: data from Southwest Oncology Group 8794. J Urol 2008;180(6):2453–7, [discussion: 2458].

22. Thompson IM, Tangen CM, Paradelo J, et al. Adjuvant radiotherapy for pathological T3N0M0 prostate cancer significantly reduces risk of metastases and improves survival: long-term followup of a randomized clinical trial. J Urol 2009; 181(3):956–62.

23. Wiegel T, Bottke D, Steiner U, et al. Phase III postoperative adjuvant radiotherapy after radical prostatectomy compared with radical prostatectomy alone in pT3 prostate cancer with postoperative undetectable prostate-specific antigen: ARO 96-02/ AUO AP 09/95. J Clin Oncol 2009;27(18):2924–30.

24. Thompson IM, Valicenti RK, Albertsen P, et al. Adjuvant and salvage radiotherapy after prostatectomy: AUA/ASTRO guideline. J Urol 2013;190(2):441–9.

25. Abdollah F, Karnes RJ, Suardi N, et al. Impact of adjuvant radiotherapy on survival of patients with node-positive prostate cancer. J Clin Oncol 2014; 32(35):3939–47.

26. Da Pozzo LF, Cozzarini C, Briganti A, et al. Long-term follow-up of patients with prostate cancer and nodal metastases treated by pelvic lymphadenectomy and radical prostatectomy: the positive impact of adjuvant radiotherapy. Eur Urol 2009; 55(5):1003–11.

27. Briganti A, Karnes RJ, Da Pozzo LF, et al. Combination of adjuvant hormonal and radiation therapy significantly prolongs survival of patients with pT2-4 pN+ prostate cancer: results of a matched analysis. Eur Urol 2011;59(5):832–40.

28. Lin CC, Gray PJ, Jemal A, et al. Androgen deprivation with or without radiation therapy for clinically node-positive prostate cancer. J Natl Cancer Inst 2015;107(7), [pii:djv119].

29. Messing EM, Manola J, Sarosdy M, et al. Immediate hormonal therapy compared with observation after radical prostatectomy and pelvic lymphadenectomy in men with node-positive prostate cancer. N Engl J Med 1999;341(24):1781–8.

30. Touijer KA, Mazzola CR, Sjoberg DD, et al. Long-term outcomes of patients with lymph node metastasis treated with radical prostatectomy without adjuvant androgen-deprivation therapy. Eur Urol 2014;65(1):20–5.

31. Boormans JL, Wildhagen MF, Bangma CH, et al. Histopathological characteristics of lymph node metastases predict cancer-specific survival in node-positive prostate cancer. BJU Int 2008; 102(11):1589–93.

32. Duchesne GM, Woo HH, Bassett JK, et al. Timing of androgen-deprivation therapy in patients with prostate cancer with a rising PSA (TROG 03.06 and VCOG PR 01-03 [TOAD]): a randomised, multicentre, non-blinded, phase 3 trial. Lancet Oncol 2016;17(6):727–37.

33. Sweeney CJ, Chen YH, Carducci M, et al. Chemohormonal therapy in metastatic hormone-sensitive prostate cancer. N Engl J Med 2015;373(8): 737–46.

34. Fizazi K, Tran N, Fein L, et al. Abiraterone plus prednisone in metastatic, castration-sensitive prostate cancer. N Engl J Med 2017;377(4):352–60.

35. Antonarakis ES, Lu C, Wang H, et al. AR-V7 and resistance to enzalutamide and abiraterone in prostate cancer. N Engl J Med 2014;371(11):1028–38.

36. Mateo J, Carreira S, Sandhu S, et al. DNA-repair defects and olaparib in metastatic prostate cancer. N Engl J Med 2015;373(18):1697–708.

37. Pomerantz MM, Spisak S, Jia L, et al. The association between germline BRCA2 variants and sensitivity to platinum-based chemotherapy among men with metastatic prostate cancer. Cancer 2017;123(18):3532–9.

38. Le DT, Uram JN, Wang H, et al. PD-1 blockade in tumors with mismatch-repair deficiency. N Engl J Med 2015;372(26):2509–20.

39. Choueiri TK, Motzer RJ. Systemic therapy for metastatic renal-cell carcinoma. N Engl J Med 2017; 376(4):354–66.

40. Tsui KH, Shvarts O, Smith RB, et al. Prognostic indicators for renal cell carcinoma: a multivariate analysis of 643 patients using the revised 1997 TNM staging criteria. J Urol 2000;163(4):1090–5, [quiz: 1295].

41. Zisman A, Pantuck AJ, Dorey F, et al. Improved prognostication of renal cell carcinoma using an integrated staging system. J Clin Oncol 2001;19(6): 1649–57.

42. Patard JJ, Kim HL, Lam JS, et al. Use of the University of California Los Angeles integrated staging system to predict survival in renal cell carcinoma: an international multicenter study. J Clin Oncol 2004;22(16):3316–22.

43. Ravaud A, Motzer RJ, Pandha HS, et al. Adjuvant sunitinib in high-risk renal-cell carcinoma after nephrectomy. N Engl J Med 2016;375(23):2246–54.

44. Haas NB, Manola J, Uzzo RG, et al. Adjuvant sunitinib or sorafenib for high-risk, non-metastatic
renal-cell carcinoma (ECOG-ACRIN E2805): a
double-blind, placebo-controlled, randomised,
phase 3 trial. Lancet 2016;387(10032):2008–16.

45. Michaelson MD, McKay RR, Werner L, et al. Phase
2 trial of sunitinib and gemcitabine in patients with
sarcomatoid and/or poor-risk metastatic renal cell
carcinoma. Cancer 2015;121(19):3435–43.

46. Oudard S, Banu E, Vieillefond A, et al. Prospective
multicenter phase II study of gemcitabine plus platinum salt for metastatic collecting duct carcinoma:
results of a GETUG (Groupe d'Etudes des Tumeurs
Uro-Genitales) study. J Urol 2007;177(5):1698–702.

47. Shah AY, Karam JA, Malouf GG, et al. Management
and outcomes of patients with renal medullary carcinoma: a multicentre collaborative study. BJU Int
2017;120(6):782–92.

48. Armstrong AJ, Halabi S, Eisen T, et al. Everolimus
versus sunitinib for patients with metastatic non-
clear cell renal cell carcinoma (ASPEN): a multicentre, open-label, randomised phase 2 trial. Lancet Oncol 2016;17(3):378–88.

49. Tannir NM, Jonasch E, Albiges L, et al. Everolimus
versus sunitinib prospective evaluation in metastatic non-clear cell renal cell carcinoma (ESPN): a
randomized multicenter phase 2 trial. Eur Urol
2016;69(5):866–74.

50. Motzer RJ, Barrios CH, Kim TM, et al. Phase II randomized trial comparing sequential first-line everolimus and second-line sunitinib versus first-line
sunitinib and second-line everolimus in patients
with metastatic renal cell carcinoma. J Clin Oncol
2014;32(25):2765–72.

51. Choueiri TK, Vaishampayan U, Rosenberg JE, et al.
Phase II and biomarker study of the dual MET/
VEGFR2 inhibitor foretinib in patients with papillary
renal cell carcinoma. J Clin Oncol 2013;31(2):181–6.

52. Choueiri TK, Plimack E, Arkenau HT, et al.
Biomarker-based phase II trial of savolitinib in pa-
tients with advanced papillary renal cell cancer.
J Clin Oncol 2017;35(26):2993–3001.

53. Koshkin VS, Barata PC, Vogelzang NJ, et al. Nivolumab treatment for patients with non-clear cell
renal cell carcinoma: a multicenter retrospective
analysis. J Clin Oncol 2017;35(15_suppl):4586.

54. Motzer RJ, Bacik J, Murphy BA, et al. Interferon-
alfa as a comparative treatment for clinical trials
of new therapies against advanced renal cell carcinoma. J Clin Oncol 2002;20(1):289–96.

55. Heng DY, Xie W, Regan MM, et al. Prognostic factors
for overall survival in patients with metastatic renal
cell carcinoma treated with vascular endothelial
growth factor-targeted agents: results from a large,
multicenter study. J Clin Oncol 2009;27(34):5794–9.

56. Coppin CM, Gospodarowicz MK, James K, et al.
Improved local control of invasive bladder cancer
by concurrent cisplatin and preoperative or definitive radiation. The National Cancer Institute of Canada Clinical Trials Group. J Clin Oncol 1996;14(11):
2901–7.

57. James ND, Hussain SA, Hall E, et al. Radiotherapy
with or without chemotherapy in muscle-invasive
bladder cancer. N Engl J Med 2012;366(16):1477–88.

58. Grossman HB, Natale RB, Tangen CM, et al. Neoadjuvant chemotherapy plus cystectomy compared with
cystectomy alone for locally advanced bladder cancer. N Engl J Med 2003;349(9):859–66.

59. International Collaboration of Trialists, Medical
Research Council Advanced Bladder Cancer
Working Party (now the National Cancer Research
Institute Bladder Cancer Clinical Studies Group),
European Organisation for Research and Treat-
ment of Cancer Genito-Urinary Tract Cancer
Group, Australian Bladder Cancer Study Group,
National Cancer Institute of Canada Clinical Trials
Group, Finnbladder, Norwegian Bladder Cancer
Study Group, Club Urologico Espanol de Trata-
miento Oncologico Group, Griffiths G, Hall R,
Sylvester R, et al. International phase III trial as-
sessing neoadjuvant cisplatin, methotrexate, and
vinblastine chemotherapy for muscle-invasive
bladder cancer: long-term results of the BA06
30894 trial. J Clin Oncol 2011;29(16):2171–7.

60. Winquist E, Kirchner TS, Segal R, et al, Genitourinary Cancer Disease Site Group CCOPiE-bCPGI.
Neoadjuvant chemotherapy for transitional cell carcinoma of the bladder: a systematic review and
meta-analysis. J Urol 2004;171(2 Pt 1):561–9.

61. Advanced Bladder Cancer (ABC) Meta-analysis
Collaboration. Neoadjuvant chemotherapy in invasive
bladder cancer: update of a systematic review and
meta-analysis of individual patient data advanced
bladder cancer (ABC) meta-analysis collaboration.
Eur Urol 2005;48(2):202–5, [discussion: 205–6].

62. Lee JK, Havaleshko DM, Cho H, et al. A strategy for
predicting the chemosensitivity of human cancers
and its application to drug discovery. Proc Natl
Acad Sci U S A 2007;104(32):13086–91.

63. Williams PD, Cheon S, Havaleshko DM, et al.
Concordant gene expression signatures predict
clinical outcomes of cancer patients undergoing
systemic therapy. Cancer Res 2009;69(21):8302–9.

64. S1314, Co-expression Extrapolation (COXEN) Program to Predict Chemotherapy Response in Patients with Bladder Cancer (COXEN). Available at:
https://clinicaltrials.gov/ct2/show/NCT02177695.
Accessed April 1, 2018.

65. Shariat SF, Passoni N, Bagrodia A, et al. Prospective evaluation of a preoperative biomarker panel
for prediction of upstaging at radical cystectomy.
BJU Int 2014;113(1):70–6.

66. National Comprehensive Cancer Network. Bladder
Cancer (Version 3.2018). Available at: https://www.

nccn.org/professionals/physician_gls/pdf/bladder. pdf. Accessed April 1, 2018.

67. Reardon ZD, Patel SG, Zaid HB, et al. Trends in the use of perioperative chemotherapy for localized and locally advanced muscle-invasive bladder cancer: a sign of changing tides. Eur Urol 2015; 67(1):165–70.

68. Stein JP, Lieskovsky G, Cote R, et al. Radical cystectomy in the treatment of invasive bladder cancer: long-term results in 1,054 patients. J Clin Oncol 2001;19(3):666–75.

69. Madersbacher S, Hochreiter W, Burkhard F, et al. Radical cystectomy for bladder cancer today–a homogeneous series without neoadjuvant therapy. J Clin Oncol 2003;21(4):690–6.

70. Shariat SF, Karakiewicz PI, Palapattu GS, et al. Outcomes of radical cystectomy for transitional cell carcinoma of the bladder: a contemporary series from the Bladder Cancer Research Consortium. J Urol 2006;176(6 Pt 1):2414–22, [discussion: 2422].

71. Bassi P, Ferrante GD, Piazza N, et al. Prognostic factors of outcome after radical cystectomy for bladder cancer: a retrospective study of a homogeneous patient cohort. J Urol 1999;161(5):1494–7.

72. Dalbagni G, Genega E, Hashibe M, et al. Cystectomy for bladder cancer: a contemporary series. J Urol 2001;165(4):1111–6.

73. Advanced Bladder Cancer (ABC) Meta-analysis Collaboration. Adjuvant chemotherapy in invasive bladder cancer: a systematic review and meta-analysis of individual patient data Advanced Bladder Cancer (ABC) Meta-analysis Collaboration. Eur Urol 2005;48(2):189–99, [discussion: 199–201].

74. Leow JJ, Martin-Doyle W, Rajagopal PS, et al. Adjuvant chemotherapy for invasive bladder cancer: a 2013 updated systematic review and meta-analysis of randomized trials. Eur Urol 2014;66(1): 42–54.

75. Galsky MD, Stensland KD, Moshier E, et al. Effectiveness of adjuvant chemotherapy for locally advanced bladder cancer. J Clin Oncol 2016; 34(8):825–32.

76. von der Maase H, Sengelov L, Roberts JT, et al. Long-term survival results of a randomized trial comparing gemcitabine plus cisplatin, with methotrexate, vinblastine, doxorubicin, plus cisplatin in patients with bladder cancer. J Clin Oncol 2005; 23(21):4602–8.

77. Bellmunt J, von der Maase H, Mead GM, et al. Randomized phase III study comparing paclitaxel/ cisplatin/gemcitabine and gemcitabine/cisplatin in patients with locally advanced or metastatic urothelial cancer without prior systemic therapy: EORTC Intergroup Study 30987. J Clin Oncol 2012; 30(10):1107–13.

78. Sternberg CN, de Mulder P, Schornagel JH, et al. Seven year update of an EORTC phase III trial of high-dose intensity M-VAC chemotherapy and G-CSF versus classic M-VAC in advanced urothelial tract tumours. Eur J Cancer 2006;42(1):50–4.

79. Balar AV, Galsky MD, Rosenberg JE, et al. Atezolizumab as first-line treatment in cisplatin-ineligible patients with locally advanced and metastatic urothelial carcinoma: a single-arm, multicentre, phase 2 trial. Lancet 2017;389(10064):67–76.

80. Balar AV, Castellano D, O'Donnell PH, et al. First-line pembrolizumab in cisplatin-ineligible patients with locally advanced and unresectable or metastatic urothelial cancer (KEYNOTE-052): a multicentre, single-arm, phase 2 study. Lancet Oncol 2017;18(11):1483–92.

81. Powles T, Duran I, van der Heijden MS, et al. Atezolizumab versus chemotherapy in patients with platinum-treated locally advanced or metastatic urothelial carcinoma (IMvigor211): a multicentre, open-label, phase 3 randomised controlled trial. Lancet 2018;391(10122):748–57.

82. Rosenberg JE, Hoffman-Censits J, Powles T, et al. Atezolizumab in patients with locally advanced and metastatic urothelial carcinoma who have progressed following treatment with platinum-based chemotherapy: a single-arm, multicentre, phase 2 trial. Lancet 2016;387(10031):1909–20.

83. Apolo AB, Infante JR, Balmanoukian A, et al. Avelumab, an anti-programmed death-ligand 1 antibody, in patients with refractory metastatic urothelial carcinoma: results from a multicenter, phase Ib study. J Clin Oncol 2017;35(19):2117–24.

84. Patel MR, Ellerton J, Infante JR, et al. Avelumab in metastatic urothelial carcinoma after platinum failure (JAVELIN Solid Tumor): pooled results from two expansion cohorts of an open-label, phase 1 trial. Lancet Oncol 2018;19(1):51–64.

85. Powles T, O'Donnell PH, Massard C, et al. Efficacy and safety of durvalumab in locally advanced or metastatic urothelial carcinoma: updated results from a phase 1/2 open-label study. JAMA Oncol 2017;3(9):e172411.

86. Sharma P, Callahan MK, Bono P, et al. Nivolumab monotherapy in recurrent metastatic urothelial carcinoma (CheckMate 032): a multicentre, open-label, two-stage, multi-arm, phase 1/2 trial. Lancet Oncol 2016;17(11):1590–8.

87. Sharma P, Retz M, Siefker-Radtke A, et al. Nivolumab in metastatic urothelial carcinoma after platinum therapy (CheckMate 275): a multicentre, single-arm, phase 2 trial. Lancet Oncol 2017; 18(3):312–22.

88. Bellmunt J, de Wit R, Vaughn DJ, et al. Pembrolizumab as second-line therapy for advanced urothelial carcinoma. N Engl J Med 2017;376(11): 1015–26.

89. Galsky MD, Mironov S, Iasonos A, et al. Phase II trial of pemetrexed as second-line therapy in

patients with metastatic urothelial carcinoma. Invest New Drugs 2007;25(3):265–70.

90. Ko YJ, Canil CM, Mukherjee SD, et al. Nanoparticle albumin-bound paclitaxel for second-line treatment of metastatic urothelial carcinoma: a single group, multicentre, phase 2 study. Lancet Oncol 2013; 14(8):769–76.

91. McCaffrey JA, Hilton S, Mazumdar M, et al. Phase II trial of docetaxel in patients with advanced or metastatic transitional-cell carcinoma. J Clin Oncol 1997;15(5):1853–7.

92. Powles T, Necchi A, Rosen G, et al. Anti-programmed cell death 1/ligand 1 (PD-1/PD-L1) antibodies for the treatment of urothelial carcinoma: state of the art and future development. Clin Genitourin Cancer 2018;16(2):117–29.

93. Cheng ML, Iyer G. Novel biomarkers in bladder cancer. Urol Oncol 2018;36(3):115–9.

94. Plimack ER, Bellmunt J, Gupta S, et al. Safety and activity of pembrolizumab in patients with locally advanced or metastatic urothelial cancer (KEY-NOTE-012): a non-randomised, open-label, phase 1b study. Lancet Oncol 2017;18(2):212–20.

95. Teo MY, Bambury RM, Zabor EC, et al. DNA damage response and repair gene alterations are associated with improved survival in patients with platinum-treated advanced urothelial carcinoma. Clin Cancer Res 2017;23(14):3610–8.

96. Lynch SP, Shen Y, Kamat A, et al. Neoadjuvant chemotherapy in small cell urothelial cancer improves pathologic downstaging and long-term outcomes: results from a retrospective study at the MD Anderson Cancer Center. Eur Urol 2013;64(2):307–13.

97. Siefker-Radtke AO, Dinney CP, Abrahams NA, et al. Evidence supporting preoperative chemotherapy for small cell carcinoma of the bladder: a retrospective review of the M. D. Anderson cancer experience. J Urol 2004;172(2):481–4.

98. Siefker-Radtke AO, Kamat AM, Grossman HB, et al. Phase II clinical trial of neoadjuvant alternating doublet chemotherapy with ifosfamide/doxorubicin and etoposide/cisplatin in small-cell urothelial cancer. J Clin Oncol 2009;27(16):2592–7.

99. Vetterlein MW, Wankowicz SAM, Seisen T, et al. Neoadjuvant chemotherapy prior to radical cystectomy for muscle-invasive bladder cancer with variant histology. Cancer 2017;123(22):4346–55.

100. Meeks JJ, Taylor JM, Matsushita K, et al. Pathological response to neoadjuvant chemotherapy for muscle-invasive micropapillary bladder cancer. BJU Int 2013;111(8):E325–30.

101. Dayyani F, Czerniak BA, Sircar K, et al. Plasmacytoid urothelial carcinoma, a chemosensitive cancer with poor prognosis, and peritoneal carcinomatosis. J Urol 2013;189(5):1656–61.

102. Galsky MD, Iasonos A, Mironov S, et al. Prospective trial of ifosfamide, paclitaxel, and cisplatin in

patients with advanced non-transitional cell carcinoma of the urothelial tract. Urology 2007;69(2): 255–9.

103. Hussain M, Vaishampayan U, Du W, et al. Combination paclitaxel, carboplatin, and gemcitabine is an active treatment for advanced urothelial cancer. J Clin Oncol 2001;19(9):2527–33.

104. Siefker-Radtke AO, Gee J, Shen Y, et al. Multimodality management of urachal carcinoma: the M. D. Anderson Cancer Center experience. J Urol 2003;169(4):1295–8.

105. Mortensen MS, Lauritsen J, Gundgaard MG, et al. A nationwide cohort study of stage I seminoma patients followed on a surveillance program. Eur Urol 2014;66(6):1172–8.

106. Oliver RT, Mason MD, Mead GM, et al. Radiotherapy versus single-dose carboplatin in adjuvant treatment of stage I seminoma: a randomised trial. Lancet 2005;366(9482):293–300.

107. Travis LB, Curtis RE, Storm H, et al. Risk of second malignant neoplasms among long-term survivors of testicular cancer. J Natl Cancer Inst 1997;89(19): 1429–39.

108. Wanderas EH, Fossa SD, Tretli S. Risk of subsequent non-germ cell cancer after treatment of germ cell cancer in 2006 Norwegian male patients. Eur J Cancer 1997;33(2):253–62.

109. Zagars GK, Ballo MT, Lee AK, et al. Mortality after cure of testicular seminoma. J Clin Oncol 2004; 22(4):640–7.

110. Powles T, Robinson D, Shamash J, et al. The long-term risks of adjuvant carboplatin treatment for stage I seminoma of the testis. Ann Oncol 2008; 19(3):443–7.

111. Warde P, Specht L, Horwich A, et al. Prognostic factors for relapse in stage I seminoma managed by surveillance: a pooled analysis. J Clin Oncol 2002;20(22):4448–52.

112. Zengerling F, Kunath F, Jensen K, et al. Prognostic factors for tumor recurrence in patients with clinical stage I seminoma undergoing surveillance—a systematic review. Urol Oncol 2017, [pii:S1078-1439(17)30331-9].

113. Mortensen MS, Bandak M, Kier MG, et al. Surveillance versus adjuvant radiotherapy for patients with high-risk stage I seminoma. Cancer 2017; 123(7):1212–8.

114. Chung P, Daugaard G, Tyldesley S, et al. Evaluation of a prognostic model for risk of relapse in stage I seminoma surveillance. Cancer Med 2015;4(1):155–60.

115. Aparicio J, Maroto P, Garcia del Muro X, et al. Prognostic factors for relapse in stage I seminoma: a new nomogram derived from three consecutive, risk-adapted studies from the Spanish Germ Cell Cancer Group (SGCCG). Ann Oncol 2014;25(11): 2173–8.

116. Tandstad T, Stahl O, Dahl O, et al. Treatment of stage I seminoma, with one course of adjuvant carboplatin or surveillance, risk-adapted recommendations implementing patient autonomy: a report from the Swedish and Norwegian Testicular Cancer Group (SWENOTECA). Ann Oncol 2016;27(7): 1299–304.

117. Aparicio J, Maroto P, del Muro XG, et al. Risk-adapted treatment in clinical stage I testicular seminoma: the third Spanish Germ Cell Cancer Group study. J Clin Oncol 2011;29(35):4677–81.

118. Chung PW, Gospodarowicz MK, Panzarella T, et al. Stage II testicular seminoma: patterns of recurrence and outcome of treatment. Eur Urol 2004; 45(6):754–9, [discussion: 759–60].

119. Classen J, Schmidberger H, Meisner C, et al. Radiotherapy for stages IIA/B testicular seminoma: final report of a prospective multicenter clinical trial. J Clin Oncol 2003;21(6):1101–6.

120. Albers P, Siener R, Krege S, et al. Randomized phase III trial comparing retroperitoneal lymph node dissection with one course of bleomycin and etoposide plus cisplatin chemotherapy in the adjuvant treatment of clinical stage I nonseminomatous testicular germ cell tumors: AUO trial AH 01/94 by the German Testicular Cancer Study Group. J Clin Oncol 2008;26(18):2966–72.

121. Tandstad T, Stahl O, Hakansson U, et al. One course of adjuvant BEP in clinical stage I nonseminoma mature and expanded results from the SWENOTECA group. Ann Oncol 2014;25(11): 2167–72.

122. Read G, Stenning SP, Cullen MH, et al. Medical Research Council prospective study of surveillance for stage I testicular teratoma. Medical Research Council Testicular Tumors Working Party. J Clin Oncol 1992;10(11):1762–8.

123. Vergouwe Y, Steyerberg EW, Eijkemans MJ, et al. Predictors of occult metastasis in clinical stage I nonseminoma: a systematic review. J Clin Oncol 2003;21(22):4092–9.

124. Nicolai N, Pizzocaro G. A surveillance study of clinical stage I nonseminomatous germ cell tumors of the testis: 10-year followup. J Urol 1995;154(3):1045–9.

125. Freedman LS, Parkinson MC, Jones WG, et al. Histopathology in the prediction of relapse of patients with stage I testicular teratoma treated by orchidectomy alone. Lancet 1987;2(8554):294–8.

126. Stang A, Jansen L, Trabert B, et al. Survival after a diagnosis of testicular germ cell cancers in Germany and the United States, 2002-2006: a high resolution study by histology and age. Cancer Epidemiol 2013;37(4):492–7.

127. Alvarado-Cabrero I, Hernandez-Toriz N, Paner GP. Clinicopathologic analysis of choriocarcinoma as a pure or predominant component of germ cell tumor of the testis. Am J Surg Pathol 2014;38(1):111–8.

128. Verrill C, Yilmaz A, Srigley JR, et al. Reporting and staging of testicular germ cell tumors: the International Society of Urological Pathology (ISUP) Testicular Cancer Consultation Conference Recommendations. Am J Surg Pathol 2017;41(6):e22–32.

129. International Germ Cell Consensus Classification: a prognostic factor-based staging system for metastatic germ cell cancers. International Germ Cell Cancer Collaborative Group. J Clin Oncol 1997; 15(2):594–603.

130. Korkola JE, Houldsworth J, Dobrzynski D, et al. Gene expression-based classification of nonseminomatous male germ cell tumors. Oncogene 2005;24(32):5101–7.

131. Korkola JE, Houldsworth J, Feldman DR, et al. Identification and validation of a gene expression signature that predicts outcome in adult men with germ cell tumors. J Clin Oncol 2009;27(31):5240–7.

132. Motzer RJ, Geller NL, Tan CC, et al. Salvage chemotherapy for patients with germ cell tumors. The Memorial Sloan-Kettering Cancer Center experience (1979-1989). Cancer 1991;67(5):1305–10.

133. Fossa SD, Stenning SP, Gerl A, et al. Prognostic factors in patients progressing after cisplatin-based chemotherapy for malignant non-seminomatous germ cell tumours. Br J Cancer 1999;80(9):1392–9.

134. Einhorn LH, Williams SD, Chamness A, et al. High-dose chemotherapy and stem-cell rescue for metastatic germ-cell tumors. N Engl J Med 2007; 357(4):340–8.

135. Beyer J, Kramar A, Mandanas R, et al. High-dose chemotherapy as salvage treatment in germ cell tumors: a multivariate analysis of prognostic variables. J Clin Oncol 1996;14(10):2638–45.

136. Moch H, Cubilla AL, Humphrey PA, et al. The 2016 WHO classification of tumours of the urinary system and male genital organs—part a: renal, penile, and testicular tumours. Eur Urol 2016;70(1):93–105.

137. Idrees MT, Ulbright TM, Oliva E, et al. The World Health Organization 2016 classification of testicular non-germ cell tumours: a review and update from the International Society of Urological Pathology Testis Consultation Panel. Histopathology 2017; 70(4):513–21.

138. Bertram KA, Bratloff B, Hodges GF, et al. Treatment of malignant Leydig cell tumor. Cancer 1991; 68(10):2324–9.

139. Young RH, Koelliker DD, Scully RE. Sertoli cell tumors of the testis, not otherwise specified: a clinicopathologic analysis of 60 cases. Am J Surg Pathol 1998;22(6):709–21.

140. Hammerich KH, Hille S, Ayala GE, et al. Malignant advanced granulosa cell tumor of the adult testis: case report and review of the literature. Hum Pathol 2008;39(5):701–9.

141. Scully RE. Gonadoblastoma. A review of 74 cases. Cancer 1970;25(6):1340–56.

Urologic Pathology
Key Parameters from a Urologist's Perspective

Alex Borchert, MD, Craig G. Rogers, MD*

KEYWORDS

- Prostate cancer • Bladder cancer • Kidney cancer • Renal cell carcinoma

Key points

- Prostate cancer, bladder cancer, and kidney cancer form a heterogenous group of disease processes, with a wide range of pathologic features.
- Accurate and detailed pathologic reporting is essential to optimize treatment for urologic patients.
- The recent changes in pathologic reporting and pathologic classification systems necessitate that all members of a multidisciplinary urologic oncology team have an up-to-date understanding of the specific pathologic parameters of various urologic malignancies.

ABSTRACT

Prostate cancer, bladder cancer, and kidney cancer represent the 3 most common urologic malignancies, and form a heterogenous group of disease processes, with a wide range of pathologic features. As a urologist, a strong understanding of the pathologic features of urologic malignancies is essential to prognosticate and counsel patients and to determine the most effective course of treatment. This review discusses the pathologic features of prostate, bladder, and kidney cancer, and examines how detailed pathologic reporting is critical to today's practicing urologist.

OVERVIEW

In 2018, there will be an estimated 315,040 new cases of prostate, bladder, or kidney cancer in the United States, with an estimated 52,540 deaths.[1] These cancers represent the 3 most common urologic malignancies and form a heterogenous group of disease processes, with a wide range of pathologic features. Accordingly, effective and efficient care requires a multidisciplinary team of urologists, pathologists, medical oncologists, and radiation oncologists. As a clinician, a strong understanding of the pathologic features of urologic malignancies is essential to prognosticate and counsel patients, and to determine the most effective course of treatment. In this review, we discuss the pathologic features of prostate, bladder, and kidney cancers and examine how detailed pathologic reporting is essential to today's practicing urologist.

PROSTATE CANCER

Prostate cancer is the most common malignancy among men, estimated to account for nearly 1 in 5 new cases of cancer in 2018.[1] After the widespread adoption of prostate-specific antigen (PSA) testing as a means of screening for prostate cancer, the incidence of prostate cancer diagnosis on prostate needle biopsy (PNB) dramatically increased. This advance led to a marked increase in prostate cancer treatment, including radical prostatectomy and radiation therapy, with associated morbidity, including incontinence and sexual impotence. However, prostate cancer is generally

Disclosure Statement: None.
Vattikuti Urology Institute, Henry Ford Health System, 2799 W Grand Boulevard, Detroit, MI 48202, USA
* Corresponding author.
E-mail address: crogers2@hfhs.org

Surgical Pathology 11 (2018) 893–901
https://doi.org/10.1016/j.path.2018.07.012
1875-9181/18/© 2018 Elsevier Inc. All rights reserved.

a slow-growing disease and the majority of men who are diagnosed will experience no symptoms and will ultimately die of some other cause. Although there is a clear need for the early detection of high-risk disease, there is a risk of overtreatment associated with increased screening. As a result, there has been a renewed effort to identify those patients with cancer in need of prompt intervention, while simultaneously refining management strategies for patients with lower risk disease, for whom strategies characterized by periodic surveillance can be successful.

Depending on patient age, comorbidities, and disease characteristics, low-risk and intermediate-risk prostate cancer can be managed by several options, including (1) no treatment, (2) active surveillance, or (3) definitive treatment with radical prostatectomy (RP) or radiation therapy. Active surveillance entails close monitoring of biopsy-proven prostate cancer, through a combination of regimented PSA screening, digital rectal examinations, and repeat prostate biopsy and/or prostate MRI. If the disease progresses or is discovered to be more aggressive than initially anticipated, definitive treatment can be recommended. Determining if a patient is appropriate for active surveillance, and subsequently determining when to recommend treatment for a patient on active surveillance, remains a challenging task for today's urologist. Risk stratification is critical to determining an appropriate management strategy for these patients. Disease risk is determined primarily by PNB specimen characteristics, with additional information provided by digital rectal examination findings (clinical stage) and serum PSA. PNB reports should include Gleason grade, the number of positive cores, the volume of cancer within each core, presence/absence of perineural invasion, and presence/absence of lymphovascular invasion.

Key Features
IMPORTANT PATHOLOGIC PARAMETERS IN PROSTATE CANCER

Prostate Needle Biopsy	Radical Prostatectomy
Gleason grade	Gleason grade
Number of positive cores	Pathologic stage
Volume of cancer within each core	Margin status
Presence of perineural invasion	Presence of lymphovascular invasion
Presence of lymphovascular invasion	Lymph node positivity (if sampled)

Gleason grade remains the most useful tissue-based parameter for prognostic stratification.[2] As pathologic diagnosis of prostate cancer and treatments have evolved, the Gleason grading system has been revised. A new prostate cancer grading system was developed during the 2014 International Society of Urologic Pathology Consensus Conference. This new system is characterized by the organization of pathologic specimens into Gleason grade groups (1–5), derived from Gleason score, and was developed with the goal of providing better prognostic information to patients.

Key Features
PROSTATE CANCER GRADE GROUPS

- Grade group 1 out of 5 is more relatable to patients as the best possible grade, compared with 3 + 3 = 6 out of 10

- Groups 2 and 3 discriminate Gleason score 3 + 4 = 7 (grade group 2) from Gleason score 4 + 3 = 7 (grade group 3)

A 2015 study validated the 2014 International Society of Urologic Pathology Gleason grade grouping, demonstrating 5-year biochemical recurrence-free progression probabilities for Gleason scores of 6 or less, 3 + 4, 4 + 3, 8, and 9 to 10 of 96%, 88%, 63%, 48%, and 26%, respectively.[3] Subsequent studies have demonstrated the utility of this grading system in predicting cancer-specific mortality and bony metastasis.[4,5] As a result, the National Comprehensive Cancer Network (NCCN) guidelines adopted Gleason grade grouping into its recommendations. At our institution, we have found this new grade grouping to be particularly helpful when counseling a patient regarding a new prostate cancer diagnosis. Patients often find it easier comprehend a grading scale of 1 to 5 and this understanding can make it easier for an individual to be agreeable to active surveillance.

Key Features
GLEASON GRADE GROUPING

Grade Group 1	Gleason Grade 3 + 3 = 6
Grade group 2	Gleason grade 3 + 4 = 7
Grade group 3	Gleason grade 4 + 3 = 7
Grade group 4	Gleason grade 4 + 4 = 8
Grade group 5	Gleason grade ≥ 9

Pathologic parameters including the number of positive cores and the volume of cancer within each core have become increasingly important in distinguishing patients eligible for active surveillance. Gleason 6 disease or lower has very low metastatic potential and exceptional survival outcomes.[6] In a 2012 retrospective study evaluating 14,123 cases of Gleason 6 disease or lower, only 22 cases (0.1%) had positive lymph nodes. Upon review of these positive samples within the new International Society of Urologic Pathology scoring criteria, all were upgraded to at least Gleason 3 + 4, demonstrating that not a single case of contemporary Gleason 6 tumor or lower was associated with metastatic disease.[7] In the absence of adverse clinical parameters, Gleason 6 (grade group 1) disease places a patient into 1 of the 2 lowest NCCN risk groups and, although definitive treatment can be considered, these patients are generally considered good candidates for active surveillance. However, patients with favorable intermediate risk prostate cancer are increasingly being considered for active surveillance. These patients have organ-confined Gleason 3 + 4 = 7 disease, with a PSA of less than 20 and fewer than 50% positive cores. A 2013 retrospective study of 1024 patients treated with external beam radiation therapy determined that intermediate risk patients with primary Gleason 4, percentage of positive cores of more than 50%, or more than 1 intermediate risk factor (cT2b-c, PSA 10–20, or Gleason score 7) had a significantly increased risk of metastasis. Additionally,

primary Gleason 4 and percentage of positive cores of more than 50% independently predicted an increased cancer-specific mortality.[8] Accordingly, the percentage of positive cores becomes paramount in evaluating patients with Gleason 3 + 4 = 7 (grade group 2) disease, because the burden of tumor seems to have significant prognostic implications. A greater percentage of Gleason 4 within Gleason 3 + 4 = 7 (grade group 2) or Gleason 4 + 3 (grade group 3) within a biopsy specimen can also influence treatment decisions. Current NCCN guidelines use a combination of pathologic and clinical parameters to determine patient risk and the NCCN has incorporated these findings into the current guidelines, and recommends that patients with favorable intermediate risk prostate cancer be considered for active surveillance.

Notably, PNB Gleason grade commonly does not correlate with RP Gleason grade. There is a significant risk of upgrading or change in Gleason grade between PNB specimen and RP specimen. This outcome is especially true for low-risk disease (Gleason 3 + 3 = 6, grade group 1), with upgrading occurring in approximately 36% to 67% of patients.[9–11] Although the majority of Gleason 3 + 3 = 6 patients who are upgraded are upgraded to Gleason 3 + 4 = 7 (grade group 2) disease, 10% to 15% of patients may be upgraded to Gleason grade group 3 or higher. Studies have demonstrated that age, PSA density, cT stage, and percentage of positive cores are independently associated with a higher risk of upgrading.[12,13] The cause of these relatively high rates of upgrading is not completely understood. Transrectal PNB provides only a sampling of the prostate gland and can miss areas of disease, particularly in the anterior zone, which is difficult to technically access from a transrectal approach. The number of cores sampled on transrectal biopsy has increased over time, from 6, to 12, and now commonly to 14 (with the additional 2 cores sampling the anterior zone). Transperineal saturation biopsies may be considered as a means to overcome the sampling error associated with the transrectal approach. Additionally, the widespread adoption of multiparametric prostate MRI and image-guided biopsy techniques will likely lead to increased diagnostic accuracy.[14] Nevertheless, the clinical implications of upgrading remain largely unknown and long-term survival data are not available. Accordingly, urologists should be aware of the risk of upgrading when interpreting biopsy results.

Key Features
FAVORABLE INTERMEDIATE VERSUS UNFAVORABLE INTERMEDIATE RISK GROUPS

Favorable intermediate	T2b-T2c OR Gleason score 3 + 4 = 7/ grade group 2 OR Prostate-specific antigen 10–20 ng/mL AND Percentage of positive biopsy cores <50%
Unfavorable intermediate	T2b-T2c OR Gleason score 3 + 4 = 7/ grade group 2 or Gleason score 4 + 3 = 7/grade group 3 OR Prostate-specific antigen 10–20 ng/mL

Adapted from 2018 NCCN Prostate Cancer Guidelines.

The presence or absence of perineural invasion is commonly reported on PNB. Some studies have demonstrated that perineural invasion in PNB specimens is an independent risk factor for aggressive pathology on RP and is independently associated with extraprostatic extension and seminal vesicle invasion, as well as an increased risk of biochemical recurrence.[15–17] Similarly, it has been demonstrated that lymphovascular invasion is also an independent risk factor for biochemical recurrence.[17] However, other studies have reported that perineural invasion is not associated with adverse pathologic outcomes.[18] Ultimately, current NCCN guidelines do not incorporate the presence or absence of perineural invasion into risk stratification.

Determining adjuvant therapy after RP is largely guided by the presence or absence of disease within lymph nodes, surgical margin status, and pathologic staging. Positive lymph node involvement remains the most important prognostic factor after RP. Not only does an extended lymph node dissection lead to more accurate clinical staging, but an extended pelvic lymph node dissection has been associated with improved mortality in select patients.[19] Patients with positive lymph nodes are often treated with adjuvant androgen deprivation therapy. However, adjuvant radiation therapy has demonstrated benefits in certain patients. A recent study has identified that patients with 1 to 2 positive nodes, pathologic Gleason score 7 to 10, and pT3b/4 disease or positive surgical margins, as well as patients with 3 to 4 positive lymph nodes, regardless of local tumor characteristics, had improved overall mortality when treated with adjuvant radiation therapy.[20] Additionally, surgical margin status and presence of any seminal vesicle involvement must be reported, because it can help to guide patient counseling postoperatively. Adjuvant radiation therapy in patients with extraprostatic extension or involvement of the seminal vesicles has been demonstrated to lead to improved biochemical failure-free survival.[21,22]

The presence of variant pathology, such as neuroendocrine prostate cancer, is associated with significantly lower overall survival as compared with traditional prostate adenocarcinoma. This variant pathology is commonly found in patients with a low or moderately increasing PSA, but extensive local or metastatic disease.[23] These patients should be managed by multidisciplinary care teams, and aggressive therapy should be recommended.

Although our understanding of prostate cancer continues to improve, the appropriate treatment for patients with localized low and intermediate risk prostate cancer remains in question. The organization of Gleason grading into grade groups has increased the prognostic power of PNB. Additional pathologic parameters including the number of positive cores, the volume of cancer within each core, and perineural invasion will likely become increasingly important as our ability to predict long-term outcomes improves. Particularly as the role of active surveillance expands, fastidious pathologic reporting and open collaboration between pathologists and clinicians will continue to improve risk stratification and ensure the identification of ideal candidates.

BLADDER CANCER

Bladder cancer is most commonly diagnosed as a result of either gross or microscopic hematuria and is characterized by a wide range of clinical presentations, from a small, solitary, superficial, papillary lesion, to widespread carcinoma in situ (CIS) with no discrete cystoscopically appreciable lesions, to a large, solid-appearing, invasive bladder mass with resulting hydronephrosis and renal failure. However, cystoscopic or radiographic diagnosis alone is insufficient, and accurate pathologic analysis of bladder tumor specimens is crucial to determining and optimizing treatment strategies.

Pathologic reports of bladder biopsies and transurethral resection of bladder tumor (TURBT) specimens should include information regarding histologic subtype, tumor grade (high grade or low grade), depth of tumor invasion (stage), presence or absence of muscle within the specimen, presence or absence of CIS, and presence or absence of lymphovascular invasion. Notably, it is crucial that pathologists, when reporting the findings of TURBT specimens, distinguish between invasion of the muscle (pTa or pT1 vs pT2) and invasion of the lamina propria (pTa vs pT1), because the difference has significant prognostic and management implications.

The presence of variant pathology in bladder tumor specimens is of critical importance and should always be reported, including the percentage of

Key Features
SELECTING PATIENTS FOR ADJUVANT
THERAPY AFTER PROSTATECTOMY

- Lymph node involvement
- Margin status
- Pathologic stage (extraprostatic extension and seminal vesicle invasion)

> ## Key Features
> ### IMPORTANT PATHOLOGIC PARAMETERS IN BLADDER CANCER
>
> Histologic subtype
>
> Tumor grade
>
> Tumor stage (depth of invasion)
>
> Presence of muscle within specimen
>
> Presence of CIS
>
> Presence of lymphovascular invasion

histologic variant. Variant pathologies, such as micropapillary, plasmacytoid, or small cell, are associated with a higher risk of disease progression and as such are often managed with a more aggressive treatment approach. Although small cell bladder cancer may respond to chemotherapy, micropapillary and plasmacytoid bladder cancers often require aggressive surgical intervention. Micropapillary and plasmacytoid bladder cancers are often progressed to advanced stage at the time of diagnosis and mortality rates are generally high, with a 5-year overall survival for patients with micropapillary cancer of 54% and a 5-year overall survival rate in patients with plasmacytoid bladder cancer of less than 30%.[24] As a result, cystectomy is often recommended for these patients, regardless of the presence of muscle invasion.

The most important pathologic parameter in determining treatment for bladder cancer is the presence of, or absence of, muscular invasion. As a result, bladder cancer is broadly categorized into 2 groups: non–muscle-invasive bladder cancer (NMIBC), and muscle-invasive bladder cancer (MIBC).

NMIBC is characterized by multiple decision points for both the clinician and the patient,[25] and the American Urological Association uses 3 risk groups to help guide decision making. Approximately 75% of bladder tumors present as NMIBC and, because this entity is characterized by relatively high rates of recurrence and disease progression, NMIBC represents a significant burden to the patient, and can present management dilemmas for the treating physician.[26]

Tumor stage and grade represent the most important pathologic parameters in guiding the management of NMIBC. Although histologic grading is highly subjective in nature, grade represents one of the most powerful prognostic factors in bladder cancer. A 2013 study on 3633 patients with low-grade cTa bladder cancer, examined the rates of recurrence and progression. The study reported an approximate 28.5% rate of recurrence at a median of 13.5 months and a rate of progression of 4.7% at a median time of 35.7 months.[27] Disease-specific mortality was only 2.4% at a median of 55 months.[27] Given the low rates of cancer-specific mortality and relatively low rates of progression, patients with low-grade cTa disease can be managed with observation. However, metaanalyses have demonstrated a reduction in recurrence rate for patients who receive immediate after TUR chemotherapy.[28] Conversely, presence of high-grade disease is associated with a higher risk of recurrence and progression. Intravesical BCG is widely recommended as the first-line therapy for high-grade, non–muscle-invasive disease, largely owing to a decreased rate of recurrence as compared with TURBT alone.[29]

Additionally, for patients with cT1 disease (regardless of grade) or for those in whom no muscle was present in the initial resection specimen, it is recommended to undergo repeat TURBT within 6 weeks of the initial resection. Repeat TURBT is associated with significantly improved recurrence-free survival rates, with 3-year recurrence free survival rates of 68.72% and 37.01% for patients undergoing repeat TUR and those who did not, respectively.[30] The presence of residual high-grade disease, lymphovascular invasion, or presence of CIS in repeat TURBT specimens, particularly in patients with high-volume disease, can influence the decision between cystectomy or intravesical BCG, and as such, accurate reporting of lymphovascular invasion and CIS is of particular importance.

> ## Key Features
> ### INDICATIONS FOR REPEAT TRANSURETHRAL RESECTION OF BLADDER TUMOR
>
> - Absence of muscularis propria in original TURBT
> - Any pT1 disease

> ## Key Features
> ### IMPORTANT PATHOLOGIC PARAMETERS IN REPEAT TRANSURETHRAL RESECTION OF BLADDER TUMOR
>
> - Residual high-grade tumor
> - Lymphovascular invasion
> - Presence of CIS

For patients with Tis, cTa, or cT1 disease recurrence after initial intravesical treatment, management with either repeat intravesical therapy or cystectomy can be considered. In particular, patients who have failed 2 courses of intravesical therapy should be considered for cystectomy. Additionally, the timing of disease recurrence is important in determining management. In 1 study of 90 patients undergoing cystectomy after recurrence after intravesical therapy, the 15-year disease-specific survival rate was 69% in those patients undergoing cystectomy within 2 years of recurrence, compared with 26% in those patients who underwent cystectomy after 2 years.[31]

For those patients with MIBC (≥pT2), recommended treatment involves radical cystectomy with or without prior neoadjuvant platinum-based chemotherapy. Although radical cystectomy has long been considered the gold standard in treatment for these patients, the surgery carries high morbidity and high rates of associated complications. Accordingly, bladder preservation with maximal TURBT and concurrent chemotherapy and radiation has been considered an option for carefully selected patients. Notably, clinical series have demonstrated a similar 5-year overall survival between patients undergoing radical cystectomy and those undergoing maximal TURBT with chemotherapy and radiation, with rates of 40% to 60%.[32,33] However, this finding should be tempered by the fact that certain patients are not eligible for bladder preservation therapy. Patients with cT3-4, N+, or M+ disease; presence of CIS; multifocal lesions; or variant or aggressive histology can be considered high risk and should not be considered candidates for bladder preservation therapy.[34–36]

Although much of this decision making is based on clinical features found on either computed tomography scan or during operative resection, accurate pathologic reporting of CIS and any variant histology is essential for specimens with MIBC, because the presence of either of these entities may preclude bladder preservation therapy as a management option. Additionally, for patients who may be candidates for orthotopic neobladder creation, a prostatic urethral biopsy should be sent to rule out urethral disease. For patients with 2 or more areas of disease, the onus is on the operating urologist to correctly label specimen location at the time of resection, because as there may be a role for partial cystectomy in patients with localized muscle-invasive disease.

RENAL CELL CARCINOMA

There will be an estimated 65,340 new cases of kidney and renal pelvis cancers in 2018, and renal cell carcinoma (RCC) will account for more than 90% of these.[1] The lifetime risk of developing this cancer is estimated to be between 1.2% and 2.1%.[1] RCC is a heterogenous disease, representing a collection of distinct types of tumors, each derived from various parts of the nephron, each possessing unique genetic characteristics and tumor biology.[37] Although tumor stage and grade are important prognostic factors, the diagnosis of RCC is largely imaging based, the management of RCC is predominantly surgical, and the decision to treat is commonly made with no information regarding tumor pathology.

With the dissemination and widespread use of computed tomography, the incidence of RCC has dramatically increased, and the majority of new cases are diagnosed at an earlier stage. Accordingly, there has been an increasing incidence in the diagnosis of small renal masses (SRMs), defined as a contrast-enhancing mass within the kidney, with the largest dimension of 4 cm or less.[38] The gold standard for treatment for SRMs is surgical removal. However, SRMs have shown relatively low rate of metastasis, with less than 2% of SRMs progressing to metastatic disease when monitored by serial imaging, with the majority of cases of metastasis thought to arise in tumors greater than 3 cm. Additionally, the growth rate of SRMs is variable—in a retrospective analysis evaluating SRM growth kinetics over a mean of 1.83 years, only 17% of SRMs grew at a rate of more than 0.5 cm/y, and 35.4% of SRMs became smaller.[39] Most importantly, 20% to 25% of radiologically suspicious SRMs are benign.[38]

Over the past decade, in light of this evidence, we have seen an expanded interest in renal mass biopsy (RMB) as a tool to potentially avoid unnecessary treatment and support treatment decisions. Consequently, the role of pathologists in the management of SRMs has expanded. The reported sensitivity and specificity of RMB is 86% to 100% and 100%, respectively. The accurate assessment of Fuhrman nuclear grade is more difficult, with accuracy rates between 63% to 76%.[38] A 2016 systematic review of RMB including 20 studies with 2979 patients and 3113 biopsies demonstrated high sensitivity (97.5%; 95% confidence interval, 96.5–98.5) and specificity (96.2%; 95% confidence interval, 90.7–100.0), but an overall nondiagnostic rate of 14.1%.[40] This significant rate of nondiagnostic biopsy may be owing to a number of factors, including tumor size, location, proximity to vital structures, cystic components, inadequate quantity of specimen, or inability to definitively diagnose a tumor based on the provided biopsy specimen. However, it has been demonstrated that repeat biopsy after initial nondiagnostic biopsy yields a diagnosis in 80% of cases.[40] Pathologists at a given center can assist clinicians by providing detailed feedback regarding nondiagnostic biopsies, thereby potentially improving diagnostic yield in future biopsy specimens. Nonetheless, the majority of patients treated with surgery for SRMs do not undergo preoperative RMB. Although an RMB demonstrating benign disease can avoid a potential surgery, an RMB confirming malignancy will generally not alter management decisions. In our institution, RMB is most often used in patients who carry a high surgical risk as a means to potentially avoid a morbid surgery. Additionally, RMB is widely used when benign disease is suspected, for a patient with suspected synchronous or metachronous bilateral renal masses, or when a renal mass is identified in a patient with metastatic disease, but without a pathologic diagnosis.

> ### Key Features
> #### IMPORTANT PATHOLOGIC PARAMETERS IN PARTIAL AND RADICAL NEPHRECTOMY SPECIMENS
>
> - Pathologic stage
> - Nuclear grade
> - Presence or absence of necrosis
> - Margin status
> - Microvascular invasion
> - Lymph node involvement

Various studies have attempted to determine pathologic parameters that are associated with disease progression and clinical outcomes. A 2005 retrospective analysis reported that both microvascular invasion and Fuhrman grade were significantly associated with disease recurrence.[41] A 2018 study assessed 23,632 patients from the SEER database treated with partial or radical nephrectomy for nonmetastatic RCC, and demonstrated an increased cancer-specific mortality in patients with lymph node involvement, pT3a-b, or Fuhrman grade 3 to 4 disease.[42] Nomograms such as the UCLA Integrated Staging System and the Stage, Size, Grade and Necrosis Score, which use pathologic parameters, have been developed to assist in patient counseling and prognostication. More recently, these nomograms have been used as criteria for enrollment in clinical trials. As an example, the role of adjuvant therapy after surgery for localized RCC is currently not well-established. There is increasing evidence that pathologic parameters may assist in determining which patients would be most likely to benefit from adjuvant therapy. The S-TRAC trial randomized 615 high-risk patients with locoregional RCC to adjuvant sunitinib versus placebo. The trial demonstrated that adjuvant sunitinib significantly improved disease-free survival versus placebo.[43] As a result, current NCCN guidelines suggest that physicians consider adjuvant sunitinib for stage III RCC with clear cell histology and high-risk features.

> ### Key Features
> #### COMMON INDICATIONS FOR RENAL MASS BIOPSY
>
> - Patients with high risk of complications from surgery
> - Suspicion of benign disease
> - Suspected synchronous or metachronous bilateral renal masses
> - Renal mass with metastatic disease of unknown pathology

Although the decision to proceed with surgical treatment of RCC is usually made without pathologic information, RCC specimen pathologic findings play an important role in determining prognosis and future management. Pathologic reports on RCC surgical specimens should include tumor stage, Fuhrman grade, presence or absence of tumor necrosis, margin status, presence or absence of microvascular invasion, and presence of nodal involvement, if nodes were provided.

With respect to metastatic RCC, the role of pathologists in determining appropriate patient selection and treatment continues to expand. As new targeted therapies for metastatic RCC are developed, pathologists will be crucial in differentiating tumor subtypes and identifying molecular markers by which to guide the choice of therapeutic agent. The role of renal biopsy has continued to expand in this area, because pathologic diagnosis is increasingly able to guide selection of systemic therapy. As treatment options for metastatic RCC expand, collaboration between pathologists, medical oncologists, and urologists will be essential to optimizing patient care.

Key Features
ROLE OF RENAL MASS
BIOPSY IN METASTATIC DISEASE

- Targeted therapies continue to evolve.

- Pathologists play an increasing key role in interpreting biopsies of metastatic renal cancer.

- Histologic subtype, and, in the future, molecular markers, may be critical.

SUMMARY

Prostate cancer, bladder cancer, and renal cancer make up the 3 most common urologic malignancies. Appropriate management of each of these cancers relies on accurate and informed interpretation of urologic pathologic specimens. The pathologist plays an integral role in accurate risk stratification and treatment planning. Although both urologists and pathologists should have an in-depth understanding of the various pathologic parameters, effective and efficient care should include a multidisciplinary team of urologists, pathologists, medical oncologists, and radiation oncologists, all working together to optimize patient outcomes.

REFERENCES

1. Siegel RL, Miller KD, Jemal A. Cancer statistics, 2018. CA Cancer J Clin 2018;68(1):7–30.

2. Egevad L, Delahunt B, Kristiansen G, et al. Contemporary prognostic indicators for prostate cancer incorporating International Society of Urological Pathology recommendations. Pathology 2018;50(1): 60–73.

3. Epstein JI, Zelefsky MJ, Sjoberg DD, et al. A contemporary prostate cancer grading system: a validated alternative to the Gleason score. Eur Urol 2016;69(3):428–35.

4. Leapman MS, Cowan JE, Simko J, et al. Application of a prognostic Gleason grade grouping system to assess distant prostate cancer outcomes. Eur Urol 2017;71(5):750–9.

5. He J, Albertsen PC, Moore D, et al. Validation of a contemporary five-tiered Gleason grade grouping using population-based data. Eur Urol 2017;71(5): 760–3.

6. Eggener SE, Scardino PT, Walsh PC, et al. Predicting 15-year prostate cancer specific mortality after radical prostatectomy. J Urol 2011;185(3): 869–75.

7. Ross HM, Kryvenko ON, Cowan JE, et al. Do adenocarcinomas of the prostate with Gleason score (GS) ≤6 have the potential to metastasize to lymph nodes? Am J Surg Pathol 2012;36(9):1346–52.

8. Zumsteg ZS, Spratt DE, Pei I, et al. A new risk classification system for therapeutic decision making with intermediate-risk prostate cancer patients undergoing dose-escalated external-beam radiation therapy. Eur Urol 2013;64(6):895–902.

9. Cohen MS, Hanley RS, Kurteva T, et al. Comparing the Gleason prostate biopsy and Gleason prostatectomy grading system: the Lahey Clinic Medical Center experience and an international meta-analysis. Eur Urol 2008;54(2):371–81.

10. Epstein JI, Feng Z, Trock BJ, et al. Upgrading and downgrading of prostate cancer from biopsy to radical prostatectomy: incidence and predictive factors using the modified Gleason grading system and factoring in tertiary grades. Eur Urol 2012;61(5): 1019–24.

11. Corcoran NM, Hovens CM, Hong MK, et al. Underestimation of Gleason score at prostate biopsy reflects sampling error in lower volume tumours. BJU Int 2012;109(5):660–4.

12. Yang DD, Mahal BA, Muralidhar V, et al. Risk of upgrading and upstaging among 10 000 patients with Gleason 3+4 favorable intermediate-risk prostate cancer. Eur Urol Focus 2017, [pii:S2405-4569(17) 30148-7].

13. Audenet F, Rozet F, Resche-Rigon M, et al. Grade group underestimation in prostate biopsy: predictive factors and outcomes in candidates for active surveillance. Clin Genitourin Cancer 2017;15(6): e907–13.

14. Siddiqui MM, Rais-Bahrami S, Turkbey B, et al. Comparison of MR/ultrasound fusion-guided biopsy with ultrasound-guided biopsy for the diagnosis of prostate cancer. JAMA 2015;313(4):390–7.

15. Harnden P, Shelley MD, Clements H, et al. The prognostic significance of perineural invasion in prostatic cancer biopsies: a systematic review. Cancer 2007; 109(1):13–24.

16. Loeb S, Epstein JI, Humphreys EB, et al. Does perineural invasion on prostate biopsy predict adverse prostatectomy outcomes? BJU Int 2010;105(11): 1510–3.

17. Kang M, Oh JJ, Lee S, et al. Perineural invasion and lymphovascular invasion are associated with increased risk of biochemical recurrence in patients undergoing radical prostatectomy. Ann Surg Oncol 2016;23:2699–706.

18. Al-Hussain T, Carter HB, Epstein JI. Significance of prostate adenocarcinoma perineural invasion on biopsy in patients who are otherwise candidates for active surveillance. J Urol 2011;186(2):470–3.

19. Abdollah F, Gandaglia G, Suardi N, et al. More extensive pelvic lymph node dissection improves survival in patients with node-positive prostate cancer. Eur Urol 2015;67(2):212–9.

20. Abdollah F, Dalela D, Sood A, et al. Impact of adjuvant radiotherapy in node-positive prostate cancer patients: the importance of patient selection. Eur Urol 2018;74(3).

21. Van der Kwast TH, Bolla M, Van Poppel H, et al. Identification of patients with prostate cancer who benefit from immediate postoperative radiotherapy: EORTC 22911. J Clin Oncol 2007;25(27): 4178–86.

22. Swanson GP, Goldman B, Tangen CM, et al. The prognostic impact of seminal vesicle involvement found at prostatectomy and the effects of adjuvant radiation: data from Southwest Oncology Group 8794. J Urol 2008;180(6):2453–7, [discussion: 2458].

23. Vlachostergios PJ, Puca L, Beltran H. Emerging variants of castration-resistant prostate cancer. Curr Oncol Rep 2017;19(5):32.

24. Warrick JI. Clinical significance of histologic variants of bladder cancer. J Natl Compr Canc Netw 2017; 15(10):1268–74.

25. Harshman LC, Preston MA, Bellmunt J, et al. Diagnosis of bladder carcinoma: a clinician's perspective. Surg Pathol Clin 2015;8(4):677–85.

26. Woldu SL, Bagrodia A, Lotan Y. Guideline of guidelines: non muscle-invasive bladder cancer. BJU Int 2017;119(3):371–80.

27. Linton KD, Rosario DJ, Thomas F, et al. Disease specific mortality in patients with low risk bladder cancer and the impact of cystoscopic surveillance. J Urol 2013;189(3):828–33.

28. Sylvester RJ, Oosterlinck W, Holmang S, et al. Systematic review and individual patient data metaanalysis of randomized trials comparing a single immediate instillation of chemotherapy after transurethral resection with transurethral resection alone in patients with stage pTa-pT1 urothelial carcinoma of the bladder: which patients benefit from the instillation? Eur Urol 2016;69(2):231–44.

29. Han RF, Pan JG. Can intravesical bacillus Calmette-Guerin reduce recurrence in patients with superficial bladder cancer? A meta-analysis of randomized trials. Urology 2006;67(6):1216–23.

30. Divrik RT, Yildirim U, Zorlu F, et al. The effect of repeat transurethral resection on recurrence and progression rates in patients with T1 tumors of the bladder who received intravesical mitomycin: a

prospective, randomized clinical trial. J Urol 2006; 175(5):1641–4.

31. Herr HW, Sogani PC. Does early cystectomy improve the survival of patients with high risk superficial bladder tumors? J Urol 2001;166(4):1296–9.

32. Mak RH, Hunt D, Shipley WU, et al. Long-term outcomes in patients with muscle-invasive bladder cancer after selective bladder-preserving combined-modality therapy: a pooled analysis of radiation therapy oncology group protocols 8802, 8903, 9506, 9706, 9906, and 0233. J Clin Oncol 2014; 32(34):3801–9.

33. Stein JP, Lieskovsky G, Cote R, et al. Radical cystectomy in the treatment of invasive bladder cancer: long-term results in 1,054 patients. J Clin Oncol 2001;19(3):666–75.

34. Gakis G, Efstathiou J, Lerner SP, et al. ICUD-EAU International Consultation on Bladder Cancer 2012: radical cystectomy and bladder preservation for muscle-invasive urothelial carcinoma of the bladder. Eur Urol 2013;63(1):45–57.

35. Smith ZL, Christodouleas JP, Keefe SM, et al. Bladder preservation in the treatment of muscle-invasive bladder cancer (MIBC): a review of the literature and a practical approach to therapy. BJU Int 2013;112(1):13–25.

36. Cahn DB, Ristau BT, Ghiraldi EM, et al. Bladder preservation therapy: a review of the literature and future directions. Urology 2016;96:54–61.

37. Rini BI, Campbell SC, Escudier B. Renal cell carcinoma. Lancet 2009;373(9669):1119–32.

38. Volpe A, Cadeddu JA, Cestari A, et al. Contemporary management of small renal masses. Eur Urol 2011;60(3):501–15.

39. Uzosike AC, Patel HD, Alam R, et al. Growth kinetics of small renal masses on active surveillance: variability and results from the DISSRM registry. J Urol 2017;199(3).

40. Patel HD, Johnson MH, Pierorazio PM, et al. Diagnostic accuracy and risks of biopsy in the diagnosis of a renal mass suspicious for localized renal cell carcinoma: systematic review of the literature. J Urol 2016;195(5):1340–7.

41. Sorbellini M, Kattan MW, Snyder ME, et al. A postoperative prognostic nomogram predicting recurrence for patients with conventional clear cell renal cell carcinoma. J Urol 2005;173(1):48–51.

42. Bandini M, Smith A, Zaffuto E, et al. Effect of pathological high-risk features on cancer-specific mortality in non-metastatic clear cell renal cell carcinoma: a tool for optimizing patient selection for adjuvant therapy. World J Urol 2018;36(1):51–7.

43. Ravaud A, Motzer RJ, Pandha HS, et al. Adjuvant sunitinib in high-risk renal-cell carcinoma after nephrectomy. N Engl J Med 2016;375(23):2246–54.

UNITED STATES POSTAL SERVICE®

Statement of Ownership, Management, and Circulation
(All Periodicals Publications Except Requester Publications)

1. Publication Title	2. Publication Number		3. Filing Date
SURGICAL PATHOLOGY CLINICS	025 – 478		9/18/2018

4. Issue Frequency	5. Number of Issues Published Annually	6. Annual Subscription Price
MAR, JUN, SEP, DEC	4	$206.00

7. Complete Mailing Address of Known Office of Publication (Not printer) (Street, city, county, state, and ZIP+4®)

ELSEVIER INC.
230 Park Avenue, Suite 800
New York, NY 10169

Contact Person
STEPHEN R. BUSHING

Telephone (Include area code)
215-239-3688

8. Complete Mailing Address of Headquarters or General Business Office of Publisher (Not printer)

ELSEVIER INC.
230 Park Avenue, Suite 800
New York, NY 10169

9. Full Names and Complete Mailing Addresses of Publisher, Editor, and Managing Editor (Do not leave blank)

Publisher (Name and complete mailing address)

TAYLOR E BALL, ELSEVIER INC.
1600 JOHN F KENNEDY BLVD. SUITE 1800
PHILADELPHIA, PA 19103-2899

Editor (Name and complete mailing address)

STACY EASTMAN, ELSEVIER INC.
1600 JOHN F KENNEDY BLVD. SUITE 1800
PHILADELPHIA, PA 19103-2899

Managing Editor (Name and complete mailing address)

PATRICK MANLEY, ELSEVIER INC.
1600 JOHN F KENNEDY BLVD. SUITE 1800
PHILADELPHIA, PA 19103-2899

10. Owner (Do not leave blank. If the publication is owned by a corporation, give the name and address of the corporation immediately followed by the names and addresses of all stockholders owning or holding 1 percent or more of the total amount of stock. If not owned by a corporation, give the names and addresses of the individual owners. If owned by a partnership or other unincorporated firm, give its name and address as well as those of each individual owner. If the publication is published by a nonprofit organization, give its name and address.)

Full Name	Complete Mailing Address
WHOLLY OWNED SUBSIDIARY OF REED/ELSEVIER, US HOLDINGS	1600 JOHN F KENNEDY BLVD. SUITE 1800 PHILADELPHIA, PA 19103-2899

11. Known Bondholders, Mortgagees, and Other Security Holders Owning or Holding 1 Percent or More of Total Amount of Bonds, Mortgages, or Other Securities. If none, check box ▶ ☐ None

Full Name	Complete Mailing Address
N/A	

12. Tax Status (For completion by nonprofit organizations authorized to mail at nonprofit rates) (Check one)
The purpose, function, and nonprofit status of this organization and the exempt status for federal income tax purposes:
☒ Has Not Changed During Preceding 12 Months
☐ Has Changed During Preceding 12 Months (Publisher must submit explanation of change with this statement)

PS Form **3526**, July 2014 [Page 1 of 4 (see instructions page 4)] PSN: 7530-01-000-9931   PRIVACY NOTICE: See our privacy policy on www.usps.com.

---

13. Publication Title	14. Issue Date for Circulation Data Below
SURGICAL PATHOLOGY CLINICS	JUNE 2018

15. Extent and Nature of Circulation			Average No. Copies Each Issue During Preceding 12 Months	No. Copies of Single Issue Published Nearest to Filing Date
a. Total Number of Copies (Net press run)			261	356
b. Paid Circulation (By Mail and Outside the Mail)	(1)	Mailed Outside-County Paid Subscriptions Stated on PS Form 3541 (Include paid distribution above nominal rate, advertiser's proof copies, and exchange copies)	187	250
	(2)	Mailed In-County Paid Subscriptions Stated on PS Form 3541 (Include paid distribution above nominal rate, advertiser's proof copies, and exchange copies)	0	0
	(3)	Paid Distribution Outside the Mails Including Sales Through Dealers and Carriers, Street Vendors, Counter Sales, and Other Paid Distribution Outside USPS®	41	56
	(4)	Paid Distribution by Other Classes of Mail Through the USPS (e.g., First-Class Mail®)	0	0
c. Total Paid Distribution (Sum of 15b (1), (2), (3), and (4))		▶	228	306
d. Free or Nominal Rate Distribution (By Mail and Outside the Mail)	(1)	Free or Nominal Rate Outside-County Copies included on PS Form 3541	33	50
	(2)	Free or Nominal Rate In-County Copies Included on PS Form 3541	0	0
	(3)	Free or Nominal Rate Copies Mailed at Other Classes Through the USPS (e.g., First-Class Mail)	0	0
	(4)	Free or Nominal Rate Distribution Outside the Mail (Carriers or other means)	0	0
e. Total Free or Nominal Rate Distribution (Sum of 15d (1), (2), (3) and (4))		▶	33	50
f. Total Distribution (Sum of 15c and 15e)		▶	261	356
g. Copies not Distributed (See Instructions to Publishers #4 (page #3))		▶	0	0
h. Total (Sum of 15f and g)		▶	261	356
i. Percent Paid (15c divided by 15f times 100)		▶	87.36%	85.96%

* If you are claiming electronic copies, go to line 16 on page 3. If you are not claiming electronic copies, skip to line 17 on page 3.

16. Electronic Copy Circulation		Average No. Copies Each Issue During Preceding 12 Months	No. Copies of Single Issue Published Nearest to Filing Date
a. Paid Electronic Copies	▶	0	0
b. Total Paid Print Copies (Line 15c) + Paid Electronic Copies (Line 16a)	▶	228	306
c. Total Print Distribution (Line 15f) + Paid Electronic Copies (Line 16a)	▶	261	356
d. Percent Paid (Both Print & Electronic Copies) (16b divided by 16c × 100)	▶	87.36%	85.96%

☒ I certify that 50% of all my distributed copies (electronic and print) are paid above a nominal price.

17. Publication of Statement of Ownership
☒ If the publication is a general publication, publication of this statement is required. Will be printed
in the DECEMBER 2018 issue of this publication. ☐ Publication not required.

18. Signature and Title of Editor, Publisher, Business Manager, or Owner

STEPHEN R. BUSHING - INVENTORY DISTRIBUTION CONTROL MANAGER

Stephen R. Bushing   Date 9/18/2018

I certify that all information furnished on this form is true and complete. I understand that anyone who furnishes false or misleading information on this form or who omits material or information requested on the form may be subject to criminal sanctions (including fines and imprisonment) and/or civil sanctions (including civil penalties).

PS Form **3526**, July 2014 (Page 2 of 4)   PRIVACY NOTICE: See our privacy policy on www.usps.com

Moving?

Make sure your subscription moves with you!

To notify us of your new address, find your **Clinics Account Number** (located on your mailing label above your name), and contact customer service at:

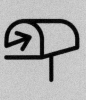

Email: journalscustomerservice-usa@elsevier.com

800-654-2452 (subscribers in the U.S. & Canada)
314-447-8871 (subscribers outside of the U.S. & Canada)

Fax number: 314-447-8029

Elsevier Health Sciences Division
Subscription Customer Service
3251 Riverport Lane
Maryland Heights, MO 63043

*To ensure uninterrupted delivery of your subscription, please notify us at least 4 weeks in advance of move.